ANCESTOR TROUBLE

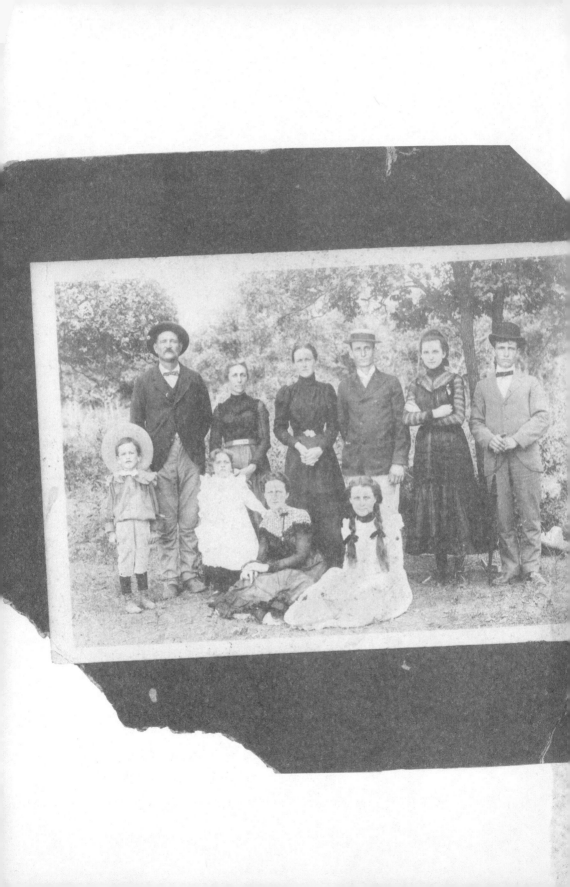

Ancestor Trouble

A Reckoning and a Reconciliation

MAUD NEWTON

RANDOM HOUSE

NEW YORK

Published in the United States by Random House, an imprint and division of Penguin Random House LLC, New York.

RANDOM HOUSE and the HOUSE colophon are registered trademarks of Penguin Random House LLC.

LIBRARY OF CONGRESS CATALOGING-IN-PUBLICATION DATA
Names: Newton, Maud, author.
Title: Ancestor trouble : a reckoning and a reconciliation / by Maud Newton.
Description: First edition. | New York : Random House, [2022] | Includes bibliographic references and index.
Identifiers: LCCN 2021025844 (print) | LCCN 2021025845 (ebook) | ISBN 9780812997927 (hardcover) | ISBN 9780812997934 (ebook)
Subjects: LCSH: Newton, Maud. | Newton, Maud—Family. | Newton family. | Genealogy. | Genetic genealogy—United States. | Racism—United States. | United States—Race relations.
Classification: LCC CT275.N5225 A3 2022 (print) | LCC CT275.N5225 (ebook) | DDC 929.20973—dc23/eng/20211108
LC record available at https://lccn.loc.gov/2021025844
LC ebook record available at https://lccn.loc.gov/2021025845

All photographs from the author's collection except page 12, bottom, from the *Delta Democrat-Times.*

Printed in Canada on acid-free paper

randomhousebooks.com

2 4 6 8 9 7 5 3 1

First Edition

Book design by Barbara M. Bachman

For my family,

LIVING AND DEAD,

KNOWN AND UNKNOWN,

INHERITED AND CHOSEN.

CONTENTS

———

MAUD NEWTON'S
Family Tree

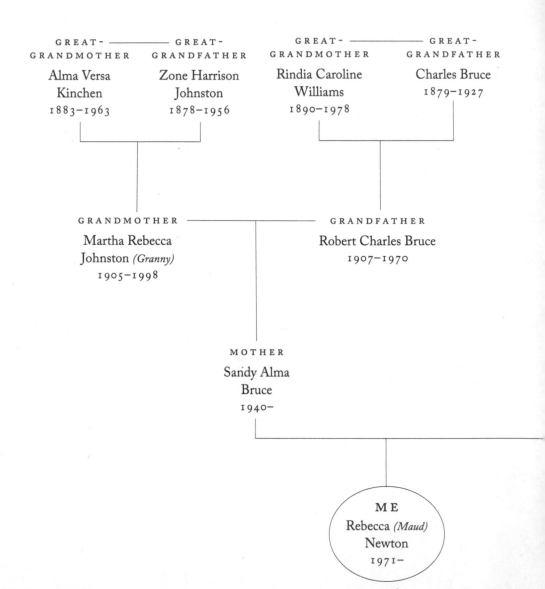

GREAT- ———— GREAT-
GRANDMOTHER GRANDFATHER

Alma Versa Zone Harrison
Kinchen Johnston
1883–1963 1878–1956

GREAT- ———— GREAT-
GRANDMOTHER GRANDFATHER

Rindia Caroline Charles Bruce
Williams 1879–1927
1890–1978

GRANDMOTHER ——————————— GRANDFATHER

Martha Rebecca Robert Charles Bruce
Johnston *(Granny)* 1907–1970
1905–1998

MOTHER

Sandy Alma
Bruce
1940–

M E
Rebecca *(Maud)*
Newton
1971–

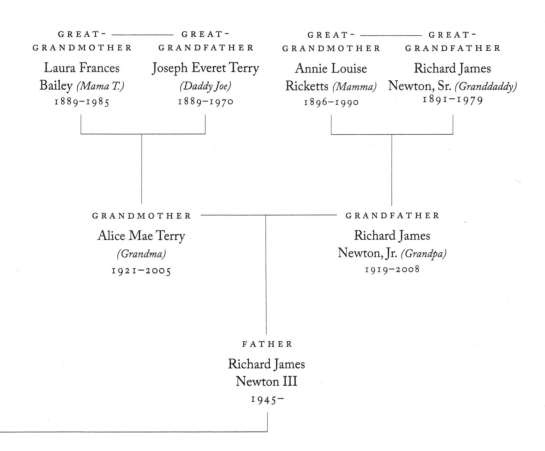

GREAT- ——————— GREAT-
GRANDMOTHER   GRANDFATHER
Laura Frances   Joseph Everet Terry
Bailey *(Mama T.)*   *(Daddy Joe)*
1889–1985   1889–1970

GREAT- ——————— GREAT-
GRANDMOTHER   GRANDFATHER
Annie Louise   Richard James
Ricketts *(Mamma)* Newton, Sr. *(Granddaddy)*
1896–1990   1891–1979

GRANDMOTHER
Alice Mae Terry
(Grandma)
1921–2005

GRANDFATHER
Richard James
Newton, Jr. *(Grandpa)*
1919–2008

FATHER
Richard James
Newton III
1945–

INTRODUCTION

———

I LOOK LIKE MY FATHER, MOVE LIKE MY FATHER, TALK like my father. When I was a child and we went places together, we were a full-size and miniature version of the same windup toy, our strides clipped and jolting, brows clenched in concentration, pale legs eerily glowing in the brilliant Miami sunlight. I am unmistakably my father's daughter, but we're estranged from each other. The last time I saw him, more than a decade ago at my grandfather's funeral, he gave me a kiss. I don't expect he'll kiss me again.

Thirteen hundred miles from me, still down in South Florida, my father is going about his day, and I can imagine it. He wakes before dawn, weighs himself, goes for a walk or a jog or rides his stationary bike. He eats breakfast if the scale permits and then he puts on a suit and drives to his law office. If he's angry about something—and he usually is—upon arriving at work, he'll pick up the phone and call around until he finds someone with the power to rectify the problem. Let's hope they fix it right away. Otherwise, maybe tomorrow morning, but probably this afternoon and quite possibly this very hour, he will ring them up again and start shouting. Eventually they will do whatever my father wants, just to be free of him.

I sympathize. I have loved my father and I have feared him, and I have lain awake in the dark late at night worrying what it means to have half his genome inside me, but I have never understood him. Sometimes I have felt that if I could just reach down far enough into myself, I would find the answers: what he wants, what he fears, what he loves. The older I get, the more I search backward, as though if I could know everyone who led to my father, who made him who he is, I would know him, too.

He always stressed to me the importance of blood—being worthy of it, showing loyalty to it, protecting what he called the purity of it. He was, by many metrics, an intelligent man. He had a master's in aerospace engineering on scholarship from an Ivy League university and was valedictorian of his law school class. But he considered slavery a benevolent institution that should never have been disbanded, and he viewed his and my fair skin as a mark of superiority.

The world being what it was in my post–civil-rights-era youth, while my sister and I were growing up in 1970s Miami, my father didn't air his prejudices in public but in private mandated separatism. "Birds of a feather flock together," he was fond of saying. He said it at the breakfast table; he said it on the way to the pool; he said it while covering the faces of brown children in our storybooks with our mom's nail polish. Sometimes he closed the pages before the paint dried so that they stuck together forever, leaving nursery rhymes unrhyming and stories filled with gaps. Once he led us onto the side porch to watch as he bashed a dark-skinned toy with a hammer until its head came off. Then he threw it in the garbage, where he said it belonged. He often recounted his triumph over being assigned, as an undergrad, to room with an Asian American student: "I marched right over to the housing office and told them that I wasn't going to live with a Chinese."

I remember being eight or nine, traipsing with him around some dismal family parcel in the Mississippi Delta. My younger sister trailed behind and chill February rain drizzled down on us as our father instructed us to pick wet cotton bolls from dead branches to fill a burlap sack he found by the side of a barn. Leading us across the acres, he stopped at some vantage point over a creek or a gully. Our forebears, Confederate soldiers, were killed on or near that very land, I seem to recall his saying. Mostly I remember wanting to go home to my mom in Miami. She had opted out of this trip, as she opted out of all family vacations toward the end of my parents' marriage, and I consoled myself by imagining her contempt.

I CAME INTO BEING through a kind of homegrown eugenics project. My parents married not for love but because they believed they would have smart children together. This was my father's idea, and over their brief courtship he persuaded my mom of its merits. Not uncoincidentally, nearly every early memory I have of my father involves letting him down in some way. He spanked me if I failed to finish everything on my plate in the half hour he allotted for each meal; he spanked me for being constipated; he spanked me for watching *Sesame Street,* because Black and white children played together on it. He didn't spank me if I made less than an A on a math test but berated me for weeks afterward and made long-division quizzes to occupy my weekends.

My dread of his wrath was a dull, continuous ache, a mental, physical, and emotional rheumatism that felt endemic to me. My mom tells me she came upon him, when I was eighteen months old, leaving a box in the middle of my room and telling me not to touch it, that I'd get a spanking if I did. She watched as he watched through a crack in the door until I did stick out my finger and make contact, whereupon he rushed in to deliver the discipline he'd promised. So I suppose the fear truly was formative.

The first time I saw a family tree, a year or two after that Delta trip, my father carried it into my bedroom with tears in his eyes to illustrate why he and my mom should not and could not split up. Flicking through pages of unfamiliar names, he explained that nowhere in our branch of his grandmother's tree, all the way back to a Revolutionary War lieutenant born in Virginia in 1755, had anyone ever divorced. It would be a terrible scandal and would bring ignominy on his mother's mother's line and on our family—on our blood, he probably said—if he and my mom were the first. I'd never seen him cry before. Though I was always begging my mom to leave him, I cried, too.

MY MOM, SANDY, WAS a blond-haired, amber-eyed whirlwind of charisma, creativity, and passion. She agreed with reluctance to date my father and then, convinced by the picture he painted, married him with pragmatic resolve six months later: They would have smart children; she would stay home and keep house; he would be a stable husband, parent, and provider, a corrective to her own fatherless childhood. My father didn't know that she'd only recently kept more than thirty cats in her small two-bedroom house and been featured in the newspaper as president of the Dallas cat club. Membership had really taken off during her term, which isn't surprising; she's always been a gifted evangelist. By the time my father started courting her, she'd found homes for all but three cats. She'd also been divorced and followed up her first marriage with a soul-crushing affair. A week before my father introduced himself at her friend's pool and asked to borrow her copy of *Time,* she downed a cocktail of iodine, sleeping pills, and lithium and climbed into the bathtub, intending to fall asleep and never wake up.

Less than a decade later, my mom started a church in our living room, ministering to downtrodden people rather than stray animals. When we went to the grocery store, she wore a blue pin with white lettering that read, I GOT IT!, "it" being Jesus, as she gladly told anyone who asked and many who didn't. She had not been raised religious, but when her conversion came, it was swift and feverish. During the first few years of my life, before we got Saved, I was the cats, I was the church, I was her all-consuming project.

She dedicated herself to grooming me for unspecified yet incontrovertible greatness. Her attention was like the sun, warm and life-giving, a little intoxicating, sorely missed when it went away.

My parents' marriage somehow lasted twelve years. My sister's birth six years in didn't halt their arguments, which overflowed into lakes of Corningware and casseroles and condiments and juices that my mom threw from the stove and fridge across the floor before roaring away in the car. Toward the end of their time together, my father would wake her in the night with a flashlight lit under his face. "And furthermore," he would say, continuing an argument they'd been having hours earlier. He took my sister and me to the Presbyterian church down the street, the one he and my mom had agreed on in the short window before salvation became the driving force of her life, rather than allowing us to attend our mom's services. Sometimes they had a screaming match in our front yard beforehand as we stood there in our Sunday finest. Once, she grabbed my father's Bible and started tearing pages from it. "Go on to that dead church, with all those hypocrites!" she shouted, flinging the paper in handfuls as the Presbyterians drove past, gaping, in their expensive cars. My father seemed confused by her intractability, and his puzzlement puzzled me. Even as a child I could see that my mom's enthusiasm rushed like water toward falls. That he could not see the futility of getting in the way made him seem naïve and vulnerable; it was one of few things that humanized him for me.

While my father idolized his ancestors, my mother saw them (and her own) as figures of fun and fascination, ripe for storytelling, and as her religious fervor gathered steam she also came to see them as harbingers of trouble manifesting in our own lives. She believed in "generational curses," an idea embraced by some evangelicals that any sinful or ungodly act, such as cheating on your spouse or on your taxes or reading horoscopes, could curse your family—yourself, your children, and your children's children, on down the line—for generations. Demons literally infiltrated you, she said, and you passed them on. She believed that she and I and everyone else had been possessed the moment we were born. Our forebears had sinned in such a way as to open the door to a generational curse. She described seeing evil spirits everywhere: sitting on shoulders, lurking in eyes, wrapped around necks like boa constrictors— shoulders, eyes, and necks including mine. Exorcisms were ferocious events, held behind locked doors in other people's houses. Sometimes, unbeknownst to my father, they were even held in ours.

In the end, luckily for us all, my parents did divorce. Their union lives on, in some sense, in me. As a child, I felt alone in this predicament. Now I tend to see its ubiquity.

Part One

GENEALOGY

Chapter 1

A DOORWAY

———

O VER TIME THE SIMPLEST FACTS OF HUMAN EXISTENCE have become to me the most unfathomable. We come from our parents, who came from their parents, who descended, as the Bible would put it, from their fathers and their fathers' fathers. We begin with the sperm of one human being and the egg of another, and then we enter the world and become ourselves. Beyond all that's encoded in our twenty-three pairs of chromosomes—our hair, eyes, and skin of a certain shade, our frame and stature, our sensitivity to bitter tastes—we are bundles of opinions and ambitions, of shortcomings and talents.

Every one of our forebears had hopes and fears, good days and bad. All of them took actions, and were forced into situations, that shaped them and that led to us. Each person on earth is a particular individual consisting of parts from other particular individuals. The alchemy between our genes and our individuality is a mystery we keep trying to solve. In the West, many of us look to science and genetics for answers to these existential questions we'll only ever answer in part. Why are some of us beautiful and some of us plain, some athletic and some clumsy, some depressive and some optimistic? How much can investigating our genes answer these questions, and what do our efforts to decode our destinies in this way say about us? In terms of DNA, we are no more related to most of our ancestors than we are to the people around us on a train or at a baseball game. And yet without each of the people who came before, who contributed to the genes that ultimately contributed to ours, we wouldn't exist as we do now.

Even as I focus on the biological family in this book, I don't idealize it. I have a complicated relationship with some of my family members and no contact with my father. I also have a blended family. My stepdaughter, my only child, is one of the most important people in my life. My sister's wonderful kids were adopted into my family. My stepfather and stepsister have both had a profound influence on me. And then there are my twin half-siblings, two of my closest biological relatives. They're my father's children, born thirty-nine years after me. I may never have the chance to know them. I share more interests and beliefs with my friends and in-laws than with many people whose genetics overlap with mine. I realize that families need not be bound by blood and also that having a blood relationship is no guarantee of affinity.

Still, the influence of our genes, our ancestors, on the people we are is undeniable. All we have to do is look in the mirror to see that. Wondering what this inheritance means for us doesn't mean we're devaluing other important family relationships—or imbuing our ancestors, or their beliefs or practices, with an assumption of supremacy.

MANY OF US TRACE our ancestors on genealogy sites that are increasingly entangled with genetic testing. But after booming for a decade, the market for consumer DNA tests seems to be bottoming out. The reduced demand has generated theories. Potential testers may be concerned about privacy; or the tests, which a user takes only once, may already have reached most interested consumers. But there's been another shift in the culture, especially among young people: a recognition that the pull toward our ancestors is at least as rooted in spiritual yearning as it is in a desire to unearth empirical fact.

Ancestor hunger circles the globe. It spans millennia. It's often been cast as a narcissistic Western peculiarity. Historically, though, it's far more usual for people to seek connection with their forebears than not to seek it. Even now, in many parts of the world, spiritual practices involving ancestors flourish. Rather than promoting self-absorption, they tend to foster a deeper sense of community, less "I" and more "we."

These traditions sound alien to many of European ancestry because we don't know our own history. True, many of the records have vanished. Accounts that survive are often muddled and contentious. But in the ancient world, the separation between the living family and the dead was not nearly as stark as many of us in the West perceive it to be. Rituals in ancient Greece and Rome were intended to bring peace to family dead in the afterlife. Ancestors shown proper reverence were spiritual allies to the living family, whereas neglected dead could wreak enormous harm. Across the ancient world, families in many cultures also venerated household gods that represented or were handed down by ancestors. (Even in the Bible, Rachel steals her father's teraphim, usually agreed to be household gods.) Ancestral practices endured in fragmented form in parts of the Christianized West until the Protestant Reformation. Vestiges survive in Catholicism, Orthodox Christianity, and the other liturgical churches, with God as the intermediary. Members of the Church of Jesus Christ of Latter-Day Saints baptize their family dead by proxy. In many parts of the world, direct spiritual connections between people and their ancestors never stopped being cultivated. To name examples is to omit far too many others, but from Korea, Japan, and China to Nigeria, Ghana, and Sierra Leone, from Mexico to Peru, ancient traditions of reverence endure. In Cuba and Haiti, in pockets throughout the Americas and the Caribbean, Indigenous and enslaved people preserved ancestor-honoring practices, often syncretizing them with Christianity so the traditions could be carried on even in proximity to the church.

In recent years, people whose ancestors lost or were robbed of this spiritual connection to their family dead have begun to reclaim it for themselves, sometimes as a wholly celebratory act, but often as a way of reckoning with family burdens and wrongs as well as the gifts of a lineage. Many people newly drawn to ancestor work see it as vital for cultural repair. It's difficult to heal intergenerational trauma if we don't understand how it began.

Modernity promises each of us the opportunity to define our own identity. It gives us the freedom, at least in theory, not to be boxed in by those who've come before us. We're no longer obliged to glorify our ancestors and take on their customs uncritically or to view their lives as destiny, which is all to the good. But in turning away from practices that encoded into familial memory the people who came before us, we've relinquished something enormous.

When I first started exploring my own family history, my interest flowed as much from fear as longing. The allure of ancestors had a lot in common with a good ghost story. Now I find myself not merely respecting traditions of ancestor reverence but advocating for them, as a doorway to something vital and sacred, accessible as earth, and natural as breath.

Chapter 2

NOT FORGOTTEN

———

GROWING UP, I ASSOCIATED GENEALOGY WITH THE BEGATS of the Bible, with that old family tree my father showed me, and with his reverence for the Old South. I aspired then to be as little like him and his branch of my family as possible. So I never expected to become interested in compiling my own family tree. When I did start researching my ancestors, slowly at first, and then in great gusts of extreme obsession, I thought of it as a kind of scattershot, backward-looking detective work. Only my mother's side interested me then: the Texan rabble-rousers, scoundrels, and misfits I'd grown up hearing about. Had my mom's grandfather, my granny's father, really been a communist in early-twentieth-century Dallas? Had my mom's father really married thirteen times? Had *his* father really killed a man with a hay hook?

Over the years, my mom and Granny had described these characters to me with the pleasure and spine-tingling finesse of girls at a slumber party. With rare exceptions—such as the account of Granny's sister, a dark-haired beauty who one day in her teens started dancing down the street naked, later pulled a knife from the bath to brandish at their mother, and eventually died in a mental institution—the stories were presented as entertainment rather than tragedy, scenes from the reportage of Mark Twain rather than the tales of Edgar Allan Poe. My mom's comic timing and flair for ironic foreshadowing tempered Granny's dry wit, her succinct and deadly condemnations. Granny had grown up poor on the outskirts of Dallas and later made her way in town, and both her origins and her tenacity were evident in everything she said. She often smelled of onions. Her pale-blue eyes flashed with warmth and sometimes icy judgment in the most dimly lit of rooms.

Someone putting on airs was, Granny would observe, "really shitting and flying now." Someone intimidated into silence was "quiet as a little mouse peeing on cotton." Her own father had been "meaner than a junkyard dog," just like (by her accounting) mine. "I wouldn't piss on him if he was on fire," she said of my father once, after I was grown. Granny was blunt, funny, and fierce, and end-lessly indulgent of my sister's and my wishes. As a child, I loved her with less complication than I've ever loved anyone.

The characters she and my mother spoke of deepened in infamy and complexity as I grew older and was thought ready to hear more details. The two of them didn't always agree on what I should be told, so I carried details back and forth, provoking each of them into divulging more. Sometimes I have trouble now remembering who told me what.

My first foray into family research came in the year 2000, shortly before my twenty-ninth birthday. I was sitting at work, eating lunch at my desk, thinking about Granny's father, Zone Harrison John-ston, the reputed Texan communist. Much later I would uncover a political petition he signed to recall the mayor and city commis-sioners, which identified him as a member of the Dallas County Local of Socialists. But that day when I idly typed his name into Google, I found nothing. So I tried Granny's mom, Alma Kinchen, and an old New England tree stretching back to 1600s Massachu-setts came right up. Until then I'd always believed all my colonial ancestors, on both sides, were Southern.

From that tree, I discovered that an ancestor of mine, Cornet

Joseph Parsons, was a founder of the town of Northampton, the very place my sister had moved to just a few years before, without knowing of any connection to it. Whenever I'd visited her there, I'd felt surprisingly at peace, a sense of belonging. I did not know then that we were on Nonotuck land.

I dabbled occasionally after that, but it wasn't until 2007, trying to make sense of the troubles in my immediate family, that I began to research in earnest at Ancestry.com, on an account I'd created a couple years earlier. There I built out my own tree, which in turn tied into other people's trees, and I began the still-unfinished work of trying to verify their research. Back then the site had a "Find Famous Relatives" feature that piggybacked on users' research and tentatively suggested I could be related—incredibly remotely— to Mark Twain, Emily Dickinson, Aldous Huxley, Jane Austen, George Washington Carver, Thomas Moore, and a host of other historical figures, including on my father's side Richard Nixon and on my mother's Lucille Ball. From the start I saw how manipulative this tool, now long-ago discontinued, was, and how unreliable. It hooked me anyway. *No wonder Lucy always reminded me of my mom!* I thought. *No wonder my dad is a charisma vacuum.*

These more-concerted explorations started during more than two years of silence between my mom and me, distance I'd initiated because of things that had happened years before. When I was twelve, my stepfather molested me. I told my mom after dinner that night. She conferred with him and blamed demons. She asked if I had any questions. I did not have any questions.

For a long time, I didn't discuss what he'd done with anyone else. As an adult, I dealt with the psychological fallout with my husband and sister, with friends and in therapy, and effectively pretended between my mom, stepfather, and me that it hadn't happened. Eventually, though, when I was in my early thirties, I sent them a letter saying that someone needed to take responsibility. My stepfather sent an expression of sorrow for my difficult childhood. My mom urged me to move on. Focusing on these "hurts, slights, etc.," was only harming me, she said. Stung by this response, I pulled away. I missed her but didn't know how to be in touch without creating more sadness, and she didn't pursue me. In her absence, I took a kind of grim satisfaction in beginning to unearth proof of my grandfather's many marriages, of my great-aunt's time in the mental institution. *These are my relatives,* I told myself. *Of course I'm crazy.*

I started posting family-history finds on my blog (which at first my mom didn't know about) every Friday. The more I uncovered, the more my curiosity burgeoned and mutated. One of the objects on which it became most intensely fixed was my great-grandfather Charley Bruce.

I CAN'T RECALL WHETHER it was my mom or Granny who told me that Charley killed a man with a hay hook in downtown Dallas. Nor do I know whether someone else claimed that he stabbed the man in a rage, in a bar, after too many rounds of bourbon, or whether I invented this scene from a bad western all by myself. Regardless, it was how I'd come to envision the "difficulty," as I later discovered the papers called it, "the trouble between the two men." I started my research expecting to find—if I could find him at all—an unapologetic swashbuckling hothead. Almost nothing I discovered about him fit the narrative arc I'd plotted.

It felt like much longer, but posts on my blog from 2007 reveal that I was less than a month into my intensive genealogical sleuthing when, breaking more than two years' silence between us, I emailed my mom about some of my findings and sent a link to my tree. Already I'd discovered things she didn't know—Charley's name, for instance. She'd referred to him rarely, only as her "daddy's father." I see now, though I didn't then, that in looking into the deep past I was trying to find a way forward for the two of us and also seeking a way to be in touch with her—to connect with her—about something safe.

We started emailing erratically, almost exclusively about dead people. As usual, she was forthcoming—delightfully, ebulliently, unexpurgatedly so. The Texan side of my family loved a good story, the more outrageous the better. What they (what we) couldn't forgive was blandness and unoriginality, which was not a problem, so far as I could tell, anywhere along the Bruce line. Still, my mom did seem a little perplexed by my fascination with Charley Bruce. He was her grandfather, true, but he was also a man she'd never known. Even her knowledge of her own father, Charley's eldest son, Robert Bruce of the alleged thirteen marriages, was limited.

Charley died more than a decade before Robert and Granny married in the fall of 1939. Robert was a handsome, magnetic guy and talented clothing designer who founded and served as president of the Dallas Ladies Garment Workers' Local union and later rose to prominence in other miscellaneous trades: mechanic, grocer, commercial real estate broker. According to Granny, he was also a drinker, who squandered so much money on whiskey, expensive suits, and other women that, she said, "I couldn't even buy your mother a goddamned toothbrush."

My mom said that Robert mentioned Charley only once, with tears in his eyes, the last time she saw him, a few months before his own death. He told her that Charley "lost his mind from grief after he accidentally ran his best friend through with a hay hook and killed him." Ultimately, Charley "died in an insane asylum," Robert said.

"I could swear somebody told me he died in prison after stabbing some guy in a bar," I wrote back. "I thought he did it on purpose."

"Who to believe?" she said. "Granny got confused at the end, but Daddy was a real 'truth-stretcher.'"

THE FACTS OF CHARLEY's life took some time to unearth. Triangulating between Ancestry.com and various newspaper archives, I learned that he was born in Georgia, in 1879. At some point, Charley made his way to the Oak Cliff section of Dallas, where, in 1906, he married Rindia Caroline Williams, then sixteen, eleven years his junior. At the 1910 census, and again in 1920, Charley, Rindia, and their children were living on rented farmland near Grand Prairie, a rural area where coyotes roamed and red hawks flew, with Rindia's family close by.

By 1930, though, Charley had disappeared and Rindia was remarried. Had the murder happened during the intervening decade? Had Charley, as Robert put it, lost his mind during those ten years?

Beyond Robert, Charley had three sons and two daughters. According to my mom, one of the sons served time. Another died in his early thirties, leaving five sons of his own. The daughters, like most of the boys, were "rounders"—excessive drinkers—she said, who didn't seem to register their niece when she met them. One son, S.E., nearly died at eighteen in a truck crash. Doctors said he'd be paralyzed. Instead, he wound up with a bad limp, difficulty controlling his limbs, and a halting manner of speaking that was hard to understand. He received an insurance settlement that he and his mother, Rindia, donated to their Pentecostal church, Bethel Temple, which went on to be the largest and most prosperous of its kind in the country, a forerunner to today's megachurches. The gift left Rindia, S.E., and the younger children exceedingly poor. They subsisted on rabbits and squirrels that S.E. hunted and on handouts. When my mom was a girl, she and Granny took them firewood. The rest of the Bruces, my grandfather Robert included, evidently couldn't or wouldn't help.

I met S.E. once, for a half hour or so, at his falling-down shack outside Dallas. I was nine, maybe ten, unnerved by his roving limbs and erratic speech while wanting to preserve his feelings and conceal mine, so I remember very little about this, my one encounter with a member of the Bruce family, except that I was careful to keep a smile on my face unless another expression was called for and, I believe, he had only one chair. (There was no question given his shaky legs that he had to be the one to sit in it.)

I put these people into my family tree at Ancestry.com and made it public. As I added great-great-grandparents and so on, the site offered "hints": matches from other family trees that seemed to overlap on Robert's lines several generations back. My tree offered reciprocal hints to users who didn't have all the information I did. Over the years, as I found and added clippings about my grandfather's many marriages and divorces and other assorted intrigues, this information became searchable on Ancestry.com, and some of the family historians whose trees tied up with mine on the site made their own research private or blocked me. I guessed they wanted to disassociate themselves from the disreputable details I was turning up.

Other subscribers were more approachable but couldn't help. Extrapolating from Texas birth records, newspaper archives, social media, and intrusive but irresistible people-locator sites and voter-registration lists, I identified a handful of my mother's first cousins, people she hadn't known existed until I told her about them. Many were dead. One was in prison, as was one of his sons. I emailed another. He replied, briefly, to ask what I wanted. I mentioned Charley and never heard back.

THE DALLAS MORNING NEWS archives yielded a short item, published June 15, 1916, concerning "a preliminary hearing for Charles Bruce, charged by affidavit with murder in the death of George Grimes," who "received an abdominal wound in a difficulty on June 6 and died Monday night." So at least part of the story was true. From articles in other papers I learned that Charley had driven a wagon full of hay into downtown Dallas to sell the bales to a feed store, and that's where the "difficulty" unfolded.

According to witnesses, Grimes attacked. Depending on which newspaper you believe, the fight happened inside or outside a feed store on Commerce Street, in the vicinity of the courthouse, a pretty red sandstone building that is now a museum. Charley parried with a hay-hook jab to Grimes's abdomen. The police pulled them apart, with Grimes's brother landing one last blow over an officer's shoulder. At first Grimes ignored his wounds, believing they weren't serious, but "the sharp point [had] penetrated some distance into the [intestinal] cavity," according to the *Daily Times Herald*. Six days later, Grimes was dead and Charley was arrested and detained for murder.

Neighbors came to his aid. They told *The Dallas Dispatch*—and, presumably, the court—that Grimes had repeatedly threatened Charley's life in the past and had, that day at the feed store, forced him into the fight. They said Charley's "testimony in [Grimes's] trial caused the bitter feeling between the two." Grimes had been sentenced to five years for "mistreatment of a 'female relative'" in that trial, but he'd been pardoned after serving less than two years.

Charley spent a few nights in jail. Ultimately, the grand jury found that the evidence didn't support a murder charge against him and ordered his release. He had been acting in self-defense.

I'D COME TO THINK of Charley as the trump in my deck of notorious-ancestor playing cards, a sort of combination joker and king. Even after my mom had told me Robert's version of events, that Charley had accidentally killed his best friend with the hay hook and then been so grieved he'd ending up dying in a mental institution, I'd clung to my vision of some small-time Jesse James. A hay-hook killing doesn't tend to suggest a sympathetic scene, obviously, and Robert was not the most reliable of narrators, but I had been offered an alternate story, from someone in a position to know, and I'd rejected it. Now I felt ashamed.

I wondered what Grimes had done to the female relative, who the relative was, and what Charley had said at the trial, exactly. Almost a century later, though, how would I ever find out?

I called the jails and I called the courthouses. They couldn't help. I searched various newspapers' archives. Nothing turned up. And then, eventually, incredibly, several years later, I happened to think to search the law books, and I discovered that the Texas Court of Criminal Appeals had considered, and ruled on, Grimes's case—twice.

In August 1909, nearly seven years before the attack on Charley, Grimes assaulted his stepdaughter, Bessie Smith, with the intent to rape her. The girl's testimony, quoted at length in the first appeal, in 1911, is harrowing stuff. She said that Grimes sent her brother away and her mother to the barn to feed the mules so he could force Bessie to, as she put it, "go to the bottom with him." When her mother came back, Bessie recalled, Grimes told the woman to go back outside "and stay until I tell you to come in the house," and then "he commenced after me," telling Bessie that if she didn't cooperate, he would break her neck.

> He grabbed me by the arms and took me behind the door and pulled my dress up. When he got me behind the door he hit me in the mouth and choked me. He said to me, "If you don't shut up somebody will come in here and take me out," and I told him I wanted loose, and he tried to turn me round, and I wouldn't do it. He had his person out, and put it up against me—behind me. He would try to turn me around, and every time he would get me around I would jerk loose, and he would just keep on trying. He never did get me turned around good. After I got loose from him I ran out to the barn where my mother was, and told her about it. I told my mother about it in the presence of my sister.

Bessie and other witnesses spoke of bruises. At trial her mother denied asking, as Bessie testified she had, whether her stepfather had "ruined" her. All of this evidence, said the court, was admissible, unlike the testimony that, a few hours earlier, Grimes "whipped her with a rope" to stop her from accompanying her mother to Grand Prairie for groceries, which "might, perhaps, have a tendency to prejudice the jury against him."

All those years I'd joked about Charley and his hay hook, when he'd only gotten involved in the brawl because he stood by a vulnerable young woman. He'd defended her in a way that no one had defended me.

I'LL NEVER KNOW CHARLEY'S precise role in the trial. All the players are dead and the briefs and pleadings long gone. But I do have a theory. A section of the first appeal mentions a witness who claimed that Grimes "had come to him and stated, 'If you had testified like I wanted you to do at the trial you would have been twenty-five dollars better off.'" If true, said the court, this "was an indirect way of offering the witness a bribe." I suspect Charley was this witness, because it feels like the kind of thing a bad-news friend might say, the kind of thing you might worry over later. *What did he mean, offering me money like that? Did he do what his stepdaughter said? Should I tell the judge?*

After fleeing her house, Bessie stayed a few nights with women who could have been related to the Bruces: a Mrs. Haddock and a Mrs. Morris, both surnames in the broader family. Perhaps not only Grimes and Charley had been friends. Maybe the families had been close.

Whether or not it's true that, as Robert told my mom, Charley "lost his mind from grief and died" over the incident, the death certificate I eventually unearthed confirms that he did suffer a breakdown that proved fatal. For a year and nine months beginning on October 7, 1925, Charley was a patient at the Northwest Texas Insane Asylum, renamed the Wichita Falls State Hospital during his time there.

Texas Monthly writer and area native Skip Hollandsworth has written that the town of Wichita Falls was given a choice between a university and a mental institution and chose the latter because, as an amateur historian put it, "they figured there would never be a shortage of crazy people." Sure enough, the doors of the place opened just four years before Charley's arrival and within months, Hollandsworth writes, "dozens of patients began arriving, some of them dropped off at the front gates by their families." Because the doctors didn't understand mental illness or know how to treat it, they subjected patients "to a variety of peculiar procedures. In hopes of fighting brain infections, a 'fever machine' was used to raise a patient's body temperature to at least 104 degrees. Hydrotherapy, involving steam baths and wet packs, was used to calm excited patients." Many patients died. Those whose bodies went unclaimed were buried out back.

CHARLES BRUCE DIED ON July 13, 1927, at the age of forty-eight. The cause, according to the death certificate, was "exhaustion from manic depressive insanity." After a little back and forth, the Texas Department of State Health Services confirmed to me that he's buried behind the asylum.

I'd like to think it was poverty rather than indifference or shame that led his family to abandon him in a plot marked only with the number 65. The thought of Charley's body interred in that place, unacknowledged and unvisited, gnawed at me until I decided to give him a headstone. My mom, who contends the physical self is irrelevant after death, that only the soul matters, couldn't understand why I would waste money on something like that. When she dies, she says, it's all the same to her if she's buried in a cardboard box.

Deciding to mark Charley's grave was the easy part. Choosing an epitaph took much longer. Three years passed before I settled on one, shortly before a planned visit to Dallas. The stone was laid before our arrival, and my partner, Max, and I drove north through the country, past farms and oil rigs and forbidding compounds we thought might be fracking setups, to Wichita Falls, a town very near the Oklahoma border, to see it. Because the cemetery is private, Toni Shirey, from the hospital's community-relations department, arranged to guide us on our visit. Her accent was the old North Texas kind, a twang that reminded me of sitting on the front porch with Granny and my mom, snapping beans and listening to old family stories.

The sun blazed down as we drove past the hospital's redbrick buildings toward the locked cemetery gates. Several weeks before, when I'd ordered the stone, it had snowed so much that the memorial company felt obliged to warn me the ground might be too soft to install it in time, but that afternoon in late March the high was eighty-nine degrees. To our left, piles of brush had been collected from neighboring land to prevent wildfires from raging in recent drought years. To the right were heaps of discarded equipment and furniture that the budget didn't allow the hospital to have carted away.

The cemetery itself was pretty and peaceful, with lush grass and mesquite trees and rows of orangey stones marked only with numbers. Just inside the entrance, a massive new granite monument listed the names, by number, of everyone buried there. It was thoughtful, sober, and complete, a result of community fundraising, and I could tell Toni wanted us to understand how much care had gone into it. I wasn't the first person she'd aided in this kind of pilgrimage.

She led me to Charley's marker, with the inscription I had chosen. Shadows from the trees shifted on its face as I stood there looking down. CHARLES BRUCE, it said. NOT FORGOTTEN.

Chapter 3

LIKE A
LENTICULAR PRINT

———

GENEALOGY IS ONE OF THE EARLIEST RECORDED HUMAN preoccupations, a cornerstone of knowledge and of belief. The God of Hebrew scripture promised Abraham descendants more numerous than the stars in the sky and grains of sand on the seashore. The Gospels of Matthew and Luke claim that Abraham's lineage went on to include King David, and eventually Jesus, though their accounts of how this happened contradict each other from David on. Muslims also trace the Prophet Muhammad's line back through Abraham, to Adam and Eve.

The longing of ancient humans to link their origins to the divine isn't unique to the Abrahamic faiths. The Greeks believed gods and mortals consorted freely, their unions giving rise to the demigods recorded in Hesiod's *Theogony*. The Hindu *Mahabharata* also interweaves gods and royalty, tying the ruler Prithu to the god Vishnu, just as the *Historia Brittonum* traces the Anglo-Saxon kings to the god Woden and Japanese myth holds that the imperial family descends from the sun goddess, Amaterasu. The Kongo people of Central Africa venerated ancestors as intermediaries between the living and the gods, and those who practice the traditional religion still do.

Not only is genealogy intertwined with stories humans have told themselves about their beginnings, it's also an integral ingredient of recorded human history and thought. By some reckonings, it's the oldest form of logic. The historians Staffan Müller-Wille and Hans-Jörg Rheinberger observe in *A Cultural History of Heredity* that humans have always used concepts of kinship and descent when trying to make sense of the world. Even basic components of "ancient logic such as genus and species" have "genealogical connotations," they say.

Maybe it was inevitable that humans would choose to explain the order of things to themselves in this way. With every birth, every death, genealogy has always been in the process of happening. It came into being in front of our ancestors, just as it does here and now for us. As they aged, as we age, it becomes evident how interconnected the generations are, how fleeting any individual life in the stream of time will be. Piecing together a family's lineage from this perspective can be humbling, a way of understanding oneself as a small part of a continually evolving whole. But genealogy can easily be and all too often has been the opposite: a narcissistic endeavor, steeped in self-aggrandizement, a way of making false connections and eliminating undesired ones. Kings have used it to exalt themselves, tyrants to decide which people to purge. Whether or not Jesus the man really was descended from King David, his disciples so desired him to have that pedigree that two of the gospels purport to trace it in incompatible ways. And so ridicule of genealogy also has a long history, one that over the millennia has run alongside the practice itself.

Plato mocked those who believed themselves to be "of noble birth, because [they] can show seven wealthy ancestors." Everyone, he writes in the *Theaetetus* (circa 369 B.C.), "has had countless thousands of ancestors and progenitors, among whom have been in any instance rich and poor, kings and slaves." Juvenal's Eighth Satire, written a couple of centuries later, opens by questioning the value of pedigrees. What does it matter, he asks, if you "boast a Fabius on your ample family chart" and "trace kinship through many a branch with grimy Dictators and Masters of the Horse," if you "live an evil life"? Never mind your ancestral wax portraits, he says, "virtue is the only true nobility." Fourteen hundred years after Juvenal, the Renaissance writer and humanist François Rabelais ridiculed the medieval preoccupation with lineage in his novel *Gargantua and Pantagruel*. Gargantua's pedigree is "so worn by age" it's illegible, but by "read[ing] letters unapparent to the naked eye," he identifies his forebears from "the days of Noah's celebrated ark down to the present." This kind of derision is evergreen. "Genealogy? That's like those people who believe in past lives, isn't it?" a friend of the journalist Christine Kenneally asked her, as she was writing *The Invisible History of the Human Race*. "And they're always Cleopatra, never an anonymous slave."

There's truth to these indictments, and then some. But a family tree is like a lenticular print—its most prominent features shift depending on the viewer's perspective. And while many of us who practice genealogy are drawn to the ancestors we admire, whose intelligence or talents or beauty or station we'd like to share, many of us are also in dialogue with those we ardently want not to resemble, whose traits we see in ourselves and wish we didn't or don't acknowledge in ourselves but should. Villains may fascinate us; those abandoned to institutions may haunt us; mysteries may consume us. For me, and for a not-insignificant number of family-history buffs, flawed people are often more interesting than those who led decorous lives.

With apologies to E. M. Forster, who once described fictional characters this way, some of our ancestors are flat, while others are round. Only a handful can hold leading roles in the stories we tell ourselves about our family. Most serve the plot, say a few lines, and recede into the background. Unlike a novel, though, which is finished once it's typeset and bound and released into the world, a genealogist's family tree is always evolving, as is the genealogist. Someone who seems like a major character may recede into a supporting role over the years while others become more prominent. When I started looking into my family history, I had no idea Charley would preoccupy me so much that I'd end up being the one who finally arranged his tombstone. Reflecting on his life feels a little like pondering the intricacies of a novel after I've turned the last page, except it's a novel from whose plot I sprang.

GENEALOGY IS ASSOCIATED WITH delusions of grandeur in part because—as François Weil observes in his survey of American genealogy, *Family Trees*—historically the practice of recording family history on any sustained scale was the province of royalty. Eventually it trickled down to lesser nobility and, much later, to the rest of us. Weil's pre-colonial discussion focuses on Europe, but the historical connection between genealogies and aristocracy extends back into the ancient world, far beyond the West, to the begats of the Bible, the Puranas of India, the Palermo Stone of Egypt, and so on. Griots of the Mande people sing the histories of royal clans stretching back centuries. "When a griot dies," the saying goes, "a library has burned to the ground."

Being a monarch seems not to have eradicated status anxiety in matters of lineage. Often, princes married princesses—sometimes even, as DNA testing suggests King Tut's parents did, their own siblings or close cousins. More often, royals sought to increase their power and influence by marrying into other kingdoms. Today the lineages of European royalty are so interconnected that traditional genealogical diagrams can't do them justice. To represent the relationships, an astronomer turned data-visualization artist created an electronic map that looks like a starry night sky. Each point of light represents a person. Selecting them brings a constellation of connections into view, two or three Orions jumbled on top of one another.

When lofty pedigrees didn't exist, or didn't seem impressive enough, bloodlines might be invented, or at least fudged. Ancient

Greek aristocrats saw Homeric ancestry as crucial to their prestige and position, but during the transition from oral to written genealogy, many intermediate generations between the living Greeks and their ancestors of legend were unknown. People solved this problem by making stuff up. In the Middle Ages, some French and German royal lines claimed descent from St. Anne, the mother of the Virgin Mary and so the grandmother of Jesus. Several dubious branches were drawn down from St. Anne to someone "considered historically important in the region," such as "a saint, a bishop, or a reigning family." Conversely, those thought to taint a royal bloodline—such as many children born to monarchs out of wedlock—tended not to make it onto the tree.

The novelist Alexander Chee has nine bound volumes of his family history, which were given to him as eldest son. They document his father's family in Korea and begin six hundred years ago, in the Joseon dynasty, with two of Chee's ancestors, a Korean princess and the Chinese general (and distant cousin to Genghis Khan) she married. The books are filled with names and biographical details, of course, and also with beautiful grave maps and family portraits. One bright-eyed dandy with a blue flower on his hat looks so strikingly like Chee, it could almost be a portrait of him. These records only exist, he told me, because his paternal family is aristocratic. Most Koreans don't keep such intricate documents. His family's are a particular solace to Chee, whose father died young and whose grandmother once implored his dad not to marry a "blue-eyed, blond-haired American girl," which is exactly what Chee's Maine-born mom turned out to be.

A GENERATION AFTER THE Revolution, Americans' suspicion of recorded family history had given way to an ardent but often conflicted interest that bubbled up among the writers and in the literature of the day. The transcendentalist writer Ralph Waldo Emerson claimed to "despise pedigree" and compared conversations with genealogists to "sitting up with a corpse," but he also, as Weil says, acknowledged a "debt to the 'kind Aunt' who told him 'oft of the virtues of her and mine ancestors.'"This aunt, Mary Moody Emerson, ultimately inspired him to keep his own genealogy notebook. She's one of many barely remembered single women who documented the backgrounds of early American families.

Nathaniel Hawthorne was haunted by his forebears' role in the Salem witch trials, a preoccupation that feeds into "The Custom-House," the introduction to *The Scarlet Letter*, whose narrator has a family history that tracks Hawthorne's in many ways. The narrator contemplates the great-great-grandfather, who "made himself so conspicuous in the martyrdom of the witches" that he must either have repented of his cruelties or be "groaning under the heavy consequences of them, in another state of being"—i.e., in hell. Charlotte Perkins Gilman, who like many at the end of the nineteenth century fetishized what Weil calls "Anglo-Saxon purity," touted her "extremely remote connection with English royalty," in her autobiography.

Of course, genealogical sleuthing in the nineteenth century necessitated privilege. Poverty didn't tend to go hand in hand with dabbling in archives—or, as the English scholar of working-class life Alison Light observes in her history of her family, *Common People*, with passing down Bibles, heirlooms, or memorabilia.

Being born out of wedlock also disrupted family histories. Often it meant not knowing one's father, or at least not being able to claim a paternal lineage. And many, if not most, children born into enslavement had little hope of knowing their biological families at all. So systematically did the plantation system deny the personhood of its victims that the census "slave schedules" don't even include names of those enslaved, only their age and biological sex, in a list under the name of their enslaver, who sometimes doubled as an unacknowledged father. People frequently were sold from one site of bondage to another without regard to family relationships—or, sometimes, for the express purpose of breaking up families. Some free African American women maintained memory books that included genealogical information, but these were a rarity.

The writer and abolitionist Frederick Douglass, who escaped slavery, recounted his own experience of its family-splintering effects:

> My father was a white man. He was admitted to be such by all I ever heard speak of my parentage.
>
> The opinion was also whispered that my master was my father; but of the correctness of this opinion I know nothing; the means of knowing was withheld from me. My mother and I were separated when I was but an infant—before I knew her as my mother. It is common custom, in the part of Maryland from which I ran away, to part children from their mothers at a very early age. Frequently, before the child has reached its twelfth month, its mother is taken from it and hired out on some farm a considerable distance off. . . . For what this separation is done, I do not know, unless it be to hinder the development of the child's affection toward its mother, and to blunt and destroy the natural affection of the mother for the child. This is the inevitable result.

The Civil War brought freedom and breathed new possibility and urgency into questions of family history for people who'd been freed. Many who'd been separated from loved ones before emancipation wrote to the Freedmen's Bureau, ran ads, enlisted the help of churches, and searched in person.

European colonizers also subjected Indigenous people to mass killing and forced removal from the lands of their ancestors. For those who survived and were counted, tribal rolls were taken. In the early twentieth century, descendants of white squatters on Cherokee land and other people of European ancestry began to claim Native ancestry and passed these claims on to children and grandchildren who have been taught that a fifth great-grandmother was "an Indian princess," although none of their ancestors were recorded tribal members. When the discovery of oil on Osage land made tribe members rich, white people married Osage in order to manage and inherit their wealth, sometimes secretly executing their new in-laws on the side.

Immigration often led to loss of genealogical memory, especially when it met with racist laws. The novelist Celeste Ng's great-grandfather came to the United States under an assumed name to circumvent the Chinese Exclusion Act, which barred people of Chinese descent from immigrating to the States unless they were already citizens or the children of citizens. Many became "paper sons," pretending to be sons of Chinese men already in the country. Ng learned these details of her great-grandfather's story when she requested his file from the Immigration and Naturalization Service, but the longer histories of her ancestors on that line are probably lost forever. "Traditionally, each Chinese family has a poem that records its lineage," she told me. "If you know the poem, you can tell who's in your family and which generation they're from. But we don't know our family poem anymore; it got left behind somewhere along the way."

BY THE END OF the nineteenth century, though, middle-class Americans of European origin faced few obstacles in tracing their bloodlines, and increasingly they hired researchers to produce lofty pedigrees for them. The modern idea of genealogy as a science hadn't taken hold, and inept and unscrupulous practitioners of the art flourished. Mark Twain's *The American Claimant* satirized what Weil calls "unclaimed estate fever," the widespread phenomenon of naïve Americans hoping for some windfall through a distant forgotten relative.

So much has been written, and so well, about the democratization of genealogy in recent years, I won't duplicate that history here. Suffice it to say, interest continued to grow as the twentieth century steamed forward. Research standards developed. People from all walks of life ventured into archives and pored over census data. And then, in 1977, a miniseries based on Alex Haley's *Roots* "burst upon the national consciousness," as Maya Angelou put it, giving Black Americans hope that they might, against the obstacles set by slavery, unearth their own family histories. The reach of the book—and the miniseries—was enormous. People of all ethnicities and backgrounds began their own searches. The longing uncorked then, the sense of something lost that genealogy might help recapture, mounted not just into a hobby but a kind of movement.

To a large extent, it was the Mormons who made the larger-scale practice of genealogy among Americans possible. Genealogy is so embedded in the catechism of the Latter-Day Saints that the church requires members to routinely produce names of dead relatives for posthumous baptism. Over time, to achieve its mandate of baptizing all forebears of Mormons, the LDS has collected records from a vast and ever-increasing number of populations, converted them into millions of reels of microfilm and microfiche, and stored them in a massive climate-controlled vault carved out of the Granite Mountains in Utah.

It was the Internet, and particularly the rise of Ancestry.com, that transformed genealogy into the mainstream hobby it has become. The site had LDS ties when it launched in 1996 as an offshoot of a small publishing company. In 2012, it sold for $1.6 billion. In 2020, it sold to Blackstone Group, a financial-sector company, for $4.7 billion. Over the last few decades, the genealogical Internet has become vast and complex and, especially after its marriage to genetic testing, a fraught development. Through this immense family-history complex, people can—as critics often charge—seek to establish or burnish lofty bona fides. They can try to prove that they really are descended, as they've always been told, from King Henry VIII or Pocahontas. But they can do much more than that. With all the tools at their disposal, contemporary genealogists can test rumors passed down like pocketknives. They can also rebut lies, expose secrets, and heal fractures.

No one has done more to show the transformational power of genealogy than Henry Louis Gates, Jr., whose brilliant TV show, *Finding Your Roots,* has acquainted guests—often actors, musicians, politicians, and thinkers—with astounding details of their family backgrounds. Many of the best episodes reckon with and attempt to mitigate the erasure of family history brought about by American slavery. In my favorite episode, Georgia congressman John Lewis, who risked his life marching for voting rights with Martin Luther King, Jr., learns that some of his ancestors freed after the Civil War were among the first Black people to register to vote in Georgia—before their right to do so was rescinded. It's an unbelievably poignant moment, the most moving thing I've ever seen on television.

PLENTY OF PEOPLE ARE uninterested in the people their DNA comes from. Obviously that's fine, and understandable. My friend Michael Aaron Lee, a painter, doesn't know who his birth parents were and doesn't intend to spend time looking. "If someone came up to me and dropped a manila folder on my desk marked MIKE LEE—BIRTH PARENTS, I'm sure I'd look at it, though," he told me. The author Sarah Miller has written that she doesn't wonder about her ancestors—maybe, she says, because her dad doesn't wonder. He didn't know his father growing up, professed never to be curious about him, and continued not to be intrigued after learning that the man his mother had claimed to be his father—Carl Miller—did not actually exist. For Sarah Miller, her last name is interesting only because it shows "all of us could so easily have been someone else."

For those of us who do feel driven to explore our ancestry, compiling a family tree is often about rediscovering something that's been lost. The tools for approaching ruptures in families are new, but the ruptures themselves are not. Ancient literature is filled with lost ancestors and wayward children, with shunnings and estrangements and gerrymandered lineages. More than two thousand years after Sophocles wrote *Oedipus*, we're still horrified by the predicament of the man who, not knowing his own family history, fulfilled the oracle's prophecy that he would kill his father and marry his mother.

Growing up, I was troubled by the biblical story of Ishmael, Abraham's eldest son, child of an enslaved woman, Hagar. As the Book of Genesis tells it, Abraham's wife, Sarah, can't conceive. She gives Hagar to Abraham so he can have a child. Then Sarah has a son, Isaac, and demands that Ishmael and Hagar be cast out, so that only Isaac will inherit Abraham's riches. Abraham hesitates, but God intervenes, saying that Abraham's crucial legacy will be through Isaac, so Abraham should do as Sarah says. The Lord forms "a covenant" with Isaac. "As for the son of the slave woman," the Lord says, "I will make a nation of him also, because he is your offspring." And so Ishmael and Hagar are banished with a loaf of bread and cask of water, nearly dying in the wilderness before an angel steps in.

In Islamic tradition, it is Ishmael rather than Isaac who's the favored son, chosen by Allah. Hagar learns that Allah himself told Abraham to leave her and the infant Ishmael in the desert, and she is unafraid. For both faiths, Ishmael becomes a patriarch of the Arab world, a forefather of the Prophet Muhammad, while Isaac is grandfather to the twelve tribes of Israel. Which of these peoples the God of Abraham favors most is a question still very much alive for some Jews, Muslims, and Christians today. And yet Isaac and Ishmael sprang from the same man.

MOST PEOPLE IN THE West are taught to value the history of a nation or place, of a battle or disaster, of a monarch, politician, artist, or criminal, but to consider the history of our own ancestors unworthy of serious attention. In intellectual circles during modernity, active interest in family history has generally been regarded as, at best, embarrassing, if not a sign of narcissism and pitiable aspiration. The late critic and satirist H. L. Mencken, whose diary reveals his racism and Nazi sympathies, considered genealogy as practiced in the United States to be "directed almost exclusively toward establishing aristocratic descents for nobodies," with its "typical masterpiece" a "discovery that the wife of some obscure county judge is the grandchild, infinitely removed, of Mary Queen of Scots." Amateur genealogists would be "much more profitably . . . employed in tracing the lineage of truly salient and distinguished men," he argued. Given his preoccupation with tracing his own ancestors, Mencken evidently considered himself to qualify.

In recent years, historians, anthropologists, and scholars of religion have drawn attention to (in their parlance) "ancestor cults" of yore, studying their prevalence in family and household religions across the ancient world. It's still a niche area of scholarship, one only now moving beyond the fringes of Western popular awareness. In the context of the academic, ceremonies revolving around ancestors have typically been framed through the lens of the distant past, far-off lands, exotic cultures, or suspect pagan revivalism. In connection with Ancestry.com, 23andMe, and the rest of the genetic-genealogy complex, this history, until recently, hasn't been discussed at all.

The stories we tell ourselves about our ancestors have the power to shape us, in some ways nearly as much as our genetics do. Many of these stories are ones we know well, while others are sublimated—hard to identify, much less articulate, more pattern-based than conscious. They can expand our sense of possibility, but they can also confine us. This idea flows from Freud and Jung, and from psychodynamic psychology, and it treads into the terrain of countless self-help books, but those credentials don't invalidate it. How we imagine our ancestors, and ourselves in relation to them, can have a powerful effect on the way we live. If our lives have been circumscribed because of the way we've viewed our family, confronting our ancestors as complicated human beings rather than distant archetypes can suggest different ways of being ourselves.

Part Two

GENETIC GENEALOGY

Chapter 4

SKELETONS AND
MAGNOLIAS

———

I GUESS IT'S NORMAL TO KNOW, FROM A FAIRLY YOUNG AGE, some of the ways your parents hope to see themselves reflected in you and some of the ways they don't. Maybe your mom is happy you have her fine alto voice but wishes you'd inherited your dad's equilibrium. Maybe your dad laments passing down his bad teeth but revels in your shared love of history. Maybe your relationship with the parent you most resemble complicates your perception of yourself: You'd prefer to be a big-boned extrovert like your mom, say, rather than reedy and introverted like your dad. If you're adopted, or were conceived with a contribution from a donor, or for whatever reason you don't know one or both of your biological parents, maybe you fantasize that they, unlike the parents who raised you, are as creative as you are, or as nerdy, or that they'd sympathize with being the tallest kid in school. Or maybe you don't wonder about them much at all.

GROWING UP IN A family like mine, it's hard to know which childhood concerns exist on the same planet as normal ones and which lie farther out in the solar system. I'm not sure when most kids start thinking about the relationship between heredity and parents' aspirations, but my own anxiety about it goes back almost as far as I can remember.

I was a very young child, three or four, the first time I asked my mom why she married my father. We were in the car, on the way to my nursery school, and I was still at the stage when small, intimately familiar things were the center of my world—my mom's elegant fingers; her long coral nails; her keychain, an etched sterling-silver globe that bobbed and glinted in the sunlight and jingled against the keys as we stopped in traffic and started again. My mom put a cigarette to her mouth and drew in the smoke. Blowing it out, she turned to me matter-of-factly. "We wanted to have smart children," she said.

I'd expected her reply to be about their feelings for each other. I wanted to understand why she'd liked him enough to choose him. "But did you love him?" I asked. She took another drag. "Love isn't very important," she said, exhaling again. "We got married because we knew we'd have smart children together, and now we have you."

As the globe shifted and twirled, I contemplated her answer. Its aloof practicality was hard to reconcile with the swirl of my mom's ideas, the thrill of her company. Knowing that the plan to create me had united my parents, that being their progeny came with these expectations, changed my view of myself. Or it confirmed something I—the sort of toddler who took my wooden puzzles under the sofa to work on them and brought them out when complete for praise—had already in some way intuited. Decades later, on a hunch, I asked my mom if this breeding project had been my dad's idea. "Oh yes," she said, without hesitation.

I GOT INTERESTED IN researching my father's family when I learned there were things they didn't want me to know. My sleuthing began in a spirit of gleeful defiance shadowed by a grimly obstinate self-righteousness. I wanted to root out every secret, lie, and hypocrisy and parade their skeletons up and down the block, to refute my dad's mythology about what he called "our blood," his view of it as an honor and an obligation, his depiction of our predecessors as inherently good and correct, never to be questioned, only emulated. When I'd failed him by (among other things) not being as smart as I was expected to be, I'd also had the sense of failing to measure up against the yardstick of our forebears. I viewed my paternal clan as a club that might reject you even if you were born into it, and deep down I resolved to reject them first.

In part my childhood sense of non-belonging must have flowed from my Texan mom's indictments of my grandma's (my father's mother's) Mississippi Delta ways—her bless-their-hearts digs at the neighbors, the tiny portions she served to women at dinner, and her way of following behind me with a dusting cloth when we visited. In that era she always wore red lipstick, expertly applied, and frequently had a smart silk scarf tied at her neck. She usually wished I was wearing something more suitable than whatever casual dress or shorts set I'd put on that morning.

"I'm not a Southern shrinking violet like your mother, honey," my mom would parry in the midst of fights with my dad. "I'm a *Texan*. With me, you get what you see."

My mom lacked any aspiration to be—or to raise either of her daughters to be—a Southern belle. The gold standard of this species was Grandma's mother, Mama T., whom my mom admired but couldn't relate to. As my mom described it, Mama T. awoke every morning and got dressed up to spend the day directing servants, jotting correspondence onto engraved stationery, and waiting for visitors to come calling.

I didn't know Mama T. well. The times I remember seeing her, she was kind to me, and she was adored by those in my family who knew her intimately. She sent me a book of nursery rhymes that my father disapproved of because it depicted Black and white children playing together. He couldn't defy the family matriarch by getting rid of it, so instead he presented these illustrations as an oversight on her part and painted over all the children of color. Only once did I visit Mama T. at her house when I was old enough to remember details. I was eight or so and we spent the weekend. Mama T.'s eyes were sharp and wise, and she seemed to enjoy talking with me. She was thoughtful, too: She'd arranged for a neighbor's daughter to come over and play. And she appeared to disapprove of my father's parenting, quietly persuading him not to spank me on our last day there for failing to finish my lunch.

But the caste system of the Old South was intact in Mama T.'s home. I'd been served the meal by Mama T.'s cook, Geneva, who was Black. I was alone at the table when she placed the pimento cheese sandwich Mama T. had called for in front of me, on china, alongside a cloth napkin and a crystal glass of juice. Though Geneva went about her duties with friendly matter-of-factness, I felt awkward being catered to in this way, and I noticed that my fingernails had grime under them.

Like my mom, I felt incompatible with the life of a Southern belle. As did Granny: Although usually impeccably polite about my paternal grandparents, she slipped once and said of Grandma—whose newsy updates arrived by mail every week or two: "I've never seen anybody write so many letters that don't say *anything at all.*"

SO MY MOM WAS an incisive, entertaining detractor, and my dad was a poor ambassador, and I myself tended to experience the older generation on my dad's side of the family as dull and disapproving, not nearly so harsh as my dad himself but somewhere on the way to that neighborhood, and thus did I resolve to be as unlike them as possible. Rebellion in families is rarely simple, though, no matter how we frame it to ourselves. Even when I was a young child, my narrative of mutual condemnation was complicated by my affection for my grandfather.

Grandpa was gruff but funny and handsome, with a dashing silver-white pompadour. He dispelled the gloom at the start of every childhood visit by chasing my sister and me around the house, brandishing his bare feet, threatening our calves with his dexterous and formidable "pincher toes." Later, when we were in our teens, Grandpa opened our trips to their small Gulf Coast town with a tour of the local sewage plant, driving along the reeking periphery of the vats with mock pride as Grandma waited at home. He had a wry sense of humor and some appreciation for irony and eccentricity—which my mom and my granny had taught me to prize—while Grandma had neither. It was she who seemed to control the annals of family lore.

From my dad, I learned about a pre-Revolutionary ancestor through Grandma, and our connection by marriage, through Grandpa's mother, to the Mannings of football fame. Grandma herself enjoyed reminiscing about growing up in the Delta, about living so near her redheaded aunts, who were her mother's sisters and also relations of her father. When asked, Grandma would acknowledge that her parents, Mama T. and Daddy Joe, were second cousins once removed, though she did not volunteer this.

Eventually I realized that Grandma avoided talking as much about the Newtons—most of all my great-grandfather, Granddaddy, Grandpa's father. Meanwhile, my mom had, as is her way, amassed many stories. Granddaddy scheduled the days of his wife, my great-grandmother Mamma, down to bathroom breaks, my mom said. He ridiculed Mamma and berated her. And when Grandpa was a boy, Granddaddy made him pull a plow on hot summer days while Granddaddy sat in the shade, drinking lemonade and ridiculing his son. But Grandma did have one Granddaddy story, edgy for her. Apparently he had a habit of clearing his throat so loudly and relentlessly through the day and the night that once, when he stayed in a hotel, a woman from the neighboring room confronted him on the landing the next morning. "Ho ho ho humn," she said, in a precise imitation. This was an unusually unflattering family story coming from Grandma, and she told it in a delighted, conspiratorial way that suggested great sympathy with the hotel neighbor. But when I alluded to my mom's stories about Grand-daddy, Grandma fell silent.

IN MY LATE TWENTIES or early thirties, I started asking about Maude Newton, Granddaddy's sister and Grandpa's aunt. My dad had told me when I was a child that Maude trained as an architect and designed her own house, surprising accomplishments for a woman of her generation in the Mississippi Delta. He never re-ferred to her merely as Maude but always as Maude Newton, the two names together, as though she was a person of distinction, a woman of note, a family counterpart to Amelia Earhart or Lucille Ball.

My interest in Maude had grown over the years as my relation-ship with my dad disintegrated and my nonconformity solidified into something that could no longer be ascribed to youth. I married an artist and moved to Brooklyn. I left the practice of law. I in-tended, as I always had, to be a writer, although I paid the bills by writing about tax law. By 2002, my dad and I were estranged, though I wasn't sure whether the estrangement was permanent when I started a website devoted to personal stories about Miami. On a whim, in an homage built on some combination of irony, perversity, projection, and a desire to shield the innocent, I decided to post my writing there as Maud Newton. (My given name is Rebecca.) My sister and husband knew about this, but the rest of my family did not. While most of my friends and some family members call me Maud nowadays, and I like it, I didn't foresee actually answering to the name when I chose it as a pseudonym.

Around that time, my sister and I traveled to see our grandpar-ents in Mississippi, as we did most years. I waited until the four of us were settled into the car for a drive home from dinner. Then I met Grandpa's eyes in the rearview mirror and asked about Maude. Was she really an architect? Did she really design her own house?

"Well," said Grandpa, his silver-white hair picking up the glow of the streetlights. He spoke slowly, in part because of his drawl but equally due to his deliberation. He was precise. "The thing they used to say about Maude was—"

"Oh, Richard." Grandma's hands fluttered to her handbag and then back into her lap. "They don't want to hear that old story." She flicked open the passenger mirror to check her lipstick. Her mouth was turned down; her dark eyes looked worried.

"Yes, we do," I said.

"Yes," said my sister, whose expression of interest in their family was a rarity, "we do."

Grandpa hesitated, then went rogue. Great-Aunt Maude did indeed design her own house, he said. Not just that, but she sat in a lawn chair and called out corrections as it was being built.

"Just look at those magnolias—*aren't they beautiful?*" Grandma's voice had risen an octave.

No one looked at the magnolias. Instead, Grandpa told us that Maude had been married but didn't like it and so "she threw pepper in her husband's eyes until he stopped coming around."

Pepper in his eyes until he stopped coming around. This revelation exceeded all my imaginings. There were difficult women on my father's side, too.

Grandma reached for Grandpa's shoulder and jogged it a little. "I just *can't believe* how the neighbors have let their hedges go!" she said.

Grandpa said we'd have to talk more about Maude "some other day." We never did.

Chapter 5

FAMILY SECRETS

——

MY INTEREST IN THE REST OF THE NEWTONS TOOK time to develop. I'd focused on my mom's family when I set up my tree and only cursorily entered what I knew of my father's genealogy. On Grandma's side, there was the line going back to colonial Virginia, the one that my father had showed me while mulling divorce from my mom. But I didn't know much about my father's father's line, the Newtons. When I did start tracing them, living sources were limited: Grandpa had Alzheimer's and would pass on the following year; Grandma had died a couple of years before; my aunt couldn't trace the line back further; my father and I weren't in touch.

As I worked my way through a box from my mom packed with old family photos, documents, and Granny's scrawled genealogies, I found some notes about the Newtons in my mom's handwriting, notes that trailed off. Eventually I asked what she knew. Not much, she said. Early in her marriage to my father, she'd asked about them and had her inquiries rebuffed. What surprised me was that the resistance came from Grandpa's father, Granddaddy, the Newton patriarch himself. He told my mom to stop asking. "Why would you ask about that?" she remembers him saying. His resistance was curious. Ordinarily, Granddaddy really liked to hold forth. He was the kind of man who told the women at a restaurant table what they were going to eat and then ordered for them. "Louise, you'll have the catfish," he'd say, as the server jotted down the entrees, "and, Sandy, you'll have the cheeseburger."

Granddaddy's wife, Louise—my great-grandmother Mamma (Grandpa's mother), who is not the same person as Mama T. (Grandma's mother), in case the Delta-ness of it all is confusing—came from money but had been divorced before she and Granddaddy got together, so she entered the marriage, around 1918, not only with wealth but shame. Granddaddy claimed dominion over her resources, apparently using them to finance his farm, his whims, and his womanizing.

Unlike Mamma, Granddaddy came from poverty. A few years into my search, I unearthed a newspaper article about him, DREW'S LAST COTTON BUYER GOES OUT OF BUSINESS, published around 1976, when Granddaddy retired at eighty-four years old. He told the reporter that he grew up in "a house without a ceiling," in the Mississippi Delta. During winter, he said, "when Papa would walk through the hall to the other side of the house his mustache would freeze." One Christmas, Santa left a note that "he was a little poor this year, so there was only a wagon and candy for all to share." Granddaddy ended with a moment of self-congratulation: "I have touched the lives of many, both black and white, during this span of years. Because I have done so, it has made me a better person." I suspect the Black people who knew Granddaddy would offer a far less sanguine perspective.

It feels almost mean-spirited to tell you how mean-spirited Granddaddy is said to have been, in part because I'm mentioned in that article as his "pixieish brown-haired great-granddaughter," one of the "objects of his greatest interest." Also, in fairness, I don't remember witnessing Granddaddy's dictatorial tendencies or his racism firsthand. I visited him rarely, and he died a month before my eighth birthday. The last time I saw him, just after I turned seven and about two years after that newspaper article, he was lying in a nursing-home bed. I knew he was very ill.

I told him I loved him, which seemed true as I stood looking into his face, even though we barely knew each other. I didn't have a gift but felt I should, so I gave him the change from my pocket. This seemed to please him. He had dementia, probably Alzheimer's (based on his son's fate a few decades later). Maybe the simplicity of my offering was comforting. But my mom maintained that my father, who idolized Granddaddy, developed his love of money by example, so maybe Granddaddy was just happy to have the seventy-three cents, or whatever it was.

The most damning evidence of Granddaddy's personality is that (according to my mom) Mamma rejoiced when she started to lose her hearing. As he berated her, she turned down the volume on her hearing aid and moved through her days in silence. After he closed his cotton business in the Delta and went into the nursing home on the coast near my grandparents, Mamma moved into an apartment and refused to see him again. Only Grandpa and my dad attended his funeral.

GIVEN MY FATHER'S OBSESSION with "blood" and the extent to which he emulated and idolized his grandfather, Granddaddy's caginess on the subject of his actual ancestry amused and intrigued me. Soon I was spending weekends working backward through history in an effort to discover whatever it was we weren't supposed to know.

In a photo, Granddaddy's mother, Minnie House Newton, my great-great-grandmother "Grand Newt," is a sharp-eyed, white-haired woman with a knowing smile. Grand Newt doesn't seem to have imparted much Newton family history before passing on in 1962 at age ninety-five. But my mom's notes establish that Minnie and her husband, James Newton, were married in Arkansas, "near Monticello," a town across the Mississippi border. Digging around in the census, cemetery records, and other documents, I discovered that the family lived in Arkansas when Great-Aunt Maude, the eldest child, was born, but Granddaddy and the other children were born in Mississippi.

Long archives story short, eventually I believed I had found my fourth great-grandfather, one Jesse Newton, a farmer probably born in Duplin County, North Carolina, in 1803. He married Elizabeth Quinn there, in 1827, and they headed west, having children in Georgia and Alabama before settling and buying land in Drew County, Arkansas. There, according to historical records, Jesse served as treasurer and was "granted a license to retail spirituous and vinous liquors." He also raised nine children: five sons, three daughters, and a boy who was orphaned at the age of three. Josiah Hazen Shinn's *Pioneers and Makers of Arkansas* (1908) refers to Jesse as "an honored citizen of that bailiwick" who "came to the state at a later date" than the other Newtons in his survey.

According to the 1860 census, Jesse also enslaved six people: a thirty-six-year-old man, a nineteen-year-old woman, a twelve-year-old boy, and three girls, ages seventeen years, twelve years, and six months old. I don't know their names because the forms, called "slave schedules," recorded only the age and biological sex of the people held in bondage, and listed them under Jesse. This wasn't the first time I'd discovered an ancestor on these rolls, nor would it be the last. I'd hoped to find that my father's family exaggerated our involvement in slavery, that they invented a plantation after the fact. I found the opposite. But Jesse's enslavement of human beings wouldn't have been something Granddaddy wanted to hide. He and Mamma both were openly, unremittingly—"jubilantly" is not too strong a word—racist. They passed along to my dad the idea that the slave system was humming along perfectly until Northern "bleeding hearts" started meddling and destroyed a good thing that had been working for everyone. The day Martin Luther King, Jr., was assassinated, Mamma was happy, and said so.

WHATEVER THE NEWTON SECRET was, I wasn't finding it. And so, in 2009, I tracked down one of Grandpa's first cousins, Wallace Dolphin Newton, Jr., then eighty-three. I asked if he could verify that Jesse Newton was in fact my fourth and Wallace's second great-grandfather. He could not. "We had the same problem that you had," he told me. "It was as if the Newton family began with Minnie. We just could not get anyone to give us information."

His daughter had theorized that we're related to the Newton Boys, the notorious bank robbers, which would have delighted me. Despite robbing eighty-five banks and half a dozen trains, they never killed anyone and, according to *Texas Hill Country Magazine,* even the bank tellers thought they were charming. But while that family descended from a Jesse Newton of Arkansas, and ours did, too, they weren't the same man. I didn't find any ties between the lines, just some similar names and close proximity. Maybe they were cousins. Still, knowing my dad's family, it seemed possible my Newtons suppressed their history because they were afraid our Jesse would be *mistaken* for someone disreputable, that people might not understand that Arkansas could have produced two Jesse Newtons and the other one was the forefather of the Newton Boys. I was going to have to approach the search from some other angle.

Chapter 6

DNA SLEUTHING

———

I SUPPOSE I WAS HOPING FOR SOME REFUTATORY REVEAL. Having failed to find one the traditional way, I turned to DNA. What would my genome reveal about my father, the five-foot-seven-and-a-half-inch amateur eugenicist who'd bequeathed to me his poor eyesight, his unimpressive stature, his awkward, clipped way of walking, and his near-homicidal intolerance of many common noises? Could I find our Newton ancestor through my genes? In 2010, I gave it a shot. I signed up for 23andMe, spit into a tube, dropped it in the mail, and, within a couple of months, received a list of predicted relatives. The first thing I realized was that, when taking a DNA test for genealogical purposes, potential cousins are remarkably easy to come by. Even people with whom you might share a third or fourth great-grandparent aren't a particular scarcity. I had thousands of matches. Later I was also tested at AncestryDNA.

Over the years since then, many more people have joined these sites, some of them closer relations. In 2019, a predicted second cousin turned up on AncestryDNA and messaged me, asking about my family's connection to Texas. Looking at our shared matches, it took me about fifteen minutes to deduce that my match descends from my great-grandparents, Charley and Rindia Bruce. The cousin turned out to be the grandchild of my grandfather Robert's youngest brother, Hillard, and the unacknowledged son of a distant relative I'd emailed once while researching Charley. According to the cousin, two of my other closest matches on the site are his half-siblings, also children of this man.

With the rise of these tests, secret forebears can be uncovered and prestigious lineages invalidated. A new world has opened up, for adoptees, descendants of enslaved people, children of Holocaust survivors, and anyone else cut off from their roots. Figuring out exactly which ancestors you share (or may share) with people in these databases can still be a needle-in-a-haystack endeavor, though, even when relatively unusual surnames are involved, even when you and a match have both done extensive work on your family trees.

Over the years, I've identified probable common ancestors for an increasingly large number of matches, maybe a hundred, probably more, all of them classified on the sites as predominantly of European descent. One remembers visiting my second great-grandmother's house in the Mississippi Delta. Looking at photos of another, a third cousin twice removed on my dad's mother's side, I see echoes of a first cousin's smile. Kevin Kinchen, a fifth cousin on my mom's mother's side, has a background in pattern recognition, private investigation, and forensics. He calls genealogy "the ultimate puzzle box." It never has to have an end, he says. Which is also something I've thought, and it is something, given my sometimes-compulsive immersion in this world, that alarms me.

It's impossible to estimate what percentage of my predicted cousins are of predominantly African ancestry, because 23andMe only allows me to see the information each match permits and AncestryDNA shows only our shared geographic regions of origin unless the subscriber opts for further sharing, but as is the case with many if not most descendants of Southern enslavers, that percentage is bound to be considerable. Slavery did so much to erase records of the personhood of its victims that, so far, I haven't been able to identify a precise common ancestor with a single match whose "ancestry composition" is said to be largely African. But records are there to be pieced together, and, increasingly, Black Americans do. The genetic genealogist Shannon Christmas is among those working to dismantle "the myth of the 1870 Brick Wall," the idea that most Black Americans descended from people who were enslaved can't trace their families back before the Civil War. Six years ago, after years of searching, Christmas found his fourth great-grandmother listed as inventory in the estate of her enslaver, unlocking what Christmas called on his blog "an unmarked door to the world that my ancestors inhabited."

Matthew Ware, one of my predicted third to sixth cousins, is a physics professor at Grambling State University. 23andMe breaks his genome down by region, in percentages that have shifted over time. As of January 2021, the site assigns him 54.4 percent European ancestry, 44.7 percent sub-Saharan, 0.6 percent East Asian and Native American, and 0.3 percent unassigned. At first, engaging in the sort of quasi-magical associative thinking people often tend toward where DNA and ancestry are involved, I imagined that Ware was a relative through my father's side, because of their shared interest in science, a common connection to Mississippi, and even, I thought, Matthew's physical resemblance to my father himself. In reality, he matches me mostly through my mother. I say "mostly" because he and I share more DNA than he and my mother do, so he's probably a match through my father, as well. Ware has learned he's descended from a Revolutionary War hero, a person who was enslaved, and an exiled Scottish rebel.

Another possible third to sixth cousin, Deborah Hampton-Miller, is a writer. "I believe that gift runs in the family (bloodline)," she told me in an email. Hampton-Miller is of predominantly sub-Saharan ancestry (as of January 2021, 23andMe identifies her ancestral origins as 79.2 percent sub-Saharan African, 17.5 percent European, 2.6 percent East Asian and Native American, and 0.7 percent unassigned). Because she doesn't share genes with my mom, we must be related through my father, but we haven't been able to link up our trees.

According to 23andMe originally, I was 99.9 percent European and 0.1 percent North African. My mother was 100 percent European. So, I thought, the North African/Middle Eastern genes must have come from my father, an irony I doubted he would have allowed himself to enjoy.

This teeny percentage isn't worth dwelling on, except to underscore its unreliability. Several years after first signing up at 23andMe, I participated in a research study also run through the site. I ended up with two accounts, so 23andMe thought I had an identical twin and kept asking if I wanted to connect with her. The second account used a higher-quality "genotyping chip" than the original—a change the company makes periodically to incorporate improvements in technology—and initially indicated the possibility of 0.6 percent North African ancestry. After some shifts on both accounts, the percentage settled for a time at 0.1 percent Middle Eastern and North African on the first account and 0.2 percent North African and Middle Eastern on the second. Then, in 2019, the site concluded that I was 100 percent European, before reverting in 2020 to 99.7 percent European, with 0.3 percent of my genome unassigned—now evidently from my mom's side. As of January 2021, I have been assigned 0.3 percent Levantine DNA (to my mom's 0.2 percent Levantine).

That's a tiny fraction of my DNA. The closest ancestor might be something like a seventh great-grandparent, if the genes came from a single person. Over the years, though, as 23andMe has refined its research and reassessed its assignments of existing users' DNA, people with large percentages of genes traced to these regions have experienced much more dramatic and disorienting swings that they've denounced in the site's forums and on sites like Reddit. If, for instance, an adopted person is told their ancestry is 49 percent North African and later told that percentage is Spanish, it can be hard to know what to believe. The site's region-labeling practices are especially likely to result in confusing and misleading results for people whose ancestry isn't predominantly European.

AncestryDNA breaks down regions differently and never designated any of my genome as North African. At first the site fudged a little, indicating that 3 percent of my DNA originated on the Iberian Peninsula, which on their map includes not just Spain and Portugal but also parts of Morocco, Algeria, France, and Italy. ("LOL," a friend from Morocco replied, when I told them this.) Now that assignment has disappeared, too. On AncestryDNA, I see only the parts of my matches' "ethnicity estimates" that match mine, unless they select to reveal all their region assignments. While about 15 percent of adults in the United States say they've used a mail-in DNA-testing service, according to Pew Research, Americans who view themselves as white are far more likely (17 percent) than those who view themselves as Black or Hispanic/Latino (10 percent) to do so. Only 12 percent of the white DNA test-takers say the results changed the way they think about their racial or ethnic identity, compared to 24 percent of users of color.

BY NOW, MILLIONS OF us have taken these ancestry tests and had our genomes assigned to different parts of the world. The fine print warns us not to rely on those results, but they seem so precise. It's hard to resist telling friends and family that we've turned out to be 19 percent sub-Saharan African or Middle Eastern or Scandinavian. Testing with another company may yield different results, though, or we may log in to our account one day and find that the allocations have changed to something else entirely. Once again we're something other than what we thought we were.

The explanations that testing companies give for these shifts tend to be passive and blandly opaque. Identifying "ancestry-informative markers" depends on "sufficient data" from "reference populations"; errors might be "noise." These observations are taken from Alex Wagner's *Futureface: A Family Mystery, an Epic Quest, and the Secret to Belonging,* in which she recalls a testing-company CEO suggesting to her that blame for these mistakes lies with the consumer, who "wants a *yes* or *no,*" when "science is not that simple." Wagner's stinging criticism of the "flossy statistics" set out in ancestry-composition results is some of the most astute I've seen. "Possibly inaccurate to the point of uselessness," she calls them, observing that the categories themselves are suspect. Some DNA is "classified using political borders," such as "Irish," whereas for others, such as "South Asian DNA," it's defined by "regional assignments." The tests also fail to account for the permeability of borders over time. True, Burma, her maternal family's homeland, was colonized by the British in the mid-1800s, but there were much-earlier arrivals of the Pyu (200 B.C.) and the Mon (1000 A.D.). The sites don't purport to look back that far, but these historical events still raise the question: "At what point was Burmese blood considered 'unmixed' and exempt of outside influence?" (Wagner rejects "Myanmar," the name given to the country by the ruling military in 1989.)

For the *New York Times*'s Wirecutter, Amadou Diallo and Brishette Mendoza observe that the major testing companies' reference samples skew dramatically toward Europeans. Nonetheless, both AncestryDNA and 23andMe have teamed up with the travel industry to offer "Heritage Tours," designed to acquaint users with (as a 23andMe blog post puts it) their "newfound ancestral lands." AncestryDNA's tour includes "handpicked hotels, authentic cuisine, guided sightseeing," an "expert Tour Director," the site's DNA test kit, and a genealogist. As of 2019, 23andMe's data set for sub-Saharan African ancestry relies on only 1,980 "reference individuals." For Central and South Asian ancestry, composition reports rely on a data set of 1,634. For Europeans, the number of reference individuals was 6,328.

In 2018, a Twitter user, Mina II Society, excoriated these tests and their assignments in a single tweet: "Only white people can steal you, enslave you for hundreds of years, systematically oppress you for hundreds more, then charge you $99.99 to tell you where they stole you from. Visit online at ancestry dot com." People whose African ancestors were enslaved on these shores may find more-precise results from a source like African Ancestry, a Black-owned site with more than 30,000 Indigenous African DNA samples.

THE DISCOVERY THAT I was as white as I'd always appeared to be was deeply, irrationally disappointing, as though having mixed ancestry would somehow mitigate the wrongs of my forebears. I knew it was dangerous to fixate on trying to refute my father's racist bloodline grandiosity with data that even he would have to accept. His attitudes were like quicksand—the more I struggled to disprove them using these tools, the more trapped, implicated, and angry I felt. And as I continued to obsess and cogitate, to find myself sunk deep in North Carolina census archives at one o'clock in the morning, I knew I needed to change my relationship to the search, but it was unclear to me what I was looking for. What I wanted was fact and not-fact. I wanted a truth that would set me free in some way I hadn't identified yet.

I kept coming back to Jesse Newton. He would be far easier to trace genetically if he were a closer ancestor than a fourth great-grandparent—and also if Southerners hadn't intermarried so much. Trees of several matches at Ancestry.com include eighteenth- and nineteenth-century Newtons from the cluster of families in and around Duplin County, North Carolina, that I believe Jesse issues from. A George Newton and Ursula Whitehead show up often, as do an Ebenezer Newton and Elizabeth Buchanan, an Isaac Newton, and a Susannah Newton. There's a good chance Jesse is related to these people, but I don't have proof. Complicating things further, other lines of mine, on both sides, go back to that area. A Y-DNA test tracing the markers of my Newton line might provide some clues about where my paternal line originated, but, as a person without a Y chromosome, I can't take the test. Only an unbroken male line will do. Over the years, I've contacted several descendants of Granddaddy's brothers. Some of these distant cousins corresponded warmly with me, but none agreed to spit into a tube for a stranger who popped up uninvited after deducing their whereabouts—and our connection—from murky Internet sleuthing.

In 2014, I hired a North Carolina genealogist named Jason Bordeaux to take a look at the Duplin County court archives from Jesse's era. On Bordeaux's first day of searching, he discovered a "gift deed" from a Sally Newton to her son. The deed cited her "natural love and affection for my son Jesse Newton" and her wish to provide for "maintenance of him in this life." In what seemed like a bequest from Shakespeare and the Old Testament rolled into one, Sally directed that a feather bed and a calf "be delivered unto him when he arrives to the age of twenty-one years." The document was signed August 14, 1810 (or 1816), but it wasn't filed until the July court term in 1823—"a very close fit," Bordeaux observed, to Jesse's twenty-first birthday. "This is a fortunate find and a great start," Bordeaux wrote. "Most projects don't start like this."

On a subsequent dive into the Duplin County records, he found a brief entry dated January 19, 1808: "Sally Newton having been delivered of a bastard child, gave bond required by law." Jesse would have been four years old when the bond was filed, but this kind of lag wasn't unusual. According to a blog devoted to Appalachian history, the North Carolina bastardy-bond process typically started "with public knowledge or a complaint that an unwed woman was with child," but sometimes the legalities were set in motion after the birth. Either way, a "warrant was issued and the woman brought into court." A book devoted to the bonds explains that the woman was questioned under oath "and asked to declare the name of the child's father." If she did, the man was "served a warrant and required to post bond." If the woman refused to identify the father, she, her father, or someone else would post bond, or she would likely face jail time.

Was this the big secret: that my Newton ancestor was an unmarried woman? If so, would she have been shunned, forced like Hester Prynne in *The Scarlet Letter* to live outside the society while having to navigate within it? I asked Bordeaux. Sally would have been ostracized, he said, but once Jesse became a man, he would not necessarily have experienced prejudice. "Illegitimacy was very common" in the area, Bordeaux said. "There are numerous entries for every term of court," typically every quarter.

Sally Newton "made her mark" on the documents Bordeaux found, but my Jesse actually signed land documents, suggesting a literacy disparity between mother and child, if he was Sally's son. And my Jesse married, with Elizabeth Quinn, into a family of relative means. Some years after they left North Carolina, an announcement in the newspaper gave notice that, because Elizabeth and Jesse had departed the state, their claim to her father's estate would be forfeited and her share divided between the rest of his children. The only other Jesse Newton that Bordeaux or I could find in the area was much older. Despite a good deal of searching, though, Bordeaux never found definitive evidence showing a connection between Sally Newton and my Jesse. For the years before Jesse reached majority, the county-court books held no land data for her, no tax data, no apprentice bond for him. Still, Sally of the bastardy bond, the feather bed, and the calf is my best lead. Her son's name fits, as do the dates. And I like to think that my mysterious Newton "patriarch" was this one—a single mother of unusual sovereignty who gave me her genes and her surname.

As it happens, my genome reveals that my parents are distantly related to each other, maybe somewhere between seven and ten generations back. Every full biological child of a parent receives, intact, one chromosome from each parent's thirteen pairs and thus shares exactly 50 percent of the parent's DNA. My mother and I share this 50 percent, and we also share an additional 0.2 percent, a small segment of fifteen centimorgans that's identical on another chromosome. Once I realized the overlap, I enjoyed imagining that my mom and Granny and Great-Aunt Maude and Sally Newton and my sister and I all descend from the same intractable woman.

Chapter 7

A UNIVERSAL
FAMILY TREE

——

WE ORIGINATED IN AFRICA, ALL OF US, EVOLUTIONARY biologists say. Humans diversified there until eventually, around 60,000 years ago, a small group of a thousand or so exited the continent. Slowly these migrants made their way across the world, becoming the ancestors of all people—Asians, Native Americans, Europeans, and so on—outside the land they left behind. The people who stayed were a far larger and more diverse cross section of humanity than those who left. We only know of the migration because, as Christine Kenneally puts it in *The Invisible History of the Human Race,* the genomic variation of "everyone in the world outside of Africa is a subset of the genomic variation still found in Africa." The migrants created the first known human population "bottleneck": Through their small group came their descendants, a new population with limited genetic variation. They would have been extremely vulnerable to disease until nature and time intervened, bringing mutations and, with them, diversity. The gene pool did get one early infusion of newness, though. Soon after departing the continent, the migrant population had babies with Neanderthals. Kenneally imagines them standing on the threshold of the unknown world, trying to decide which way to go, when they hooked up with their distant kin.

Our understanding of our species' past is so limited, we can barely conceive of everything we don't know. Only in the last decade did we learn about the Denisovans, cousins of both the Neanderthals and modern humans. Now, with DNA testing, we're building what Kenneally calls "a library of ancient genomes," one that allows us not only to compare ourselves to our ancient ancestors but "the ancients to one another." As skulls turn up with blended traits of Neanderthals and other archaic humans, some paleoanthropologists contend that we shouldn't conceive of these groups as separate species but as part of what the scholar Erik Trinkaus calls "a unified humanity across the Old World." New discoveries raise the possibility of multiple migrations out of Africa, before the defining 60,000 B.C. trek population geneticists have posited.

Carl Sagan and Ann Druyan imagined our even-more-distant origins in their 1993 book, *Shadows of Forgotten Ancestors.* "Our family tree was rooted when the Earth was just emerging from a time of massive, obliterating impacts, molten red-hot landscapes, and pitch-black skies," they write, "when our connection with the Universe around us was manifest." They denounce our refusal to acknowledge kinship with our animal ancestors, from our close cousins, the primates, with their complex social hierarchies and their ability to wield tools and learn language, all the way back to the "microbes of the primeval sea." If we would only accept and contemplate our interconnectedness with these forebears, they argue, we would reevaluate our obligations to one another and the planet at large. But, especially in the West, many of us remain committed to our narrative of superiority and separateness.

SINCE THE START OF human history, we've been losing track of it. The longer we live, the more we see this attrition happening in real time. Beloved grandparents die, taking their memories and leaving photo albums filled with people who were integral to the clan fifty years ago but are strangers now. Migration and forgetting, in particular, often go together.

Joan Didion's *Where I Was From* recounts the move of her granddad's family "from the hardscrabble Adirondack frontier in the eighteenth century to the hardscrabble Sierra Nevada foothills in the nineteenth." On the long wagon journey, Didion's great-great-grandmother buried a child, gave birth to another, contracted mountain fever twice, and sewed a quilt, "a blinding and pointless compaction of stitches," which she must have finished en route, "somewhere in the wilderness of her own grief and illness." Throughout the book, Didion ruminates on her forebears, women "pragmatic and in their deepest instincts clinically radical, given to breaking clean with everyone and everything they knew."

In their progression across this land, settlers like Didion's ancestors—and mine—pushed Indigenous people out, by forced displacement or genocide. In *The Heartbeat of Wounded Knee,* David Treuer explains how accounts written by penitent descendants of colonizers have compounded these injuries by implying that Indigenous cultures died out with the fallen, even as their descendants live on, making art, running for office, protesting at Standing Rock. It pains Treuer to think of the Battle of Wounded Knee, and it also pains him to read Dee Brown's bestselling 1970 book, *Bury My Heart at Wounded Knee.* Treuer writes:

> What hurts is not just that 150 people were cruelly and viciously killed. It is that their sense of life—and our sense of their lives—died with them. We know next to nothing about them. Who among them was funny? Who kicked his dog? Were they unfaithful, or vain, or fond of sweets? The tiny, fretful, intricate details are what make us who we are. And they are lost again and again when we paint over them with the tragedy of "the Indian." In this sense, the victims of

Wounded Knee died twice—once at the end of a gun, and again at the end of a pen.

Memory is short. What we think we know about the people who came before us is often wrong. Even biographies of the most famous men are hotly debated, their authorship of works questioned, their lives reinterpreted. No matter how someone might toil to distinguish oneself during life, Mark Twain wrote, "Twenty little centuries flutter away, and what is left of these things? A crazy inscription on a block of stone, which snuffy antiquaries bother over and tangle up and make nothing out of but a bare name (which they spell wrong)." He imagines an encyclopedia entry from the year 5868: "'URIAH S. (or Z.) GRAUNT—popular poet of ancient times in the Aztec provinces of the United States of British America.'"

With such low odds that even major historical figures will be memorialized accurately, the chances of maintaining familial memory over centuries must be minuscule. A fantastic counterpoint is recorded in a documentary about the Gangá-Longobá people of Cuba, who still perform songs and dances passed down by a family matriarch, Josefa, on a sugar plantation where she was enslaved. The filmmaker recorded these rituals and went in search of their origins, and one man in a Sierra Leone coffee shop who saw her video urged her to visit the village of Mokpangumba. When she screened it there, the villagers were soon dancing and singing along. "They are we!" they said.

More often, ancestors lost for a generation or two have tended to remain lost. The centuries have cut us off from knowledge of our forebears, shrouded our familial places of origin in mystery. Now, with genetic testing, we've begun to sort out some of this confusion, but we've also created new dangers and uncertainties. Yes, the technology for solving genetic mysteries is available to just about anyone with a hundred bucks and access to a computer. But they may want to enlist the help of an expert like the forensic genealogist CeCe Moore.

Moore lives in Southern California, has a background in theater and music, and is a natural sleuth with a roving intelligence, quick intuition, and easy charm. I first reached out to her in 2013, when I was beginning to explore the scientific underpinnings of genetic genealogy. In our first conversation, I learned how Moore—without a background in science, long before anyone thought possible— helped invent the practice of genetic genealogy, using tools accidentally created by 23andMe. While focusing on its primary mission, health and medical research, the company had assembled all the data that ultimately fed into 23andMe's "Relative Finder," which allows predicted cousins to find one another. Moore and other genealogists on the site pushed them to make the information available to subscribers and more user-friendly. "Other companies were saying, 'You can't use autosomal DNA for genetic research,' but 23andMe did it in 2009," she told me over the phone.

Moore and I bonded over a shared fascination with the way talents and burdens pass down in families, the ways secrets have of bubbling up a couple of generations down the line. We disagreed about the potential dangers of autosomal DNA testing. She explained to me that the ultimate goal of DNA-based genealogy is to create a "Universal Genetic Family Tree" revealing exactly how everyone in the world is related to everyone else. Back in 2013, Moore called this universal tree a future "inevitability." Even then I suspected she was correct, and increasingly I can see the tree assembling itself in real time on AncestryDNA for those who've done testing. In 2018, a study reported in the journal *Science* concluded that about 60 percent of Americans of Northern European descent can be identified from consumer DNA sites using a third cousin or closer match, even if the individual hasn't been tested. The technique, they concluded, "could implicate nearly any U.S. individual of European descent in the near future."

A genomic database of this kind would eliminate false pedigrees and solve long-standing mysteries. The ultimate implications for humankind are hard to project. To Moore, transparency is an inherent good. I was tempted to agree in principle, but the mechanisms of our society, the rewards and punishments handed out, are not neutral. There are many dangerous possibilities. If each of us was as readily identifiable from our saliva as the characters in *Gattaca* are from their skin cells, how might we all be siloed? Still, my anxiety about DNA-based genealogy didn't prevent me from being tested at both 23andMe and Ancestry.com or from uploading my data elsewhere. My fear and my curiosity battled it out, and curiosity won. It wasn't much of a contest.

MOORE'S OWN FAMILY HISTORY was the gateway to her work. As an amateur genealogist and a professional musician, she was excited by the repetition of musical talents in her own family tree. Starting in 2010, she began to write about these recurrences and her genealogical discoveries on her blog, Your Genetic Genealogist. Soon she became so interested in the potential of combining genetic data with traditional genealogy that she started helping other people solve family mysteries.

Her brother-in-law, John, took a DNA test and was surprised that his results showed he's 5 percent African American. Moore started researching and soon realized that John's mother descended from Madison Hemings, the son of Sally Hemings and Thomas Jefferson. On her blog, she wrote that John had always admired Jefferson more than any other historical figure, and he'd felt a strong connection to Monticello on visiting a decade before. Still, he and Moore's sister were shocked to learn that Jefferson was his ancestor. As they started searching online to make sense of it, though, they discovered a familiar photo on a website about Monticello, a photo that had hung on the wall of John's childhood home. Eventually

John discovered that his mother had some awareness that her family was related to Jefferson or Hemings, but never told her children.

The first time the family visited Jefferson's home in Monticello, before they knew of their connection to the man and the place, John's daughter fainted. It could have been the warm day, Moore concedes, but her niece had never fainted before and never has since.

When we first got in touch, Moore mostly worked for private clients, solved adoption and other cases on a volunteer basis, consulted with 23andMe and other genealogy sites, and did a lot of speaking and teaching. She was beginning her work on Henry Louis Gates, Jr.'s *Finding Your Roots*, where she remains the genetic genealogist and is now a producer. She'd get so invested in her work that she found it hard to sleep when she thought she was getting close to solving a case. There was always a chance that she'd have to tell an adoptee not only who his birth mother was but that the mother had died a couple of months earlier. Moore's method involved triangulating between DNA matches, genetic-genealogical research databases, and other archives and resources available through Google. Using this approach, she's reunited adoptees and birth parents and solved other family mysteries. She found the birth parents of a man who as a toddler was discovered abandoned in New Jersey. She worked with an amnesiac to locate his family. She solved a century-old switched-at-birth case. And she exposed a fertility-clinic tech who had decided to "help" a couple conceive by substituting his sperm for the father's; it turned out that the tech had also substituted his sperm for other men's.

In recent years, Moore's path has taken a turn into crime-solving, a development that foregrounds some of the concerns I had when we first spoke. She's probably best known now as the star of ABC's *The Genetic Detective*, a true-crime show devoted to cracking cold cases. Her focus explicitly shifted in 2018, after researchers used forensic DNA research to pinpoint the identity of the serial rapist and murderer known as the Golden State Killer, whose trail had long been cold. Moore wasn't involved in the case but immediately knew the methods they'd used, and she was promptly hired as head genetic genealogist at Parabon NanoLabs, a company that purported to create predictive mugshots from DNA left at crime scenes and sold the resulting images to law enforcement. I was aware of Parabon's "Snapshot" product in part because it piggybacked on a Penn State DNA study, headed by an anthropology professor and funded in part by the U.S. Department of Defense, that attempted to tie genetic markers to physical characteristics, with predictably unreliable and sometimes racist results, in what were framed as "DNA mugshots." We know AI can't even accurately match a photo of a Black or brown person to another photo of that same person in a database; creating wanted posters based on genetic data has been, unsurprisingly, even less effective and at least as dangerous, if not more so.

Parabon became embroiled in controversy when the media reported that the sleuths who identified the Golden State Killer used data from GEDmatch, a free genealogy site, without informing users. Moore told *MIT Technology Review* that she viewed the Golden State Killer case as a "green light" to proceed with research in GEDmatch. Amid all the publicity, she reportedly reasoned, anyone who objected could delete their data. I had once uploaded mine, despite knowing there were risks; I deleted it after this though my genetic data is in the hands of law enforcement anyway through a research study. In 2019, GEDmatch changed its policy, protecting users' genomic data from being used to solve crimes unless the user opts in.

I have a mixed reaction to Moore's work. I'm all for accurately identifying rapists, serial killers, and other perpetrators of sexual assault and violent crime. And her efforts have exonerated wrongly accused people in addition to pinpointing culprits. But some biological relatives of violent offenders have been wrongly targeted.

And rooting around in databases where people uploaded genetic data without realizing how it might be used is ethically murky.

Back in 2013, Moore was as ardent an advocate for genetic-genealogical sleuthing as she is now. Still, she'd seen enough situations where DNA testing had "unexpectedly uncovered complex family relationships" that she warned those who test to "expect unexpected surprises." So many people have different fathers than they thought, she told me, that the incidence of misidentified paternity "must be way higher than we thought back through time." But while her clients were sometimes confronted with shocking discoveries, most of the people she worked with were happy to have the answers DNA provided, even when those answers were painful.

Moore acknowledged that some aren't in a rush to pinpoint the genetic truth of relationships. "People with a storied pedigree have a lot to lose," she said, and often refuse to risk being tested. But John, her brother-in-law, knows that Thomas Jefferson and Sally Hemings are his fourth great-grandparents; the DNA results show "tons" of Jefferson descendants; and the evidence that Hemings and Jefferson had children together is overwhelming. Moore couldn't write about her brother-in-law's discovery "officially, scientifically" without DNA data from the "pedigreed ancestors."

She'd seen this situation from the other side, too, when a friend who was proud of their descent from Benjamin Franklin took the test and waited anxiously. The lineage was confirmed, but an "NPE"—a "non-paternal event" in genetics-speak—"would've been devastating."

Chapter 8

TAKING A BITE

———

IN *THE SOCIAL LIFE OF DNA,* THE WRITER AND SCHOLAR Alondra Nelson argues that ancestry tests create the potential for honest reconciliation. They expose relationships and bolster demands for reparations. But, as she says, whether our "turn to forensic evidence" is a match for "culturally induced ignorance" remains to be seen. While genealogy is a big-tent hobby, its practitioners congregate uneasily together. The xenophobia that's geysered into the open over the past several years has always roiled in DNA-testing forums. Years ago, a 23andMe subscriber reported in site forums that one of her partner's DNA matches rejected a request to share information, saying, "There has just got to be something wrong with Relative Finder. I can't be related to either you or your 'friend'—we just don't have BROWN people in our family." Andrea Badger, who was one of the site's early "ancestry ambassadors," commented that another user had encountered a similar situation when one of his matches "thought he was Jewish and sent a message full of racial slurs." Elsewhere on the site, a user with the screen name RyanMD started a contentious thread: "Are Ashkenazi Jews and other ethnic groups really smarter than others?"

On 23andMe, users can download and compare maps of their

chromosomes to see precisely where they match with someone. If clusters of predicted relatives connect on the same segment, this knowledge can help pinpoint common ancestors. In this way, 23andMe far surpasses the other consumer genetics sites in access to genetic information. Overall, though, its weaknesses as a genealogical tool are significant. The site offers little family-tree functionality, making it difficult to figure out how the genetics connect to the people.

AncestryDNA is a different beast, an outgrowth of Ancestry. com's vast genealogical resources. Historically, in contrast to 23and-Me's customers, many of whom were interested in medical data, AncestryDNA users signed up specifically for the purpose of researching their family lines. Now the site blends its genealogical resources with test results. When users are a predicted cousin match, AncestryDNA compares their trees to see if it can automatically pinpoint their common ancestors. Unlike 23andMe, AncestryDNA doesn't let users see precisely where their chromosomes overlap with predicted relatives. No actual genetic data is available to subscribers who match. But its "Thrulines" feature looks at data even in locked trees or trees that aren't linked to users' DNA tests and surfaces predictions from that data. While I'm selfishly glad to have this information, I worry for those of the site's 18 million users who don't realize how many of their family connections the site reveals.

In predicting "common ancestors," the AncestryDNA model runs a greater risk than 23andMe's of perpetuating genealogical inaccuracies. If you and I are genetic matches who both wrongly believe we are descended from a John McElwee of Orange County, North Carolina, and we both have that error in our trees—a not-uncommon situation—the site won't help us correct the mistake. Instead, it's likely to highlight McElwee in both our trees, reinforcing the error. As Moore told me in 2013, if we can't see the underlying genetic data, we can't know the basis for their conclusions. AncestryDNA's approach results in a kind of walled garden made of our own genetic data. Why should a company have more information about our genomes and what they might say about us than we do?

FOR SOME GENETIC INDICATORS, 23andMe offers comprehensive results from tests that are at the cutting edge of preventive research—whether you're a carrier for common strains of cystic fibrosis, if you're at increased risk for Alzheimer's, how likely you are to contract tuberculosis if exposed. In the past, 23andMe also predicted fertility, longevity, skin pigmentation, and likely allergies, and it purported, somewhat tentatively, to answer more-speculative questions. Is your episodic memory "increased" or merely "typical"? Can you effectively learn to avoid errors? Do you have a high or only average nonverbal IQ? But the U.S. Food and Drug Administration temporarily ordered the site to stop providing health data in 2013. By agreement with the FDA in 2015, the site relaunched consumer genetic testing in the United States. 23andMe has added tests for breast cancer, Parkinson's, and other conditions since. But any genomic predictions that were removed from the outward-facing, customer perspective are still available to 23andMe—and its investors.

A controversial breast-cancer-risk test introduced in 2018 focuses on two BRCA gene mutations that occur in about two out of one hundred women of Ashkenazi Jewish ancestry and one out of one thousand women in the rest of the population. The test could give subscribers a false sense of security, because it doesn't analyze the more than one thousand other BRCA mutations that contribute to breast-cancer risk. And reactions to marker discoveries vary. One 23andMe user was devastated to learn she had a high-risk gene for breast cancer and wished she'd been told by a person rather than the site. Another user credited the site with identifying her propensity to Hashimoto's, a thyroid disorder her doctors diagnosed only after she'd suffered for six years.

If DNA sites improve at pinpointing ancestral origins, they

could generate important treatment insights. Alzheimer's genes manifest differently in people with African DNA and call for different approaches, for instance. Margaret Pericak-Vance, director of the University of Miami's John P. Hussman Institute for Human Genomics, advocates medical research and treatments tailored to very specific populations. She's studied the disproportionately large population of Latino children in Miami who are autistic and the surprisingly high incidence of breast cancer in young Bahamian women there. She's frustrated that doctors fail to recognize the value of research this focused. Most studies still focus on men with predominantly European ancestry.

For a time, 23andMe offered an "Inheritance Calculator," which has since been removed. As an early subscriber, I had access to those results, which predicted that if my husband (who also tested) and I had children, their genes would predispose them to being able to perceive bitter tastes, to tolerating lactose, and to having brown or black eyes. Ancestry.com, traditionally a pure genealogy destination, got into the medical game, too. AncestryDNA rolled out the public-facing portion of its health research in 2015 and offered a collection of crowd-pleaser "traits" questions, surprisingly identical to some of 23andMe's lighter fare, such as: Does your pee smell funny after you eat asparagus? As Daniela Hernandez observed at Splinter, Ancestry.com "has been collecting ancestral data about its users for decades." Through death certificates and obituaries added by subscribers, the company knows how many of our great-great-grandparents died. Longtime users who accessed Ancestry.com solely for traditional genealogical purposes may not have wanted their research to help businesses predict their health or longevity. Nor, in all likelihood, did more recent subscribers who declined DNA testing realize how their family-tree entries feed into the site's genetics research or the possibility of eugenical conclusions or consequences. In 2021, the company announced that it would discontinue the health portion of its genetic testing.

23andMe subscribers love to pore over genetics studies sensationalized by the media. I'm no exception. The "empathy gene," for example, has never been incorporated into 23andMe's own results, but it's been a popular topic since reports of it emerged in 2009. I have this marker (GG at Rs53576) but relate to the description of its typical expression only partly. I do smile and nod a lot in conversation, but no one who knows me well would say that I'm unanxious, which people with this marker also supposedly are. My empathy tends to be as free-floating as my anxiety, which is saying something. Although I possess only half the personality traits ostensibly connected to the empathy gene and I'm skeptical of these reductive approaches to genetic encoding, I often find myself effectively taking the supposed import of my genotype at face value. As I suspected, my mom is also GG. But in terms of markers, my father is as responsible for the pair as my mother is. Each of my parents contributed a G—for whatever that's worth.

Some scientists compare this kind of genetic forecasting to astrology. As someone who's more likely to remember a friend's sun, moon, and rising signs than their birth date, I'm not as insulted by the comparison as many people would be. But I do puzzle over the appetite—mine and others'—for oversimplified predictions like the empathy gene. Why, knowing how unreliable they are, do we seize on test results that confirm some fated sense of ourselves? The novelist and critic Laila Lalami, who regrets having tested, once compared signing up for these sites to the allure of the Tree of Knowledge. "You can't resist taking a bite," she told me.

Part Three

NATURE AND NURTURE

Chapter 9

IT SKIPS A
GENERATION

———

SOMETIMES GRANNY DREAMED ALL NIGHT LONG, FOR nights on end, about falling through a dark shaft. She confided this to me when I was a child, knowing I often lay awake worrying and then fell asleep into nightmares. I was surprised. Granny always seemed so strong—the decisive set of her jaw, the conviction that lit her eyes, the way she took command on her long visits from Dallas, derailing my father's diatribes with scorn. It was hard to fathom that the fiercest person I knew had a weakness, let alone one of mine. About a decade ago, I mentioned Granny's nights of plummeting to my sister. "I've had that dream," my sister said.

Nowadays when I'm brushing my hair or dressing for bed, sometimes I catch a whiff of Granny's smell in my own scent, some chemical part of her I hadn't known I was wistful for, living on in my own cells. She bequeathed her anxiety and, by some mechanism, the musk of her, too.

Long before the debates on intergenerational emotional tendencies that rage in our era, Granny worried what might be hiding in my blood. I worried, too. Even as a young girl, I felt enough kinship with my mom's feverish projects, plate-throwing rages, and weeping spells to wonder what her tendencies meant about mine. But when I was twelve, Granny warned me to watch for signs of insanity in myself, my sister, and our future children. "It skips a generation," she said. Her voice was quiet, and her eyes were a dull, distant gray. By then, Granny and I had enjoyed glooming over our shared anxious tendencies for many years, but this overt suggestion of madness in the blood stoked one of my deepest fears.

We were talking that day about Granny's younger sister, Louise, who'd been considered a great beauty, winsome as a movie star. The family hoped Louise would do well for herself. For a girl of Louise's background in those days, during the Roaring Twenties in Dallas, this would have meant marrying a wealthy boy, at least as Granny and her family saw it. Instead, Louise started dancing with scarves when she was sixteen, waving them in front of her face, sweeping them around her body. Eventually she took off her clothes and sashayed, naked, up and down the street. Later she pulled a knife on her mother in the bathtub and died in an asylum.

As I grew older, it seemed to me that Granny's bluntness, pragmatism, and refusal to suffer fools at all costs came from witnessing her sister's short, agonized life and enduring their parents' troubled marriage. She was opposed to drama, disdainful of instability, and had developed a hypervigilance about her own boundaries and behaviors that she hoped to pass on to me. But the more I learned about her life—her marriage to my grandfather in particular—the more I wondered whether her resolute guarding against a life of madness and suffering had driven her to create just that.

GRANNY'S FOLKS WERE POOR subsistence farmers in Texas. I grew up with her reminiscences of wringing chickens' necks, the stench of pigpens. "He looked at me like a calf at a new gate," she said once of someone who struck her as slow to catch on. And then she had to explain that a calf doesn't know how to exit through an unfamiliar gate until you lead it through. "Don't that just take the rag off the bush," she would say, of some particularly exasperating interference. We always laughed along with her, but after Granny's death, even my mom couldn't translate this one. A friend thought it might be referring to menstrual rags that poor women of Granny's era often left out on shrubs to dry after washing.

Granny's father, Zone, was an accomplished carpenter. When work was scarce, he drove a rickshaw. His buildings survive across Texas and beyond, and I drink my coffee in a rocking chair he made more than a century ago. He was also a drinker, womanizer, and erratic laborer. *"Mean,"* Granny called him, whenever I asked. "Meaner'n a snake." Zone dragged Granny, her sister, Louise, and my great-grandmother Alma to construction jobs across Texas— from petroleum boomtowns like Eastland to company towns like Sugar Land—and as far away as Missouri. Then he ran off with other women, leaving his family penniless, drinking his wages away. Each time this happened, Alma's brother or father hitched up the wagon to fetch her and the girls. They stayed with family in Dallas until Zone resurfaced, hat in hand, months later. Alma always took him back. "No matter what he'd done, she'd just say, 'He needs me,' and let him in," Granny told me, rolling her eyes. Her ridicule was a force that seemed to drain the room of oxygen. As with my mom, but even more so, I never wanted to give Granny reason to disapprove of me.

While Alma was often immobilized by depression, Granny relied on quick wit and hitch-up-your-britches-and-get-on-with-it spirit. She taught me never to wallow if I failed. "Pick yourself up, dust yourself off, and start all over again," she sang. She attributed her tenacity to growing up with so little and her long life to onions, garlic, and beans, the staple foods of her childhood, when she'd had food to eat at all. She'd gone hungry so often that she started losing adult teeth as a girl, had them all yanked in her twenties, and wore dentures the rest of her life. It took her two or three times as long as the rest of us to eat a meal, more if meat was served, so arduous was the chewing. At night she plunked her teeth in a glass of water and quietly nursed her gums.

Though Granny eventually became a woman of means, living in an upscale neighborhood, her lifestyle was far from luxurious. Well into her eighties, she washed her clothes in the bathtub with a toilet plunger and hung them out to dry on a backyard line. She ridiculed the washer and dryer my mom gave her, insisting "they'd just tear up my clothes." Until she was no longer able to care for herself, Granny bought her clothes at thrift stores, believed that one square of toilet paper was ample, and reused aluminum foil until it turned to ash. As a teenager, she dropped out of high school to support her family. She mastered stenography well enough that, as she often told me while extolling the value of practical skills, she always had work, even through the Great Depression. She got a job so young to put food on the table, because her father couldn't be counted on, but also to bolster Louise's marriage prospects, to buy her sister clothes and shoes that would make her more attractive to wealthy boys. Granny seemed to feel the sacrifice was natural, or at least never seemed to regret it. She adored Louise.

When I was a tiny girl, Granny told me my hair was the same color as her sister's. "Brown," she said, in an admiring tone no one else used when speaking of my hair. *"Brown."* In the photographs I have of her as a young woman, Louise is small, with dark curly hair and a disarming smile. She looks a bit like the silent film star Lillian Gish. When Louise was sixteen, after she danced naked in the street, the family committed her to the North Texas Lunatic Asylum (now known as Terrell State Hospital) in Kaufman County, about thirty miles east of Dallas. Alma had kin in the area.

Doctors diagnosed Louise with "dementia praecox," a slippery term used then to describe what we now call schizophrenia. The psychiatrist and historian of science Richard Noll characterizes it in *American Madness: The Rise and Fall of Dementia Praecox,* as "a diagnosis of hopelessness from its creation," the "terminal cancer of mental diseases." The condition was poorly defined. Diagnosis, according to Noll, was "like the experiences of recognizing a melody or a scent"; the patient needed only to evoke "an uncanny feeling of remoteness or of the 'bizarre' in a physician." Dementia praecox became an epidemic in American asylums, "the most frequently diagnosed condition" and a sentence of "incurable insanity" given to hundreds of thousands of people before it fell out of vogue in the 1950s. Granny's family despaired. They tried bringing Louise home, but then she pulled the knife from the bath and tried to kill her mother as Alma was bathing her. After this incident, Louise was institutionalized for the rest of her days. Granny visited often over the years. The visits underscored the impossibility of connecting with the sister she had known.

According to Louise's death certificate, she died of tuberculosis at age thirty-four, after seventeen years, one month, and twenty-three days in the mental hospital, on February 1, 1943. Going through Granny's papers after her own funeral fifty-five years later, I found a letter from the asylum superintendent following up with Alma about Louise's death. Its sterility shocked me out of my own grief. "We are sorry this girl could not have been mentally restored," the superintendent wrote. "We assure you we cared for her so far as she would allow us to do." Alma's draft response was exonerating, and distant. "I feel sure everyone did their duty. You may do what you want to with her clothes, for I do not want them." The obituary was brief, with no cause of death given. Louise Johnston "died at local hospital on Monday night."

LOUISE WAS THE ONLY example Granny offered of mental illness in our family, but my mom later told me that their mother, Alma, also had a history of suicide attempts, in reaction to Zone's affairs. Granny was just a girl but, with her father off gallivanting, would have had to navigate the aftermath both for herself and Louise. Maybe that's when she began to feel a responsibility for supporting her family, when she developed the idea that a rich man could save them all. After she told me about Alma, I pressed my mom further on disturbing family lore, and she mentioned rumors of an infanticide committed by Zone's mother, Granny's paternal grandmother. As the story was told, my great-great-grandmother Rebecca Johnston announced after the birth of her ninth child that she'd decided against having more. When she got pregnant again and delivered anyway, she bashed the baby's head against the back stoop. "Mammy was rather a fearsome lady," my mom said. "I don't recall she ever said a kind word to me, nor did she ever cuddle me or do any of the things grandmothers are supposed to do."

Mammy's husband, Allen—Zone's father—had been a carpenter, saloonkeeper, and house mover. They were rough folk. Allen had passed on when Granny was a girl, but dipping snuff and quarreling remained popular family activities into my mom's childhood, for the women as well as the men. "Each Johnston carried a can around to spit in, and after a meal we all would sit in the living room and each one would spit from time to time and argue and fight," my mom remembered. "Zone's family was a striving, hell-raising bunch! I hated being there." Still, she had some sympathy for Mammy. "It is not too hard to believe what she did—she was probably tired of all the children and couldn't picture another mouth to feed and another baby to take care of and rear to adulthood." Nor is it too surprising that Granny's father, raised by a mother who may have killed one of his siblings, periodically abandoned his own family. Beyond environment, was he—were all of us who came from this tangle of acrimony and mental illness—also struggling against something innate? Was Granny right that our lives should be spent in guard against it?

DESPITE GRANNY'S DISGUST FOR alcoholics and philanderers, and the women who put up with them, she married my grandfather Robert (son of Charley Bruce, who died in the mental hospital and whose headstone I placed). Robert was dangerously charming, with a striking jaw, a great sense of style, and a tall, trim frame. He was a heartbreaker, a storyteller, a clothing designer, a mechanic, a grocer, a commercial real estate agent, and an absent father who died the year before I was born. He was also, at times at least, an abusive drunk, the definition of instability. By Granny's count (relayed to my mom, and through my mom to me), Robert married thirteen times. So far I've found evidence of a mere ten marriages, to nine women, but there could easily be more.

Only one image survives of Robert and Granny alone together. It's a large black-and-white print from a Dallas restaurant called Italian Village. I'd guess it dates to the early days of their courtship, sometime in 1939. Robert sits, urbane and elaborately casual, with one elbow on the table and one foot up on the seat beside him, handsome enough to break the rules. His eyes are not those of a man who's having a good time. Across the table, Granny is almost, if not actually, glowering. She purses her lips and directs her gaze away from Robert and the photographer both. The jaunty floral wallpaper and shiny tabletop jukebox are a hilarious contrast with the grimness of the occasion. Whenever I mention the photo to my mom, she laughs, too. Later in life, Granny rarely drank, but here beer bottles sit open alongside their meals. She looks as disgusted as she does miserable. I couldn't fathom why she had married him.

Every time I asked her, Granny told me that she'd decided to have a child in her thirties because she didn't want to be alone in her old age. Marriage, she implied, was a necessary vehicle for having the child. As when my mom described her reasons for choosing my father, Granny dismissed love as a factor in her marriages to Robert and to her second husband. The child was the goal. So I had difficulty imagining her tied to or constrained by any man, or even desiring one, although my mom says Granny was in love once, before Robert, with a man who married someone else.

Among Granny's papers after her death, we found a newspaper clipping noting the date she and Robert got their marriage license.

The item was bracketed. None of us paid much attention to it in the midst of our grief. Almost a decade later, though, I started putting information into my family tree and counted the months between the date in October 1939 and my mother's birth in June the following year. Then I counted them again. The time between the dates was less than eight months. Neither Granny nor my mom had ever suggested that my mom was premature, whereas they often reminisced about my early birth, my stint as an incubator baby, how tiny I was when I was allowed to go home at two weeks and five pounds. And Granny had been candid about the hardships of mothering, her difficulty nursing. On the phone years later, my mom confirmed that she wasn't born early.

"So Granny must have been pregnant when they got married," I said.

"I just can't imagine it," said my mom. "But I guess she must have been."

I also had trouble reconciling this fact with Granny as I'd known her. She wasn't prudish, but in my memory she was so impervious to bullshit, frippery, and the attention of men, it was hard to comprehend her decision to sleep with Robert. Was it lust? Some fundamental misunderstanding of him? A way to have the child she wanted? On the one hand, it felt borderline disrespectful to puzzle over my grandmother's sex life like this, but on the other hand, she'd circled the date in the newspaper and left it for us to find. She must have known we'd wonder, or at least that I, always drawn to old papers, would wonder. I asked my mom how she thought Granny had gotten involved with Robert. "He could charm anyone," she said, and paused. "As long as they didn't know him."

MY GRANDPARENTS MET WHILE they were both working for Justin McCarty, a prominent Dallas clothing designer and manufacturer. Granny was McCarty's office manager. Robert, my mom says, "was their most outstanding designer and pattern drafter. Mr.

McCarty would say of my dad that he was a real genius of the business and would go far if he would leave the bottle alone." But how did they go from being colleagues to sitting across from each other at that grim dinner and having a child together?

Researching further, I discovered that they didn't marry for seventeen days after they got their marriage license, seven months and ten days before their baby was born. Not only was my mom conceived before their wedding, everyone must have known it. I also learned that Robert had already been married and divorced three times and that the last of these marriages ended just six months before he and Granny wed. Before that split became official, a court issued an injunction in the case of *Rose Marie Bruce v. Robert Bruce,* forbidding Robert to go "in or about or upon the premises" where his third wife lived, raising the possibility of domestic abuse. I wondered how much Granny knew before getting involved with Robert and how much she found out at the courthouse when their license was issued. Had she known he'd been married less than a year before? That he'd had multiple wives? That the most recent of them had taken out a restraining order? Did the lag between the license and the wedding suggest that Granny considered raising their child alone?

At some point Robert wept and confided to Granny that he'd had a baby who died, according to my mom, who believes this tragedy was key to their relationship. I agree that Granny would have felt a kinship with Robert's losses. Knowing how stricken she was by her sister's deterioration in the mental hospital, I suspect the death of Robert's father in the same kind of institution was a major factor in Granny's decision to commit herself to a partner who turned out to be as unstable as her own father had been. She loved her sister but didn't want to be judged by her sister's madness. Nor should Robert be judged by his father's mania, I imagine her deciding in her fair-minded way. And perhaps she had truly fallen for him, against all her better judgments, letting down her guard in the hopes of finding a true soul mate. Thus was the cocktail of volatile tendencies and abusive marriage poured from the shaker for the next generation.

Granny said that Robert drank throughout their time together, that he ran around on her, hit her, and squandered their money on other women. Apart from these details, she avoided discussing him with me, no matter how much I pestered. I remember her mentioning bouts with yellow fever and warning me that "men don't like sick women," but I didn't understand the context or severity. Later my mom told me that Granny suffered intensely from malaria after giving birth and that the disease receded and returned for years.

Many nights during her earliest years, my mom hid under the covers while her parents argued and hit each other. She said Robert often called Granny at the end of his workday and told her "to cook him a steak and draw him a bath and he'd be home in fifteen minutes." Then he wouldn't come home at all. Even now it's difficult for me to imagine Granny responding to his eventual return with anything other than incredulous laughter and sass before slamming the door in his face, but she was a debilitated woman with a baby, and for a time at least, she tolerated this behavior. One night, she drove with my mom to a parking lot in downtown Dallas, where they stopped and waited—for Robert, my mom assumed. He never turned up.

When my mom told this story, I thought of one of her own, from her time with my father. Throughout their marriage, my father left the house each night after dinner, ostensibly to do research at the nearby university, where he was an adjunct. Early one evening, not long after my sister was born, he disappeared more abruptly than usual. My mom had a bad feeling. Leaving my sister and me alone for a few minutes, she dashed down the street and onto the campus. There she glimpsed him walking around the lake with a young woman, holding her hand. When my mom called his name, my father rushed over to her and claimed that he was comforting a distraught student. "Go home and take care of the baby," he ordered my mom, and she did. As with Granny, I'm surprised that my mom tolerated treatment like this. But, then, Granny's mom, Alma, did, too—forever, with occasional suicide attempts. And Alma's great-grandmother was abandoned by her French husband in Louisiana before dying in childbirth at the age of twenty-two.

THREE LETTERS I FOUND among Granny's papers establish how her marriage to Robert eventually ended. The first, to Robert from Christine, the woman who would become his next wife, reveals their affair. "Sweet heart, I cannot bear to leave you," she writes. "I want you to believe that if we were married I would rather die than trifle on you. . . . I know that we have had a lot of scraps, but . . . If you & Martha [Granny] don't go back together & you still want me, just say the word & I will be there as fast as I can make it."

Next came Robert's letter to Granny, care of her dad, postmarked September 11, 1943. He urges Granny to leave her parents' place, where she'd fled with my mom, and return to him. "I am so lonesome for you both," he writes. "I am sure you are a little fast about everything. . . . You jump at conclusions too quick." They should work things out, he says, and "give Sandy the kind of home she is entitled to have." The letter grows increasingly self-pitying and unhinged; I imagine he was drinking as he wrote. "Tell Sandy Dad[d]y loves her and will take her to the zoo if she comes home at once and if not she may never see me again. You took all her pictures and also there are no sheets for the bed. The one on the bed now stinks." In a postscript, he adds: "Give Sandy my love and you can have it to[o] if you want me instead of shit." At first, I imagined Granny's outrage as she read all of this—her eyes at their most blazing, contemptuous blue—but nowadays I think of her anguish. Her sister had died earlier that year. The unraveling of the marriage to Robert must have been all the harder to bear following that loss.

For the third letter, I only have Granny's handwritten draft to

Christine's husband, Ernest, who I think was in California, conva-
lescing in a Navy hospital. I don't know for certain that Granny
mailed the letter, but her tone is urgent. "I was told of your knowledge of the 'affair,'" she writes, but "I could not believe you knew
about it because as soon as I found it out my first impulse was to let
you know. However, since familiarizing myself with your background I can readily see that your silence in the matter for this
length of time is only one of the sterling qualities that you possess."
Evidently, Granny had already *wired* Ernest by the time she drafted
this, and I gather his lack of reply prompted her to beseech him at
more length: "It has been impossible for me to find a handle to this
situation without consulting with you, and I may be presumptive in
thinking that you will ever discuss this with me, but believe me that
I am only appealing to your sense of fairness and consideration in
trying to eliminate the hurt you and I alone are suffering." Her tone
is both familiar and mysterious to me. I recognize her sense of fairness in: "Regardless of what Christine has done I blame her no
more than the man. I am a great believer in the 'Single Standard.'"
But Granny seems to hope that Ernest will help bring the affair to
a close. It had never occurred to me that she might really have loved
Robert, but here she claims that she does. Taking the same tack she
denounced Alma for taking with Zone, she says she intends to work
things out with Robert. He is already trying to be a better husband,
she writes, before getting in a dig that's very Granny: "Believe me
when I say that there has always been room for improvement."

Whatever Ernest did or did not reply, the goal of reconciliation
was short-lived. Granny divorced Robert on February 10, 1944. My
mom was three and a half years old. Robert, who did not appear for
the proceeding, was granted visitation "at all reasonable and season-
able times" and ordered to pay five dollars per week in child support,
which Granny must have known she'd never see. By then I imagine
she would have felt, in addition to bereft and mortified, relieved to
be rid of a philandering alcoholic spouse who'd turned out to be no
more reliable than her own father. Until the war ended, she ran a

boardinghouse. Once soldiers started coming home, she went to work in an office again.

MY BEST CLUES TO Granny's emotional state in the years after her divorce are my mom's memories, a tricky source. Apparently, Granny was so convinced that she would succumb to malaria and leave my mom an orphan that she began to prepare my mom, age four, for that fact. Granny took my mom to the bus depot downtown and said she would need to be able to navigate the city alone when Granny died. She'd have to understand transit schedules and do everything else on her own, too. My mom rode home by herself on the bus that day. By age five, she was going downtown alone every Saturday with a dollar. A dollar was a lot of money, money they didn't really have, but Granny always indulged my mom, I think both to atone for my mom's fatherlessness and to correct for Granny's own childhood deprivation. So every week my mom went to a movie and the soda fountain. Afterward, she had enough money left over to choose an animal at the pet store.

The stories about their menagerie—the cats and dogs and rabbits and chickens and ducks and turtles, and especially the alligator, who got loose in the neighborhood and wound up being adopted by the zoo—were my favorites as a girl. "Tell me about the alligator again," I would beg my mom and Granny as we snapped beans on the front porch. It sounded like heaven to me then, unlimited animal companions. (My high school and college years, when my mom amassed several hundred birds and at least sixteen dogs, were a pointed lesson in being careful what you wish for.)

In the way of children and their parents, I didn't understand the heart of my mom's Saturday trips until I was much older. The animals my mom gravitated to in the pet store were sick. She took them home and fed them through eyedroppers. If they died, she gave them a funeral, with a eulogy from the minister at the Presbyterian church across the street. Later she would become a preacher

herself, of the tongues-speaking fire-and-brimstone variety, but
these were her first sermons, delivered standing in the yard, last
rites for dead kittens and hamsters and whatever strays she took in.
She was giving them the tenderness she wished for herself and the
healing she wished for her mother.

Direct expressions of love were never easy between Granny and
my mom, just as they've often felt fraught between my mom and
me, but animals were a proxy from my mom's earliest years. One
afternoon, when she was four years old, before all those trips to the
pet store, my mom found her cat, Katy, dangling lifeless from a tree
limb by her collar. She knew what to do. Granny repaired my mom's
dolls, patched her dresses, nurtured the plants and animals, rigged a
fix for anything in the house that broke. So my mom carried Katy's
body in to Granny and asked her to mend the cat. Decades later,
when I was the same age my mom had been, Granny told me the
story with tears in her eyes over the memory of having to explain
that Katy could not be resurrected.

WHILE GRANNY WAS AT work, my mom was left with a housekeeper, or sometimes alone. After the divorce, she saw her father
maybe twice a year, to stay the weekend with him and, as my mom
put it once, "whatever wife he was married to at the time." And
then, not long after her tenth birthday, my mom stopped seeing
Robert at all. She's often told me she doesn't recall feeling any real
sense of loss when Robert left, because he'd been around so rarely
anyway. I've pressed her on this: Wasn't she sad? Confused? Angry?
No, she's said, it was just her and Granny. Later she resented her
stepfather for taking some of her mother's attention away.

Even as Granny taught my mom to fend for herself, she also
transmitted competing messages. In 1949, Granny married an older,
well-off man named Smith, another alcoholic. She did this, she always said, for my mom. Smith was a jealous man who didn't let
Granny so much as run errands without him. Being controlled was

a bitter pill for an independent woman, but Granny swallowed it, as she did his doting and his tantrums. Sometimes he shouted and flailed, and in later years it took Granny and her housekeeper, Carrie, to wrestle him to bed. But Smith had money. He provided stability and, to some degree, respectability for my mom, a child of divorced parents, at a time when divorce was the most scandalous thing anyone could think of. The neighbors still forbade their children to play with her, but Smith showered my mom with gifts and gave her his last name, which she used until college, an expensive private school that he paid for.

One of the things that surprised me most among Granny's belongings at her death was a prefilled scrapbook she gave my mom for Christmas at age nine, in an apparent effort to rewrite history, a few months after Granny and Smith got married. The first tableaux is of idealized baby pictures and toys cut from magazines. "Sandy Baby Days," it reads at the bottom. Spreads labeled "Childhood" and "Growing Up" feature children in beautiful clothes. On a page labeled "Helping Mother," a woman and girl in matching dresses smile and wind yarn together. Names of my mom's dogs and cats and dolls are sprinkled here and there, but the images aren't much like the life she and Granny described leading together. The last two pages are devoted to young women on a college campus and then wearing caps and gowns. "Happy Days in College," reads one caption. "Sandy Graduates," says the other. To some extent, this narrative unfolded. My mom became a sorority girl. She got an undergraduate degree, then a master's. She married and tried to be interested in social climbing. And she made decisions that, in some ways, despite her determination to do the opposite, echoed Granny's. Both my mom and Granny resisted seeing these common threads.

Several years ago, I wrote to Robert's stepson, Ray Lee, Christine's child, by letter. I didn't expect to hear back, but, though bemused, Ray Lee rang me up and was fully willing to revisit those days. He called Robert a great businessman, smart and talented and charming, good at making money—"really a good guy," Ray Lee was for some reason at pains to say, except when Robert drank. It was a big "except." Ray Lee once awoke to the sound of his mother screaming as Robert slapped her around in the next room. Ray Lee ran in, picked up an empty whiskey bottle lying next to the bed, and hit Robert over the head with it, knocking him out. My mom had never put much stock in Granny's assertions that Robert had hit her, just as Granny didn't give credence to my mom's claims that her first husband had been violent. Each of them took the position that the other woman was the difficult one. Granny thought my mom was overdramatic, unreliable, and obstinate, whereas my mom viewed Granny as sour and joyless, a melancholic stick-in-the-mud weighing down Robert's ebullience. It confused me that their similar experiences didn't deepen the understanding between them. Later I enmeshed myself in a combative college relationship. I remember the sense of fated doom I felt each time I returned yet again to the apartment I shared with that boyfriend.

It seems to me that my mom and Granny tried to build their lives as bulwarks against family patterns. Then each of them chose partners with whom they were guaranteed to generate new, spectacularly terrible iterations of those patterns. Later, I did this, too, despite resolving as a child to chart my own destiny by never having children, never being dependent on a man for money, and never getting married.

To some degree, we reenact the patterns we watch unfold in our own childhoods. Sigmund Freud posited that trauma begets a repetition compulsion: We re-create traumatic scenarios and dynamics from our early lives in the hope of a different outcome. The late psychoanalyst Anne Ancelin Schützenberger argued that families reenact "hereditary structures," not just genes but dynamics, so we replay dramas out of an unconscious loyalty to family.

Is there some deeper, more elemental pull toward this reenactment? Researchers in a 2014 study on genetics and intimate partner violence contended that "genetic variants do not *cause*" this kind of violence, but certain variants may "increase the risk or probability of violence" through their interplay with other factors, such as impulsivity. An earlier study of identical twins in the UK suggested that infidelity could have a heritability rate of about 40 percent, "similar to heritability for divorce." The genetic epidemiologist Tim Spector posits some evolutionary and genetic basis for the tendencies investigated in the twin study but observes that they can also be affected by changes in the expression of an individual twin's genes based on experiences. This research is tricky; whether the twins are raised together or apart, the influence of nurture is difficult to quantify. And, conversely, so is the part that's innate.

Chapter 10

AN IMPULSE TO LEAP

—

As my mom's child, I saw from a young age how the absence of her own father propelled her toward mine, though she never connected the two and always resisted my efforts to persuade her. I came up against my mom's emotional blankness toward Robert as I did Granny's three rote quips about his awfulness and her unsentimental denunciation of her own father, Zone. Much later, in my mid-thirties, I recognized a similar numbness toward my father in myself. Like Granny and my mom, I thought it was strength not to feel sadness. I buried those feelings so deep, I didn't know they were there.

From my earliest years, my parents' marriage perplexed and troubled me. Strangers confided to my mom in parking lots, laughed at her stories in checkout lines, sympathized with her grumbling in waiting rooms. She was fun, charming, and, in most ways, indomitable. And yet she'd chosen to tie herself to someone like my dad, who has never to my knowledge charmed anyone. Just as Granny once had, my mom intended to be a stay-at-home mother. Yes, she disliked that my dad shouted at all of us, sometimes for hours; that he spanked my sister and me if we didn't finish our meals in the time he allotted; that he grounded me for weeks if I got anything less than an A on a math test; that he woke my mom in the night with a flashlight to lecture her; and that he was cruel to the animals. Even so, she had little personal experience of dads and considered him vastly better than no father at all. "At least he's invested," she would say. "At least he cares about you." Unlike her dad, he was there for breakfast and dinner, for reviewing our math homework. He was, in his way, devoted to us.

But the society my dad wanted to cultivate bored her, as did cooking each night, driving her daughters to and from school, supervising field trips. "I'm not interested in being *supermom*," she would say, whenever I was sent home with some flyer soliciting volunteers to bake cupcakes. Because of his late-night research at the university library, my dad was rarely around to spend time with her after we went to bed, which depressed her, but his presence depressed her more. Over the years, she became less sanguine about their union, more critical, mocking, and defiant.

All day long she'd give herself pep talks, reflect on how fortunate she was to have a husband so dependable, how good it was for her children to have a father so "invested"—that was the word she often used. Then his car would pull into the driveway, and, as she gleefully dramatized it to her friends at the time and still says now, the parakeets stopped singing, the cats slunk under the sofas, the dogs tucked their tails between their legs and crept out of sight, and my sister and I hovered anxiously near the hallway, waiting to gauge his mood when he came through the door. At the time, this description struck me as exaggeration to underscore our unhappiness. I was too fearful of my father to see it was accurate. Just as my mom said, he berated us if we didn't greet him when he got home but also if we did. On occasion, if he was in a bad mood and deemed the dogs too rambunctious, he'd kick one. I remember our boxer, Sam, yelping as he skidded into the wall. I'd forgotten about this until my mother sent me her file of papers from various disputes following their divorce. The memory rushed back with painful clarity.

THE LONGER MY PARENTS were married, the more often my mom's anger boiled over. Dinnertime was a common flash point. Her resentment would already be at a low simmer over the time spent paring potatoes, minding the pot roast. She'd call my father to the table and he'd dawdle over his work in the study. We weren't allowed to eat until he sat down. Two minutes passed, then five, then sixteen, and then, on occasion, she started throwing things. She lobbed drinking glasses, frisbeed dishes, hurled hot pots of peas and bubbling sauce, flung condiments and juices and other make-shift grenades from the refrigerator. Shattering glass made the most dramatic explosion against the marble tile of the Florida room, so she pitched it hard in that direction, out the kitchen door, occasion-ally taking a running start as if she were bowling. Sometimes the entire meal ended up in a lake across the floor. When she was really livid, she threw some of their gilded wedding china, so the whole mess gleamed as the sun went down.

Then she roared off in the car, leaving my dad to put my sister and me to bed before he headed to the law library. A few times my mom disappeared for a night, once for several. My father drove my sister and me to school each morning and took us to Burger King for dinner. The house stank of rancid orange juice and putrefying meat amid broken plates that we all sidestepped and did not dis-cuss. The mood was grim, our future uncertain, the marble stained. Eventually my mom returned and cleaned things up, and for a day or two everyone was contrite, grateful, even pleasant.

Once they had an argument on a Sunday afternoon—always a tricky time, what with their ongoing fights about church. My mom threw a plate at the wall, and when it shattered, a shard flew back and hit my father's cheek. Blood ran down his face as he grabbed my hand and my sister's and hustled us into the car. The wound turned out to be superficial, but the tissue he held to it quickly turned red and dripped. Usually I was as thrilled as I was terrified by Mom's displays of fury, but on that day my dad had my sympathy.

I suspect my sister felt the same way. I joke sometimes that my parents knew from the time I was a very small child that I wanted to be a writer and they chose to carry on as they did anyway, whereas my sister did nothing to court the misfortune of having a memoirist for a sibling. She has her own point of view, her own experiences to process. While we've always been close, she's far more private than I am, and her small footprint in this book is intentional. At times even telling my own story feels like an encroachment.

I was fiercely protective of my sister when she was a young girl, but we also fought. I remember once, after one of our parents' arguments, when they'd careened off in their cars and left us alone, the two of us standing on opposite sides of my room screaming "I hate you" at each other. I picked up a heavy old rotary phone and heaved it in her direction. It missed her head by a foot, a foot and a half at most, before crashing against the wall. I must have been nine or ten, more than old enough to know better. She was four or five. I rushed to her and pulled her to me and told her how much I loved her, how sorry I was. I was shaking, terrified to find something like my mom's rage boiling over in me and to think what I might have done.

TEN MONTHS BEFORE SHE met my dad, my mom was officially divorced from her first husband, Tom, a striver who'd cheated on her through their marriage, belittled her as she supported him through law school, and locked her out of the house in her pajamas one night when it was extremely cold. She was dating a lot, glad to be free of Tom, but she was also adrift, unsure what course her life would take next. She'd gone on some dates with a municipal judge who'd decided a case against a man caught stealing my mom's underwear off her clothesline. The judge "gave me back my bras and panties and asked for my number," my mom said.

She also had a serious beau, "Mr. Nord," whom she'd met through her work as a secretary. She loved Mr. Nord, who claimed he was separated from his wife and getting divorced and that he would marry my mom. The split never seemed to be finalized, and he kept giving excuses. Meanwhile, my mom had lost interest in pursuing a doctorate in English literature, which wasn't going to help her pay the bills. She hated her new job as a secretary for the Society of Petroleum Engineers. A vacation to Puerto Rico with her sorority sister, Linetta, didn't raise her spirits much. They flew back to Dallas just after Hurricane Camille, in August 1969. From the sky they could see the overturned boats and mowed-down houses the storm had left behind.

The next day, Mr. Nord's wife called my mom. Contrary to what he had said, they were neither divorcing nor separated. "You can have him if you want him," Mrs. Nord said. Mortified, my mom apologized. She had no idea they were still together, she explained, and didn't want to break up their marriage. She confronted Mr. Nord at her friend's apartment, which had often been their love nest. "Well, I figured you'd find out sooner or later," he said. And then my mom leapt from the third story of the building into the dumpster below.

Mr. Nord ran down to find her banged up and shaken but not seriously hurt. He coaxed her into his car, to take her to her psychologist. On the way, my mom asked to stop at the lake. There she bolted into the water, twice, with the intention of drowning herself. Finally, they made it to the office of the psychologist my mom had been seeing for a year. Dr. Miller chose to release my mom rather than commit her because he believed she would "be good and not try it again." He told her that Mr. Nord had turned out to be "exactly the sort of man he'd thought he would be" based on my mom's descriptions. She spent the night at her friend's place, where only hours before she'd jumped into the dumpster.

The next morning, a Saturday, Linetta picked my mom up and took her home. My mom sent Linetta out to fetch three, possibly more, bottles of sleeping pills. Once alone, my mom ran a warm bath. She drank a bottle of iodine and took all the sleeping pills and a bottle of lithium (she says she doesn't remember why it was in her house or whose it was except that it wasn't hers). Then she lowered herself into the water and waited to lose consciousness and drown. She awoke on the floor the next morning, to the sound of knocking. Her memory of what happened before she answered the door to find Linetta standing there is hazy. Linetta drew back in horror. My mom's hair and face were red with blood. Neither of them understood where the blood had come from; my mom hadn't cut herself. They concluded that it was from vomiting. "I must have had seizures all night," my mom says.

Linetta apparently called Granny, who stoically set about cleaning up, seeing to details. She'd been through this with Alma. My mom thinks Louise attempted suicide, too. And Granny herself had those dreams about falling, dreams I trace to a terror that if she stopped driving herself, if she dropped her defenses and allowed herself to feel her despair and depression and anxiety in all its fullness, she would lose her mind or try to kill herself, too.

That night, Granny went home. She tried sending her housekeeper, Carrie, to stay with my mom overnight rather than doing it herself. But my mom says Carrie was drunk and weeping over my mom's condition—I suspect manifesting feelings Granny couldn't or wouldn't access. My mom sent Carrie home to rest and asked Granny to come back instead. She did. I don't get the impression her manner was particularly nurturing.

A week later, my mom met my father at Linetta's pool.

MY MOM FIRST TOLD me most of this—apart from the proximity of her suicide attempt to meeting my father—on the phone one night a decade ago, well into my genealogical explorations. My gut sank with a terrible sense of confirmation.

I felt I had known somehow, long before her telling me, that she had tried to kill herself. I had always known. And now, hearing her

story, I was struck by echoes. I had once threatened, wildly and in-
explicably, to leap from a window while arguing with a college boyfriend. He'd pushed me. Rageful anxious impotence had bubbled
up. I'd brandished a dull kitchen knife at him and then at myself and then moved to jump. Even then I wasn't sure whether
or not I meant to do it. The impulse seemed to come from some
part of myself I wasn't really acquainted with that suddenly got
switched on.

Beyond his ideas of the repetition compulsion, Freud maintained that "the archaic heritage of human beings" includes
"memory-traces of the experience of earlier generations." In her
1998 book, *The Ancestor Syndrome,* Anne Ancelin Schützenberger
connected these threads to a phantom or haunting, not from the
dead but from their painful and unresolved secrets. While working
with cancer patients, she found that sometimes they fell sick at exactly the same age as an ancestor. Things like car accidents, too,
sometimes repeated dates and details of an ancestor's accident. She
began to work from the assumption in her practice that "psychological heredity" may be possible, through "unconscious family loyalty and a kind of anniversary syndrome." Finding Schützenberger's
work a decade ago didn't so much influence my thinking as re-
inforce it.

A year or two later, I learned of epigenetics—biological factors
that affect the way our genes are expressed rather than altering the
DNA itself—and hotly debated theories suggesting a possible epigenetic role in trauma that repeats through families. When I encountered reports of a (disputed) study suggesting that children
and grandchildren of Holocaust survivors might tend to become
depressed and anxious because of epigenetic changes passed down
by the survivor, I thought, *Aha!* Efforts to broach intergenerational
trauma and epigenetics wholly through psychology haven't satisfied
me so far. The most popular book for casual readers, Mark Wolynn's
It Didn't Start with You, marshals psychoanalytic theories and advocates "family constellation" role-playing while tying clients' issues to

scientific theories, often imprecisely. Wolynn also maintains that cutting oneself off from an ancestor inevitably results in repetition of generational patterns that can only be halted by resuming ongoing contact, regardless of the circumstances that led to estrangement. To put it mildly, I disagree. Insisting on a relationship with a relative who might be unsafe can have damaging consequences, in some cases even deadly ones. But I agree with Wolynn that ignoring toxic family patterns can cause them to fester and manifest in new (or old) ways.

I asked my mom how she felt when she decided to kill herself. "It was the best thing to do at the time, I thought," she said. "There weren't many options for a thirty-year-old divorced woman." And how did this connect to her feelings about my dad? "There wasn't much left to choose from," she said. "That's just the reality when you're a thirty-year-old divorcée."

LONG BEFORE I LEARNED how many reasons I had to worry about losing my mind, I worried about losing it. I didn't know Louise had danced down the street naked or tried to kill her mom or died in a mental institution, or that Alma had tried to commit suicide, or that my mom had. I didn't know Rebecca was said to have killed her baby by banging its head against a rock or that Charley had succumbed to exhausted mania. I knew that my father could be cruel, but the potential of his wrath was ever-present as the weather or the judgment of God. As a child I didn't worry too much about what he might have passed on to me. I was too busy worrying that I might set him off.

I remember being four years old, sitting on the floor of my bedroom. I was in trouble, I don't recall what for. My mom's tomato pincushion sat before me, stuck all over with needles and pins. Experimentally, I pulled one out and pricked the inside of my upper lip, right behind the fleshy center, until it bled. The pain gave me focus. When the skin grew back, I did it again. Later I secretly bit the insides of my cheeks, dug my fingernails into my palms, banged my head against the wall.

My mom enjoys recounting how she vanquished my first tantrum, when I was just over two years old. My godmother, Nana, warned her it was coming and instructed her to keep a jar of water in the refrigerator. The very first time I started to buck and kick, my mom was ready. Fetching the jar, she tossed the water into my face. My crying stopped. "You just blinked your eyes and stood up," she says, "and you never threw a tantrum again." The ease and practicality of this triumph is a source of great pride for her. There was the problem of the tantrum, and she solved the problem. If only other people had some gumption and common sense, they could quash their own children's outbursts, too. Their children would grow up to be fine, considerate people, just as (in her view) I did. But while my toddler tantrum phase apparently ended the very day it began, my anxieties ballooned and my palms bled sometimes where I dug my fingernails in.

Granny didn't throw cold water on my mom, as far as I know, but the trip to the bus depot, the message that she needed to be able to handle herself like an adult when she was still a small child, must have had the same effect. Once, when I was seven or so, my mom found me beating my arm with the hard bristles of a hairbrush. I say she "found me" as though I had been doing it in secret, when in fact I had positioned myself so she was bound to notice me. She was raging through the house, furious because I needed a pilgrim costume for a school pageant. Though she'd known the deadline, as a busy mom and Bible-study leader, she'd put off making the costume and now was livid to have to interrupt her evening for something so pointless. She was a talented seamstress and often took in sewing for spending money but wanted to be spending her time reading scripture and preparing her lesson, not putting together some effete costume for a religious school that she had once been very gung-ho about but that did not approve of her new spiritual practices, such as speaking in tongues.

I sat on my bed crying, hitting my arm with the hairbrush, until she came into the room. She looked on with scorn. "I hope you don't expect me to feel sorry for you," she said, or something like that. "You're *choosing* to beat your own arm." I saw her point. Maybe that was the lesson she took from Granny's response to her suicide attempt: You did this to yourself. You need to pull yourself together, live a normal life, conform like the rest of us.

AFTER GRANNY LEFT ROBERT in 1943, she and my mom stayed with Zone and Alma. The four of them often spent the night out-doors, on the sleeping porch. One night, Robert rolled up, drunk, and rattled the screen door, trying to get in. Everyone stayed quiet until he went away. After my mom moved out of my dad's place in 1981, he would call her up and fill the answering-machine tape with commands and denunciations. Back then you could hear messages as they were being left, so we'd turn down the volume and let him rant. Sometimes the tape would click off a half hour later and we'd realize he'd been blustering all that time. When that one college boyfriend and I argued in 1992, things would reach a crescendo and I would storm off. A couple of times, like my mom, I disappeared for a night or two. He tracked me down, apologized, made me din-ner, suggested a future life together in which he would support me while I worked on my writing.

All the while I was wandering that codependent hellscape, in the tradition of my mom and Granny, I *acted* pretty sassily indepen-dent. Nights I lay awake worrying what I might have inherited from my biological family, and by day I railed against determinist ideas. In coffee shops and bars and women's studies classes, I argued that everyone's personhood—our temperaments, our talents and shortcomings, nearly all of our attributes—flowed from environ-ment rather than biology. My crusade for the proposition that nur-ture always triumphs over nature was short-lived, a popular argument in academia at the time that I latched on to because I was and had always been terrified that the opposite might be true. I worried that I might have a religious conversion and start a church in my living room. I worried that I might have a child as lacking in empathy as my father. I worried that I might go crazy. I often went without sleep, occasionally for days in a row.

The influence of Granny and my mother is a riddle, in the way inclinations that flow from both nature and nurture are. I've always ascribed my independence and determination to their influence. More privately, I treasured the anxious melancholia I associated with Granny. I cultivated my depressive fear as if it were a fire on a winter day, feeding and fetishizing it. And as a young woman, I was often proud of barn-burner rages that rivaled my mother's. Traits I liked less, traits I didn't like to acknowledge in myself, I traced to my other ancestors. But Granny wasn't exactly the person I idolized, the fierce solitary sun I saw her as being. And repeating my mother's insistence on expressions of fury rather than quiet acceptance of painful feelings didn't make those feelings go away. It made them more excruciating and impossible to ignore. Contemplating all these tendencies has freed me up to be more honest with myself about my own habits and desires, about what exactly I fear and how much I, like everyone, want love. Both Granny and my mom were imperfect. Of course, I am, too.

Chapter 11

THE IDEA OF
HEREDITY

———

HUMANS HAVE ALWAYS STRUGGLED WITH THE IDEA THAT
our ancestors might determine our destiny, that they could
bless us by passing along longevity or sex appeal or doom us with
dementia, baldness, or gout. Over the past century, we've often
thought in terms of genes versus environment. We've sought to
know what our parents transmit through the raw material that pro-
duces us and what comes from the way we're raised. The either-or
view of nature and nurture may be giving way to a more nuanced
view, in some ways an older view. The hope and anxiety are timeless.

The French Renaissance writer and philosopher Michel de
Montaigne was twenty-five years old when he witnessed the onset
of his father's gallstones. His father had been in "a happy state of
health" until taking ill at age sixty-seven, Montaigne recalls in his
1580 essay "Of the Resemblance of Children to Fathers," but his
father's last seven years were excruciating. Montaigne himself feared
gallstones more than any other malady he associated with old age.
He writes that even as a child (and thus long before his father took
ill) he held them "in greatest horror." At age forty-five he, too, began
to suffer from the dreaded disease and was confounded.

Where, he wonders, was "the propensity to this infirmity hatching all this time?" His father had been fit and virile at the time of Montaigne's birth. None of Montaigne's brothers or sisters showed signs. So how did that one particular drop of his father's sperm, "this slight bit of his substance, with which he made me," contain "so great an impression" of the disease as to inflict it on Montaigne? And how did it "remain so concealed that I began to feel it forty-five years later"? Contemplating this uncanny coincidence, he decides that the "seed from which we are produced bears in itself the impressions not only of the bodily form, but of the thoughts and inclinations of our fathers!" Where do all these possibilities hide in a single dash of fluid, he asks. "And how do they convey these resemblances with so heedless and irregular a course that the great-grandson will correspond to his great-grandfather, the nephew to the uncle?"

For relief from his condition, Montaigne didn't turn to doctors. His father had lived to age seventy-four, his grandfather to sixty-nine, and his great-grandfather nearly to eighty years old, and none of them, according to Montaigne, had ever taken a single doctor's prescription. They "had an aversion to medicine by some occult natural horror," an aversion he shared, one he half-jokingly called "hereditary." His tone is familiar to any of us who've offhandedly ascribed some idiosyncratic trait, talent, or opinion to our genes. Just like us, he's kidding and he's not kidding.

MY FATHER WAS SURE that his genes guaranteed my sister and me superior intellects and good health, that any issues with our achievement or fitness could be blamed on our mom or us. In my mom's view, the question of what traits were innate was more slippery. She often invoked the ancient concept of the four humors. In the original iteration, a different bodily fluid was associated with each of four personality types: blood with sanguine temperament, black bile with melancholy, phlegm with phlegmatic, and yellow bile with choleric. A Christian reinterpretation of the scheme was popularized by Tim LaHaye, a prominent End Times preacher whose 1966 book, *Spirit-Controlled Temperament*, dispenses with the ancient scientific reasoning behind the humors but presents the "four temperaments" as more or less innate.

Together, my mom and I enjoyed classifying people in this way, considering their personalities and propensities and their particular temperamental mix and trying to predict what they might do or feel in some situation. This pastime was tricky for us, too, though, because my anxious, downbeat bent—reflective, to my mom, not just of Granny and me but the melancholic temperament in general—exasperated her so that she coined a verb and command: "Quit melling."

According to LaHaye, personality flows from "hereditary factors" that are "arranged at the time of conception." The first chapter of his book is titled "You're Born with It!" The second is "Temperament Can Be Modified!" For all my exasperation with it now, I read *Spirit-Controlled Temperament* several times, starting when I was ten or so. Some part of my fascination with the nature–nurture puzzle of personality began there. Over the years, as I realized how LaHaye stripped the four temperaments of their original context, I wondered what the ancients really thought about the relationship between our ancestors and our individuality.

Ideas about transmission of traits between the generations have shifted over the ages. Biological inheritance is a surprisingly recent concept. The word "gene" came into existence only in 1909. Until about two hundred years ago, Western thinking on the matter rested on ancient theories that are largely unknown to us. Those ideas are part of the bedrock of Western philosophy, intertwined with the development of science, inextricable from our history and in some ways from our thinking even now. Much of the source material has been lost. Authorship of what remains is frequently uncertain. Even contemporaneous secondhand accounts can be contradictory. And, of course, most of what humans have thought about reproduction in their time on the planet was never recorded.

As the historian John Waller argues in *Heredity: A Very Short Intro-duction* (2017), "We can be fairly sure that when our *Homo sapiens* ancestors emerged in Africa about 200,000 years ago they realized that like begets like." Before long, they would inevitably have no-ticed unusual traits recurring across generations of families and wondered about them.

One of the earliest records of humans musing on reproduction is a Sumerian cuneiform tablet dating to about 2450 B.C., which traces kings to "the seed of gods." Supernatural elements continued to dominate stories about human reproduction for the next two thousand years. The God of the Old Testament created Adam in his own image and then, because his creation was lonely, fashioned Eve from Adam's rib. "Verily, We created Man from a drop of mingled sperm, in order to try him," says the Qur'an, 76:2.

Rational approaches originated in classical Greece. Historians of genetics trace the beginnings of our ideas to Hippocrates, who was born sometime around 460 B.C., and to the physicians he taught and influenced. The Hippocratics rejected superstitions ascribing illness to acts of the gods. They sought to establish medicine as a discipline. It's hard to generalize too broadly about what they thought, because only a handful of their texts coalesced into the of-ficial corpus. Even those are sometimes inconsistent, and in most cases we don't know who wrote them. The writings do establish the Hippocratic belief that a baby began with sperm that came, as the unknown author of *The Seed* put it, "from the whole body of each parent, weak sperm coming from the weak parts, and strong sperm from the strong parts." Each parent contributed "both male and female sperm." Strong sperm produced male children, weak sperm produced girls, and "whichever sperm prevails in quantity" deter-mined whether the couple would have a daughter or son. "Bald parents usually have bald children," and "squinting parents," "squint-ing children." A child favored the parent "who has contributed a greater quantity of sperm to the resemblance, and from a greater number of body parts." The idea that semen came from all parts of the body was later adopted by Charles Darwin, who called the theory "pangenesis."

Some Hippocratics contended that traits people developed during their lifetimes could be passed on to children. The author of "On Airs, Waters, and Places" attributed the long heads of the Macrocephali people to generations of head-binding, for example. These features were "acquired at first by artificial means," but (the argument went) "nature collaborates with tradition," and ultimately long heads became characteristic of the population. The Hippocratics also emphasized the influence of climate, landscape, celestial bodies, and nutrition, and some made sweeping, pejorative claims about the characteristics of people from specific places. And they developed the beginnings of the humoral theory of temperament that would dominate medicine nearly until modernity.

With their conviction that both parents contributed seed, the Hippocratics departed from the stance usually attributed to Pythagoras, the mathematician and philosopher known for his triangle theorem. In *The Gene,* Siddhartha Mukherjee ascribes to Pythagoras the idea that the father's seed determined the form of his offspring by collecting instructions for building a child (an anachronistic but useful shorthand) as it moved through the father's body and by absorbing "mystical vapors from each of the individual parts." The seed "provided the essential information," while the mother's womb "provided nutrition so that this data could be transformed into a child." Essentially, Mukherjee characterizes Pythagoras as a pangeneticist, but some scholars reject this idea.

The next major explanation of how parents determine a child's traits came courtesy of Aristotle, whose ideas dominated Western thinking on the matter alongside the Hippocratics' until Darwin and Mendel displaced them. Aristotle ascribed an inert, unwitting contribution to the mother. In *Generation of Animals* (published around 350 B.C.), Aristotle argued that the male animal supplied the sperm, which carried a magical active ingredient "pneuma," a kind of spirit or soul that created "vital heat." The female animal was inherently cold and passive. Aristotle scoffed at the idea that both parents determine the form of the child. This is true, he said, "only in the sense in which a bedstead is formed from the carpenter and the wood." The carpenter's "soul" and "knowledge," like the man's semen, were the crucial fuel. It's unclear whether parents passed along acquired traits in Aristotle's scheme. He alluded to children born with "the outline of a scar in the same place where a parent had a scar," but observed that "mutilated parents" didn't always produce "mutilated children."

Aristotle did allow that women had an extremely minor role to play in determining the form of a child, insofar as a father's sperm wouldn't be able to collect knowledge from his own body for forming a daughter's "generative parts." (He also held that men with long penises were more likely to have girls because the semen cooled before it could reach the womb. This, like his misogynistic notions of the role women played in reproduction, leads me to some unkind speculations about Aristotle's feelings about his own anatomy.) Ultimately, Aristotle believed the sun, moon, and stars had more to do with the form of a child than the mother did.

Most ancient thinkers ascribed great influence to the stars. Many also emphasized climate, landscape, diet, and so forth. The Hippocratics taught that these factors affected the balance of four basic fluids, or humors, in the body and that the humors in turn determined the wellness—or sickness—of a person, as well as the kind of child they were likely to have. In *On the Nature of Man,* Hippocrates's son-in-law, Polybus, associates each humor with a season: blood with spring, yellow bile with summer, black bile with fall, and phlegm with winter. He characterizes health as a state in which these humors "are in the correct proportion to each other" and pain and disease as the result of an imbalance.

The Hippocratic writer of *On the Sacred Disease* echoes this, calling epilepsy "hereditary," while pondering its inconsistent occurrence in children of epileptics. "If a phlegmatic child is born of a phlegmatic parent" and "a bilious child of a bilious parent," why do some children of a parent "afflicted with [epilepsy] not suffer similarly?"

Humoral theory of disease reigned until the nineteenth century. Ascribing these bodily fluids so much importance sounds arbitrary now, but when blood settles in a test tube, it separates into four strata that appear to be red, yellow, black, and white. Twenty-first-century scientists understand the composition of these layers far more accurately than the ancient Greeks did, but disease really can alter their relationship to one another: the rate of separation when a sediment test is performed, and in the case of pneumonia even their proportions.

The Hippocratics saw the humors as both innate and changeable. Noga Arikha explains in *Passions and Tempers: A History of the Humours* that they considered "the humoral characteristics present with the individual from birth or even from conception" to determine personality and body types but also believed environment and the passage of time could affect the humors and their manifestation. Not only could humors ebb and flow, they might be expressed inconsistently from person to person. In *Problemata*, Aristotle (or a follower) postulated a connection between creativity and the melancholic temperament but also the possibility of "groundless despondency" if the melancholic's black bile was too cold or frenzy if it was too hot. The effect on a given individual was unpredictable, he said, because, like "wine mingling in a stronger or weaker form in the body," black bile "gives us our own special characters."

WITH SOME INTERPRETIVE ASSISTANCE, the theories of the Hippocratics and Aristotle formed the core of Western thinking about generation for nearly two millennia. Their endurance owes a debt to Galen, a Greek physician and scholar prominent in Rome in the second century A.D., who elaborated upon and attempted to reconcile their ideas. Galen held that every person's constitution and character was determined by six "non-natural things" and seven "natural things." The non-natural things—environment, nutrition, rest, exercise, excretions, and psychological states—could be changed or influenced. The natural things were spirits, elements, humors, organs, functions, capacities, and temperament and were believed "to result from the direct, physical creation of the embryo." In his thinking about disease, Galen endorsed much of the Hippocratic scheme.

Galen created the humoral system as it's remembered today, tying the humors to temperaments: blood was the sanguine (cheerful) type; phlegm was the phlegmatic (slow and steady) type; yellow bile was the choleric (spontaneous, energetic, and angry) type; and black bile was the melancholy (anxious, depressive, creative) type. Galen also brought together competing ideas about the mechanics of generation. He agreed with the Hippocratics that both parents produced sperm but with Aristotle that women produced and were the result of inferior seed.

Islamic scholars also made major contributions. The medieval Persian philosopher and physician Ibn Sina (known in the West as Avicenna) synthesized Aristotle's and Galen's seed theories and helped pave the way for genetics. He characterized the phenomenon of polydactyly (extra fingers) and other rare conditions as natural rather than supernatural and as inevitable rather than random. Classifying these "rare disorders as purely natural phenomena was a fundamental step toward the establishment of a consistently naturalistic perspective on medical phenomena." Avicenna also cited the Prophet Muhammad on the creation of the "life germ" and sided firmly with Aristotle on the principle that women do not contribute seed. (Unlike the Bible, the Prophet afforded the mother some agency. According to the hadith compiled by Bukhari, when asked why some boys resemble their father while others resemble their mother's side of the family, the Prophet answered that if a man has orgasm first, "the child will resemble the father," whereas if the woman has an orgasm first, the child resembles her.)

John Waller highlights a possible nadir of views devaluing the woman's contribution: an "anonymous late thirteenth-century text, invitingly called *Women's Secrets*," which maintained that "if a cat ejaculated on a herb that was unwittingly consumed by a man, he could have cats 'generated in his stomach.'" As a corrective, I like Kate Millett's argument in *Sexual Politics* that it would have been natural—and, judging by the prevalence of ancient fertility cults, probably was in fact natural—for early humans to view mothers and childbirth as the most "impressive evidence of creative force." But the eventual realization that men also played a role created an opening for downgrading women and ascribing "the power of life to the phallus alone."

Women were usually cast as junior players in reproduction until (and largely through) the Renaissance period. By the eighteenth century, a more superstitious and sinister view had taken hold. As Jenny Davidson explains in *Breeding: A Partial History of the Eighteenth Century*, theorists of the era tended to attribute a baby's features to the mother's imagination. The mother could unwittingly transmit to the fetus whatever she thought or witnessed; "a desire for strawberries might produce a strawberry birthmark, the sight of a mutilated beggar a child with missing limbs." A son resembled his father because of his mother's mind—and potentially her trickery. She might have slept with a lover but produced a child who looked like her husband by thinking of him at the moment of conception. Courts generally rejected resemblance as evidence in paternity cases under this rationale.

The emphasis on imagination had ancient forerunners. In a story from Genesis, Jacob's father-in-law, Laban, kept taking his sheep. Jacob had his ewes look at speckled branches, so his sheep developed distinctive markings and Laban could no longer claim them. Ambroise Paré cited this tale in his influential 1573 book *On Monsters and Marvels*. Invoking Aristotle and Hippocrates, he contended that the mother's "ardent and obstinate imagination at conception" could cause birth defects and "monstrous children." He recounted a story that Hippocrates intervened on behalf of a princess who was accused of adultery when she had a Black child. She and her husband were white, but Hippocrates attributed the child's complexion to a portrait, "similar to the child," which hung near the princess's bed. Men weren't entirely exempt from this kind of consideration. Plato argued that "while drunk a man is clumsy and bad at sowing seed, and is thus likely to beget unstable and untrusty offspring." He counseled men against acting to bring on violence or injustice, lest they be stamped "on the souls and bodies of the offspring."

In the eighteenth century, the mother's imagination became the default explanation for unwanted traits. Her uncanny influence extended to breastfeeding, by which she infused the child with "her ideas, beliefs, intelligence, intellect, diet and speech," along with "her other physical and emotional qualities." This mystical conception of maternity made the mother an easy target for perceived defects in the baby. It was also a reason to be suspicious of her curiosity and passions and to curtail her exposure to the world.

THE IDEA OF "HEREDITY" as we think of it now solidified only in the nineteenth century. While people had long known unusual traits of ancestors often reappeared in their descendants, these recurrences weren't conceptualized in terms of biologically hardcoded inheritance. Humoral medicine's emphasis on "the fundamental influence of the environment" meant, as the historian of medicine Silvia De Renzi puts it, that until the end of the eighteenth century, "nothing was so fixed in the inherited temperament that it could not be altered." (John Locke famously characterized the mind as a blank slate, comparing children to "white Paper or Wax, to be molded and fashioned as one pleases.") Conversely, the nineteenth-century conception of heredity suggested that inherited traits both "shaped the makeup of offspring" and "determined their life, diseases, and death."

Carlos López Beltrán traces the medical origins of heredity as a concept through the history of "hereditary," an adjective that appeared in antiquity and was nearly always negative. European translators probably imported the concept from Arabic treatises in translating the idea of "hereditary diseases," so the adjective was associated with unusual, typically undesirable, traits that ran in a family and were considered signs of "temperamental similarity." Montaigne stretched the concept with the joke about his "hereditary" dislike of doctors, though not with his puzzlement over how he ended up with the same gallbladder issues as his father.

Only in the eighteenth century did physicians start to characterize hereditary traits and diseases as "part of the organic constitution," something formed "before the first solidifications of the seminal humors in the womb gave rise to the new individual." Around the same time, plant and animal breeders began to think in terms of "inheritance capacity," to create hybrids in an effort to maximize desirable traits among offspring.

Charles Darwin's *On the Origin of Species*, published in 1859, was one of the first widely read books to depict heredity "as the central problem of biology," as Müller-Wille and Rheinberger put it. This is true, although he was vastly less interested in similarities among ancestors and their descendants than in the ways organisms adapt to their environment. In keeping with his evolutionary insights, he tended to view heredity as "a developmental process" rather than a question of a fixed substance being transmitted. He did contend that when a "very rare deviation" among individuals "exposed to the same conditions" appears in the parent and recurs in the child, the "mere doctrine of chances almost compels us to attribute its reappearance to inheritance."

But Darwin didn't come anywhere near gene theory. He had some sympathy, at least early on, with the ideas of Jean Baptiste Lamarck, author of the 1801 book *Theory of Inheritance of Acquired Characteristics,* who contended that a parent could pass along to their offspring traits the parent acquired during their lives. Lamarck pointed to the long necks of giraffes as evidence, arguing that with each generation, the giraffes' necks stretched longer to reach the leaves on tall trees. But ultimately Darwin was a pangeneticist. Following Hippocrates, he suggested that, as one historian of science explained it, "the true carriers of hereditary properties" weren't parents but gemmules, "submicroscopic entities that are distributed anew in each generation" and "percolate through" later generations. He believed that these percolating particles came from all parts of the body.

The work of Gregor Mendel, who was isolating inheritance factors in plants even as Darwin's ideas transformed scientific thought, wouldn't gain serious attention for some time. Plant breeders were some of the earliest people to think about heredity in a fixed naturalistic sense—and in a practical way that could affect their livelihoods. It's not too surprising that the foundation for our understanding of genes came from a botanist of sorts.

Inspired by breeders' successes with hybridization, and hoping to understand how organic forms evolved, Mendel contemplated the predictability of pea plants and tried mixing strains that had obvious differences in the same categories: height (short or tall), color (white blossoms or violet), texture (smooth leaves or wrinkled), and so on.

WHEN HE BRED THE tall and short pea plants, the second generation of plants were all tall. Clearly the tall trait was more powerful than the short. But in the third generation, some short plants appeared, suggesting hidden factors that were resurfacing. Mendel deduced that there were dominant and recessive traits. As Siddhartha Mukherjee writes, by studying the mathematical relationships between the kinds of plants that resulted from each generation in the experiments, Mendel was able "to construct a model to begin to explain the inheritance of traits." The male and female parts he spliced together each contributed one vote—a "form," as Mendel called it, and we now call it an allele—toward the trait that ulti-

mately appeared. Although Mendel didn't name the units of heredity that determined height, color, or texture in his experiments, "he
had discovered the most essential features of a gene."

Mendel published the results of his experiments in 1866, only
seven years after Darwin's *On the Origin of Species* appeared. His
findings received little attention until around 1900, and Müller-
Wille and Rheinberger emphasize that this timing was no fluke.
The "knowledge regime of heredity" had to shift before the world
was ready for genetics. There were "economic and social preconditions," such as the beginning of mass food production and the rise
of drug manufacturing and vaccines. "The omnipresent catchword
was 'purity,'" which became "a marketable quality of living beings,"
including cattle. Into this world of pedigrees, the gene was born.

Chapter 12

GENES EXPRESSING
THEMSELVES

———

NOWADAYS STUDENTS LEARN OF MENDEL AND HIS PEA plants at a young age. Even back in the 1980s, my fourth-grade class made inheritance charts focused on eye color. Our teacher explained that brown eyes were dominant, and as we all talked about our results, one classmate told another that her parents couldn't really be her parents, because they had brown eyes and hers were blue. My elementary school class was a microcosm of what happened when the concept of the gene took root. As is often the case when people get excited about the results of scientific discovery before the experimentation has been carried far enough for its limitations and dangers to be understood, a new set of half-baked principles emerged. Eugenics, which had already begun to flourish, exploded.

A century ago, the possibility of improving the human gene pool was widely accepted as a science. Today we tend to associate eugenics with Nazism, but its proponents weren't all right-wing fascists. George Bernard Shaw advocated "the socialisation of the selective breeding of Man." Bertrand Russell proposed color-coded "procreation tickets" and fines for mismatched ticketholders who dared to have children. "Three generations of imbeciles are enough," wrote the Supreme Court justice Oliver Wendell Holmes, Jr., in *Buck v. Bell,* a 1927 decision upholding Virginia's Eugenical Sterilization Act of 1924, which targeted "mental defectives."

I first learned of this case in my teens, because of my father's enthusiasm for Holmes's opinion. For a while after my parents' divorce, he took my sister and me to lunch at the same fast-food restaurant every Sunday; an elderly woman and her disabled son also ate there. Throughout these meals, my father muttered about imbeciles as the man shakily tried to feed himself. The scope of my father's censure included not merely people of other ethnicities and people with disabilities but also people he deemed overweight or unintelligent or lazy, and so on.

Twentieth-century proponents of eugenics advanced it as a remedy for a wide variety of perceived heritable shortcomings, including lack of intelligence, as defined by the eugenicists themselves. These impulses are very much with us now. Donald J. Trump, former president of the United States, credited "good genes" for his success, intelligence, and health, and the orange glow of his skin. "I always said winning is somewhat, maybe, innate," he said in an interview. "You know, you have the winning gene." Elsewhere, he observed that when you "connect two racehorses, you usually get a fast horse." And at a rally in the lead-up to the 2020 presidential election, he explicitly endorsed "the racehorse theory." Michael D'Antonio, author of a biography of Trump, contended in a PBS documentary that Trump believes "there are superior people and that if you put together the genes of a superior woman and a superior man, you get a superior offspring."

Richard Dawkins, author of *The Selfish Gene,* might agree. Writing to the Scottish *Herald* in 2006, Dawkins wondered, "If you can breed cattle for milk yield, horses for running speed, and dogs for herding skill, why on Earth should it be impossible to breed humans for mathematical, musical or athletic ability?" Although he stopped short of advocating for "designer babies," he argued that "sixty years after Hitler's death, we might at least venture to ask what the moral difference is between breeding for musical ability and forcing a child to take music lessons." Three seconds of searching YouTube will unearth much of this same sort of thinking, some of it propagated by violent white supremacists.

But our genetic inheritance is not nearly as rigid as some would have us believe. The more scientists uncover about what our genes dictate, the more we learn how much we don't know. Our DNA coding may be fixed, but its expression is not.

TAKE IT FROM A CONVERT. Tim Spector is a genetic epidemiologist and physician who spent nearly two decades closely studying identical twins and "trying to convince a skeptical public and scientific world that virtually every trait and disease had a major genetic influence." Slowly, though, he writes in *Identically Different: Why We Can Change Our Genes,* he developed "a nagging doubt that we were missing something." Even eye color—once "believed to be controlled by only three genes"—has turned out to be anything but straightforward, "influenced by at least twenty and possibly hundreds of genes." Spector has even "met a few rare identical twins with different colored eyes to each other—a phenomenon that was said to be impossible." Spector's team was frustrated to find that gene markers for common diseases weren't especially useful, because "each gene is of tiny individual effect." Common diseases are controlled "not by one gene but by hundreds or even thousands."

Sharon Moalem, a geneticist, physician, and writer, compares our genes to sheet music. None of us play Mozart the way Mozart himself would have played it. The hardest thing to explain to patients about genetics, Moalem writes in *Inheritance: How Our Genes Change Our Lives and Our Lives Change Our Genes*, is that disease markers are not fate. Like Spector, he observes that so far DNA hasn't turned out to be a good predictor of whether a person will actually develop most diseases.

OUR BIOLOGICAL INHERITANCE FROM our forebears is much more flexible than was believed through the twentieth century. Over the course of each of our own lifetimes, the expression of our genes can change and change again through shifts in our epigenome. The clearest and most succinct explanation of the epigenome I've seen for the layperson comes courtesy of the writer Carl Zimmer. In *She Has Her Mother's Laugh: The Powers, Perversions, and Potential of Heredity,* he refers to the epigenome as the "collection of molecules that envelops our genes and controls what they do."

Some epigenetic modifications happen through the common process of methylation (the addition to the DNA molecule of three hydrogen atoms bonded to one carbon atom), which doesn't change the content of DNA but can result in a gene being turned on or off. Other epigenetic changes occur through histone modification, in which proteins are instructed whether to use or ignore part of our DNA coding. These epigenetic changes help determine how we respond to stress or react to an illness. They're deeply intertwined with our experiences—diet, exercise, sleep, infection, and nurturing.

While our own genes unquestionably change in these ways over the course of our lifetimes, the assertion that epigenetic marks are transmissible to the next generation is highly contentious. Some scientists contend that these changes in expression can be passed down from parent to child. Experiments with plants, worms, fruit flies, and mice suggest this kind of transmissibility is possible in other species. Opponents argue that the human epigenetics studies to date have relied on questionable methodologies and raised more questions than they've answered, and that those who want to see transgenerational epigenetic inheritance in humans are relying on conjecture and magical thinking rather than evidence. Some geneticists also ridicule the results from intergenerational epigenetics studies on other mammals and animals.

A particular contempt has arisen among evolutionary biologists toward psychologists and others in what are often called the "soft sciences." In a new afterword to his 2002 book *The Blank Slate: The Modern Denial of Human Nature,* Steven Pinker derides the common understanding of epigenetics, comparing it to "the 1990s, when blank-slaters thought it was an amazing revelation that education, or psychotherapy, or learning a new language can *actually change your brain!* (as if learning might have taken place in the pancreas)." Epigenetics, he argues, "has become the new silly putty, the shape-shifting, input-copying ingredient that gives us a license to circumvent careful analyses of heredity and environment and embrace a holistic interactionism."

Over the past decade, an ongoing study of Holocaust survivors and their children and grandchildren exploded into the public consciousness with tantalizing headlines like GHOSTS OF FAMILY TRAUMA HAUNT DESCENDANTS and CAN WE INHERIT MEMORIES OF THE HOLOCAUST AND OTHER HORRORS? The reporting often seemed to suggest that scientists knew that epigenetic changes stemming from trauma could be passed down through multiple generations.

Since then, the study has been called into question. Detractors have noted the small sample size, only twenty-two descendants of thirty-two survivors. They've pointed out that other factors can affect the kind of methylation targeted in the study and that a child of two Holocaust survivors had the opposite methylation response from children descended from only one survivor. Some critics argued that the study would show true epigenetic changes only if great-grandchildren were studied, because the eggs that made grandchildren would have been present in the mother when she was a fetus inside the grandmother, and any epigenetic changes that occurred in the grandchild could be a result of the grandmother's womb environment. The study also lacked a control for environmental factors, such as the children hearing stories of the Holocaust, and their grandparents' experiences, while they were growing up.

Another frequently cited study of transgenerational epigenetic changes in humans focuses on what's commonly called the "Dutch Hunger Winter," a famine in the Netherlands toward the end of World War II caused by a Nazi blockade. Research based on the records from that time showed that children of mothers who were pregnant during the famine were more likely to be obese, diabetic, or schizophrenic as adults. On average, they weighed more and had higher triglycerides and LDL cholesterol than other adults. (If the mothers were malnourished only at the end of the pregnancy, though, the children tended to be born smaller than average and to stay small throughout their lives.) At one time, the researchers contended that different but equally notable changes were passed on to the next generation, to the grandchildren, but these results are disputed.

In 2018, Rachel Yehuda, the lead researcher on the Holocaust study, co-authored an article in *World Psychiatry* denouncing how the media presented research on possible epigenetic mechanisms in transgenerational effects of trauma, with reports ranging from "sensationalistic claims to global dismissals." Denouncing interpretations suggesting "a reductionist biological determinism," the authors argue that the research also suggests "potential resilience, adaptability, and mutability in biological systems affected by stress." And they call for research on the epigenetic impact of historical traumas including colonization, slavery, and displacement, focused on Black and Indigenous populations.

Comprehensive epigenetics studies on Black and Indigenous populations are scant, but many health professionals and activists suspect an epigenetic component to the multigenerational trauma that the researcher and educator Joy DeGruy describes in her 2005 book, *Post Traumatic Slave Syndrome.* DeGruy explores the effects of slavery across generations and the institutional racism that has followed, with the goal of showing, as her website puts it, how the Black community can "use the strengths we have gained in the past to heal in the present."

In *My Grandmother's Hands,* the therapist and trauma specialist

Resmaa Menakem argues that nearly all of us in the United States, "regardless of our background or skin color, carry trauma in our bodies around the myth of race" and that we'll never heal racism and its legacy in ourselves or in the culture until we deal with the ways the idea of "white body supremacy" has embedded itself in our bodies. He points out that poor white Europeans emerged from the Dark Ages, from a thousand years of land theft, imperialism, colonialism, brutality, and more, and then came to this land, where they established whiteness as supreme and inflicted all those same traumas, and even more-devastating ones, on Native people and the African people Europeans kidnapped to enslave here.

THE HOLOCAUST STUDY CAPTURED the public's imagination because it suggests connections that many of us feel we have in some way intuited. But the science is still largely uncertain, and a careful writer like Carl Zimmer sidesteps the debate over the Holocaust and Dutch Hunger Winter studies by not mentioning them in his book. He does, however, cite a study conducted by a Swedish scientist that concentrated on the people of that country's remote Överkalix region, where existence was perilous during the scientist's childhood. Farmers there suffered crop failures in some years and surpluses in others, leaving them dangerously hungry through many harsh winters. As Zimmer explains, the study suggested that men "whose paternal grandfathers lived through a feast season just before puberty died years sooner than the men whose grandfathers had endured a famine at that same point in their life." A subsequent study by the same researcher of women in that period suggested that "If a woman's paternal grandmother was born during or just after a famine, she ended up with a greater risk of dying of heart disease."

Mice and rats take the brunt of the pain administered by our medical and scientific testing complex, and they figure prominently in epigenetics studies on anxiety and stress. One of the most famous was conducted by Brian Dias, a scientist whose research focuses on the neurobiology underlying stress, depression, social behavior, and fear. Dias and his colleagues taught male lab mice to fear the scent of acetophenone, which is often compared to cherry blossoms. Every time the fragrance filled the air, the researchers administered a shock. Eventually the mice came to dread the scent so that they froze or trembled whether or not a shock was forthcoming.

The researchers inseminated female mice with sperm from these male mice. Once the pups were grown, the new generation reacted negatively to the smell although they'd never been exposed to it. "Smelling it made them more likely to get startled by a loud sound." Later, the children of these mice—grandchildren of the original males—turned out to be sensitive, too. A region toward the front of the brain had grown unusually large in the males trained to fear the scent, and the researchers found that, as Zimmer puts it, the "same patch of brain tissue that was enlarged in the trained mice was enlarged in their descendants," even though the only link between the granddads and grandpups was sperm. Subsequent acetophenone studies on female mice produced similar results, but the researchers did not study the brains of these mice and their descendants in the way they did for the males.

Other notable epigenetic research on rodents has focused on nurturing. In one study, rat babies who weren't properly groomed and looked after by their mothers ended up frazzled and unkempt, and they went on to treat their own babies the same way. The result was the same when the babies were raised by mothers who weren't their biological parents. Zimmer doesn't mention that study, which has come under criticism for its methodology, but he notes other studies on young mice that show those "separated from their mothers for hours at a stretch act a lot like depressed people." These mice tend to respond to danger with passivity and helplessness—quickly giving up trying to swim when thrown into water, for example—which seems to be passed down by male mice as well as females. I thought of this while reading Morgan Jerkins's conjecture in *Wandering in Strange Lands* that the transatlantic slave trade could have generated an instinctive fear of the water for some Black Americans that began when "some Africans forbade their children from swimming" for fear of the children being lost forever.

If the experiments with mice hold up, Zimmer says, "there must be something inside sperm (and eggs, too, presumably) that can pass down these mysterious marks. And since it can be influenced by experience, it can't be genes."

ZIMMER UNDERSCORES THE HARM done by twentieth-century scientists' insistence on genetic determinism. He highlights a story written and popularized by the eugenicist Henry Goddard, which captured the imagination of the 1910s and beyond, in much the way that the Holocaust study has recently. Goddard worried that New Englanders, the country's "'best people'" and finest stock, weren't breeding nearly as much as "'the feebleminded'" were. He advocated for "'a carefully worded sterilization law'" in every state. His bestselling 1912 book, *The Kallikak Family: A Study in the Heredity of Feeble-Mindedness*, contrasted a disreputable family line resulting from a gentleman's affair with a barmaid, with the brilliant, successful, and upstanding children the same gentleman had with his wife. In *The Mismeasure of Man*, Stephen Jay Gould characterizes the Kallikaks as "a primal myth of the eugenics movement."

Goddard scoffed at a series of studies conducted a century ago, which showed that exposing guinea pigs to alcohol fumes before they mated seemed to result in higher chances of developmental disorders, among other issues. The researchers found that "the same troubles carried over for four generations of guinea pigs." Goddard denied the role of drinking—"every feeble-minded person is a potential drunkard," he said—and scuttled the research, delaying the discovery of fetal alcohol syndrome until the 1970s. More recently, scientists have demonstrated that the changes leading to fetal alcohol syndrome are epigenetic. A pregnant rat's consumption of alcohol "alters the methyl groups and other molecules around the DNA in a fetus." And while, as Zimmer says, "the evidence is thinner," it's possible "that fathers who drink before conception can contribute to fetal alcohol syndrome, too." Score one for Plato.

One appeal of epigenetics is that it offers some conceptual release from the determinism of Mendelian heredity. To a degree, we have the potential to shape aspects of our own genetic expression. Another appeal of epigenetics is that it suggests we might connect to our ancestors on some mysterious, mystical level, through feelings and tendencies that proteins encode in methyl groups and warning tags placed on our histones.

But it's important to recognize that if transgenerational transmission of epigenetic marks is possible, this scheme has the potential for reductive, eugenical applications of its own. With studies into loaded subjects like anxiety, we could wind up right back at a place where a woman's behavior or state of mind during her pregnancy could be blamed for her child's strawberry birthmark, or someone's own traumatic experience could be considered to contaminate them for life. *You were bullied in school? Sorry, you're sullied goods, I can't procreate with you.*

Part Four

PHYSICALITY

Chapter 13

GRANDMA'S EYES

———

GROWING UP IN MIAMI, I WAS THE PALEST PERSON I knew—paler than redheads, paler than fellow freckle-faces, paler than the girl in my class who was allergic to the sun. My mom could tan. My sister and Granny could, too. I could only burn, blister, and peel, and my pastiness was so profound that no one could tell even when I had sun poisoning. "Didn't you go to the beach?" friends asked. I shifted my top toward one shoulder to show my sunburn, suddenly magenta in comparison to the cadaverous line left by my bathing-suit strap.

People often thought I was sick. My elementary school principal asked for a doctor's note confirming that I wasn't anemic. "What's the matter, darling," an ex-boyfriend's father asked later, "don't you like the sun?"

My skin color, like my dark hair, came from Grandma, my father's mom, who passed her complexion along to him and, through him, to me. When I despaired over my pallor as a child, my father was indignant, insulted. My skin was a mark of distinction, he said, a signifier of supremacy. No one else I knew in Miami praised my skin, luckily. They were far more likely to mock it. The privilege inherent in being this color was invisible to me.

I was a tiny, waifish, spectral child, with circles under my eyes like bruises, and allergies to mangos, citrus rind, most pollens, and most detergents and soaps. Though evidently an early and endless talker—I believed my mother was exaggerating until I came upon the conversations she recorded in letters from the time I was two-and-a-half and three—I started walking late and lagged behind kids my age in the simplest activities: flicking switches, turning knobs, pressing doorbells. She expressed concern about these developmental delays in her letters, too.

Before I was born, my mom had resolved that I would be more coordinated than she was. Unlike her (and my father, whom she often called "Mr. Magoo," after the nearsighted cartoon character, especially when he arrived home having put yet another dent in the car), I would be able to dance and jump rope and play ball. At age three, I was enrolled in tap and ballet; after our first recital, the teacher suggested that the lessons be discontinued, a blow to my mom and a relief to me. The first time I played kickball, in fifth grade, I rushed forward to kick the ball and instead stepped on top, transforming it into a launching pad. After achieving liftoff, I landed glasses-first in the dirt.

Evidently I was diagnosed with asthma, but my mom had found Jesus by then and believed that her faith foreclosed the possibility of "an asthma demon" attaching itself to her child, so I never had an explanation for why my lungs hurt when I ran, until she mentioned this much later. As I flash back to my younger self running laps, glasses bumping up and down on my nose while I trailed half the parking lot behind my classmates, legs corpse-ily glowing, I can't say I'm sorry that the reel doesn't include my stopping to suck on an inhaler.

Based on appearance alone, everyone assumed I was weak and unathletic, which was true. From a young age, I resented this, and by extension I resented Grandma, whom I suspected to be the source of my frailty. I wanted to be like Granny, who in the western of my mind confronted adversity by hopping onto the bare back of

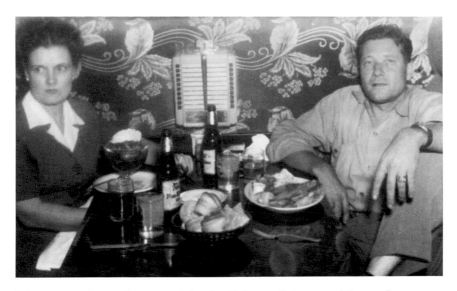

My maternal grandparents, Martha Rebecca Johnston (Granny) and Robert Charles Bruce, at dinner in Dallas, around 1940.

My great-great-grandmother Martha Caroline (Burge) Kinchen, center, with her granddaughters, Martha (Granny), at left, and Louise Johnston, at right, probably Dallas, around 1913.

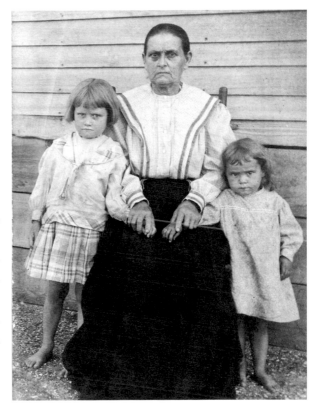

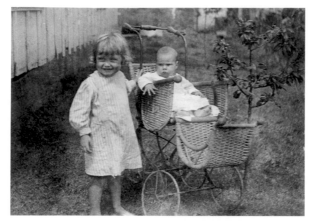

Martha (Granny) and her baby sister, Louise, in Dallas, around 1909.

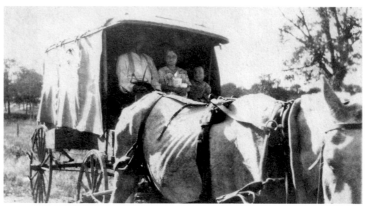

My traveling-salesman great-great-grandfather Sylvester Kinchen, with his granddaughters Martha (Granny) and Louise, and a hungry horse, around 1912.

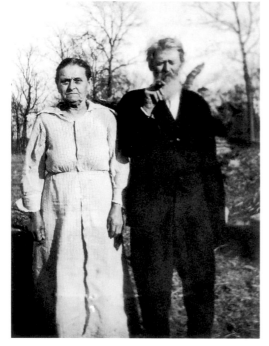

My great-grandparents Martha Caroline and Sylvester Kinchen, probably in Dallas, in the 1910s.

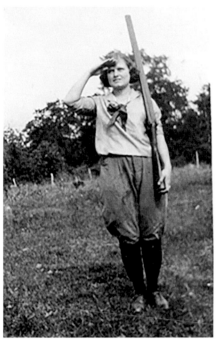

Granny as a young woman, saluting and holding a gun, probably in Dallas or Irving, or Kaufman County, maybe 1919.

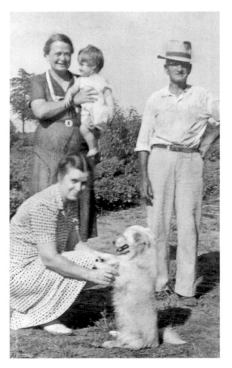

Granny, in foreground, with her parents, Alma Versa (Kinchen) and Zone Harrison Johnston; my mom, Sandy, as a baby; and one of the family dogs, around 1941.

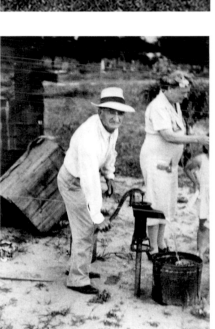

My great-grandparents Alma and Zone Johnston, on their farm in Irving, Texas, around 1950.

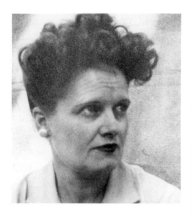

Left: Granny,
around 1950.

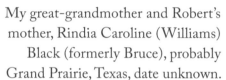

My great-grandmother and Robert's
mother, Rindia Caroline (Williams)
Black (formerly Bruce), probably
Grand Prairie, Texas, date unknown.

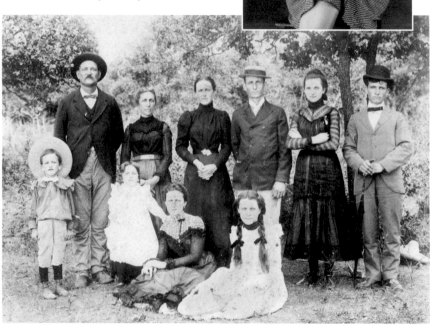

The Johnston family. Back row, left to right: my great-great-grandparents
Allen Alexander Johnston and Rebecca Ann (Smith) Johnston, followed
by Sarah Clamansy Johnston, John Allen Johnston, Maude Lee Johnston,
and my great-grandfather Zone Harrison Johnston. Front row, left to
right: James Earl Johnston, Gertie Louise Johnston, Jennie Pearl
Johnston, Mary Alice Johnston. During my mom's girlhood, long
after Allen's death, they all liked to dip snuff, the women included.

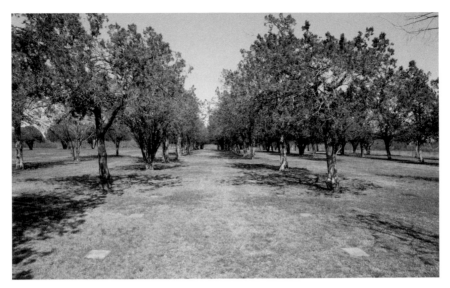

The cemetery where my great-grandfather Charley Bruce is buried, behind Wichita Falls State Hospital, a mental institution in Wichita Falls, Texas, 2015.

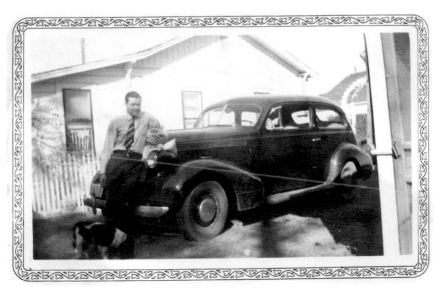

My grandfather Robert with my mom, Sandy, and their dog Bobo, in front of Granny's house in the Oak Cliff section of Dallas, around 1941.

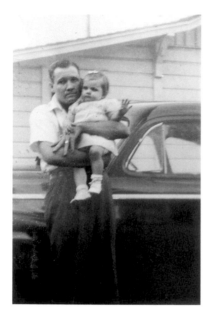

My grandfather Robert
with my mom, Sandy,
in front of Granny's
house in the Oak Cliff
section of Dallas,
around 1942.

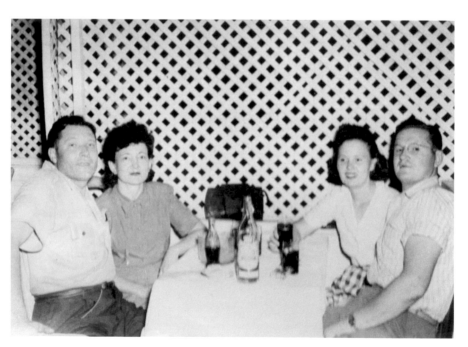

At left, my grandfather Robert with Christine (Barta) Weber,
his fifth known wife and the woman he married after Granny,
at Sivil's Drive-In, in Dallas, July 1944.

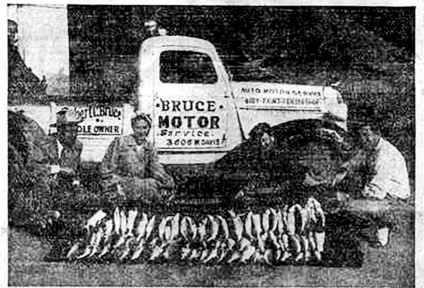

FISHING PARTY BRINGS BACK PROOF—Shown above are Mr. Spivey, Mrs. Spivey, Mrs. Bruce and Mr. Bruce, member of the Bruce fishing party which fished the waters at Aransas Pass last week and brought home proof of their catch. The waters at Aransas Pass and Rockport were great fishing favorites of the late Franklin Roosevelt. Robert Bruce, owner of Bruce Motor Service says that he is ready to go again if he can find the time. If you have any fish tales to swap drop around and have a tale-telling bee with Mr. Bruce. True to tradition the party reports that the biggest one got away.

My grandfather Robert with Christine in "Oak Cliff Shopping News," a free circular, in front of his Bruce Motor Service truck, in Dallas.

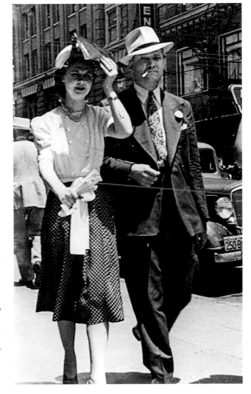

My grandfather Robert with an unknown woman, year and location unknown.

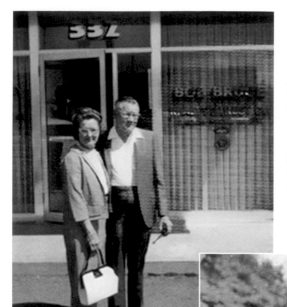

My grandfather Robert
with his last wife,
Eleanore (Havel)
Lussier, in front of
Bob Bruce Realty,
in Phoenix, Arizona.

My paternal grandmother,
Alice Mae (Terry)
Newton (Grandma),
in front of the fountain at
Belhaven University,
Jackson, Mississippi,
around 1942.

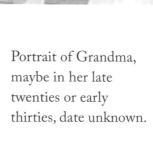

Portrait of Grandma,
maybe in her late
twenties or early
thirties, date unknown.

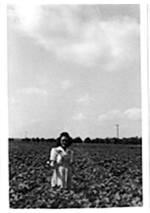
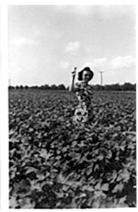

Grandma (left and center) and her older sister, Pearl (right), probably in the fields at Four Fifths Plantation, Shellmound, Mississippi, around 1943.

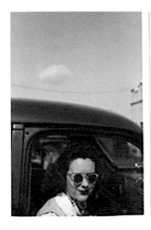

Four Fifths Plantation sign, Shellmound, Mississippi, 2007.

Mr. J. E. Terry says:

ll kinds of equipment but only one kind of tire—

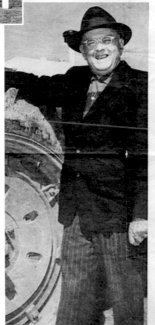

FIRESTONE
CHAMPION
GROUND GRIP."

Mr. Terry is General Manager of Four-Fifths Plantation, one of the largest and finest in the Delta, near Greenwood, Mississippi.

Running a plantation with 5,000 acres under cultivation calls for a lot of equipment, and according to Mr. Terry, "Everything on Four-Fifths runs on Firestones." And that goes for Robertson's Deadening, another 2,000-acre plantation he manages, too.

Service is the big thing, according to Mr. Terry—longer and better operating service from Firestone Tires, and continuing personal service by his Firestone Dealer, Mr. Lee "Ken" Kenneth. Matter of fact, Mr. Terry completely relies on Ken for Hydro-Flation and regular checking on the condition of all tires on his 25 tractors and other equipment.

You don't have to run 25 tractors, however, to better fit from Firestone tires and service—Firestones can also help you do any work faster and more economically. The tread on these tires was designed to last longer, and to get more work out of your tractor.

Drop in and talk it over with your Firestone Dealer or Store. He's a good man to see for all your farm tires and service.

Lee Kenneth is the Firestone Dealer Mr. Terry relies on for regular tire inspection.

My great-grandfather Joseph Terry (Daddy Joe, Grandma's father) in a Firestone Tires advertisement featuring Four Fifths Plantation.

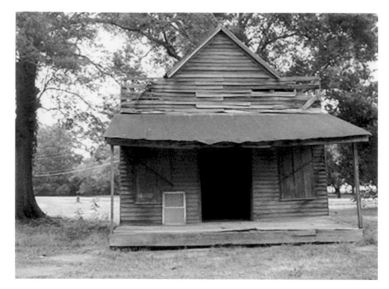

Daddy Joe's former office on Four Fifths Plantation, Shellmound, Mississippi, 2007.

Tilling machinery on Four Fifths Plantation, Shellmound, Mississippi, 2007.

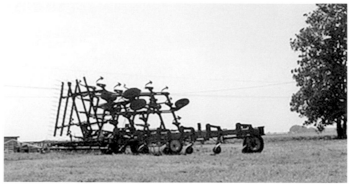

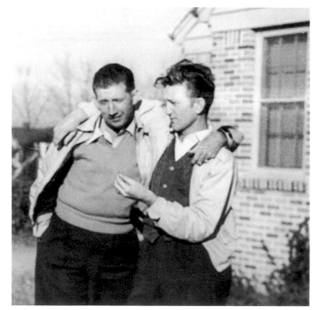

My paternal grandfather, Richard James Newton, Jr. (Grandpa), at right, as a young man, with unnamed friend, date and location unknown.

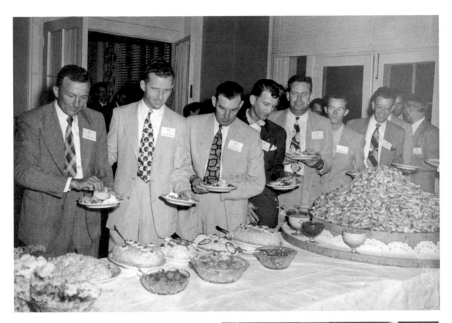

Grandpa, fourth from left, at a Junior Chamber of Commerce Convention, Buena Vista Hotel, Biloxi, Mississippi, probably 1950s.

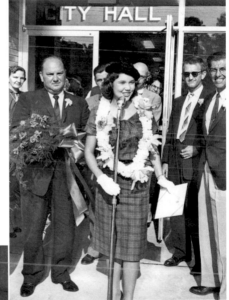

Grandpa, second from right, as part of welcoming committee for Miss America 1959, Mary Ann Mobley, on the Mississippi Gulf Coast.

Grandpa at work in Gulfport, Mississippi, maybe 1960s.

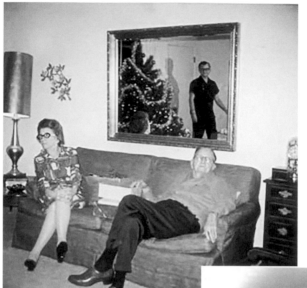

My great-grandparents
Anne Louise Ricketts
(Mamma) and
Richard James
Newton, Sr. (Grand-
daddy), on sofa, with
Grandpa (their son)
reflected in the
mirror, Long Beach,
Mississippi,
around 1972.

My great-great
grandmother Minnie
Ann (House) Newton
(Grand Newt), probably
in Drew, Mississippi,
maybe in the 1960s.

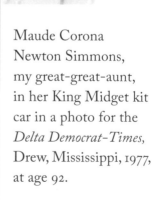

Maude Corona
Newton Simmons,
my great-great-aunt,
in her King Midget kit
car in a photo for the
Delta Democrat-Times,
Drew, Mississippi, 1977,
at age 92.

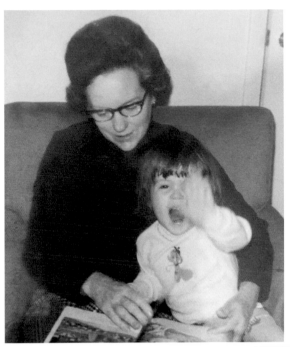

Grandma and me in
Miami, around 1974.

Grandpa and me,
probably in Long
Beach, Mississippi,
around 1973.

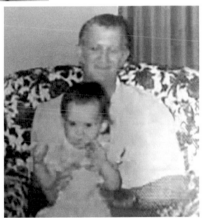

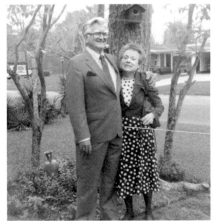

Grandma and
Grandpa, in
Nashville,
Tennessee, 1994.

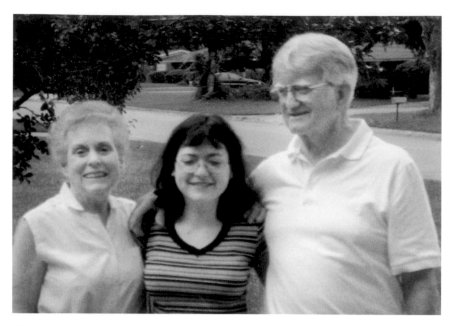

Grandma, Grandpa, and me in Long Beach, Mississippi, around 1997.

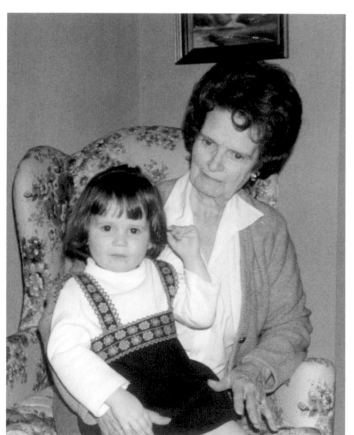

Granny
and me in
Dallas,
around 1974.

Granny and me at the dinner table, during my mom's bird-breeding era, in Miami, Florida, around 1996.

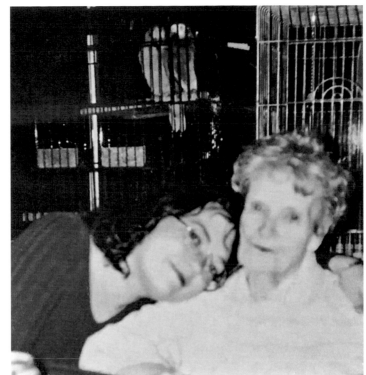

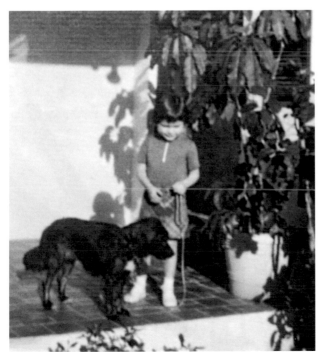

Me as a girl with our first dog, Harris, in Miami, around 1975.

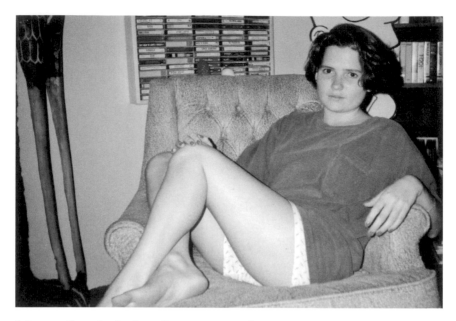

Me at a friend of a friend's apartment, Gainesville, Florida, summer 1990.

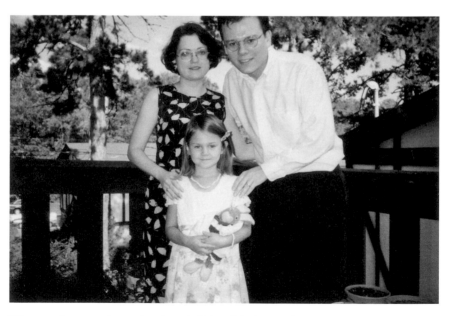

Photo of me with my husband, Max Clarke, and my stepdaughter, Autumn, in Tallahassee, Florida, spring 1999.

a horse and stampeding off to set things right. Instead, I was built like Grandma, a lady made to swoon in petticoats and be brought around with smelling salts. My appearance was an emblem of shame to me: a sign that I came from women bred to sit around on plantations and be waited on.

AS A TODDLER, I was wary of a photo of Grandma that my mom kept in a clear plastic cube with a different family photo in each of its six windows. In the picture, Grandma held the infant me and appeared to be smiling at the camera while also glaring at it. Her expression terrified me more than my toy clown's face in semidarkness, more than Willy Wonka singing, "There's no earthly way of knowing, which direction we are going," more, even, than Cruella De Vil, who wanted to make herself a coat from Dalmatian puppies, because Grandma was a real person. She would eventually be standing in the same room as me, expecting me to hug her. Between visits, I made sure to put the picture on the bottom of the cube so I couldn't accidentally see it from any vantage point.

Every time we were traveling to Mississippi to see my dad's parents, and every time they were coming to visit us, my mom picked up the cube and showed me the photo, even though she knew how I felt about it. Grandma's gaze looked so hard and angry. The expanse of white around her irises was deeply alarming, particularly in contrast with the smile on her face, which looked genuine and therefore demented, like a murderer's smile. The disjunction made my breath catch in my throat. It filled me with stomach-sinking dread.

"What's wrong with her eyes?" I'd ask my mother.

"Nothing's wrong," she'd say. "That's just how they look."

In person Grandma wasn't scary, but she was fluttery and nervous and perfectionistic, calling me "sugar" with her mouth but not, I felt, with her eyes or her heart. By the time I was in college, though, we'd grown closer, the first of several ebbs and flows. My sophomore year, I called every week or so to tell her about school and the boy I was dating. Less than a month before she was supposed to meet him, we broke up. She seemed to understand, without my saying much, how sad and unmoored I felt. By then I recognized how her own fidgety movements and frail ankles, her iron grip on her keys and the steering wheel and other everyday objects, echoed in my own. I had long since stopped seeing her eyes as anything other than part of her face.

Not long after parting ways with that first college boyfriend, in my early twenties, I started dating someone else and launched into a twisted relationship, the one during which I threatened to leap from the window. Our attraction was based, from my end at least, almost entirely on our similar dysfunctional histories. Every day we fought, and every day I cried. I was in a state of continual excitement, vacillating between anger, lust, anxiety, and sadness, raging as my mother once had and weeping like her, too. Sometimes I also starved myself, severely limiting calories for a week or two. After a couple of years of this, my hands started to shake and my palms wouldn't stop sweating. No matter how much I ate, I felt unsteady and ravenous. When I ran my fingers through my hair, it came out in my hands. I thought I was losing my mind.

Friends kept asking if I was okay. At first I thought they meant the tremors, which were unsettling even to me. If I picked up a piece of paper, it rattled audibly, like the wings of some frantic insect. Increasingly, though, my friends mentioned my eyes. "You know, your *eyes*," they would say, as though I should understand what they meant, and I didn't. My eyes, so far as I was concerned, so far as I had always been concerned, were narrow and nondescript, a dark nearsighted hazel, not one of my better features but the least of my worries just then.

This had been going on for several months before I graduated from college, moved back home with my mom and stepdad, and went to renew my driver's license. When the clerk pressed the laminated card into my shaky hands, I almost gasped. There in the photo, a greatly exaggerated version of my grandmother's stare glared back at me from my own face. The whites of my eyes were enormous, my irises disquieting islands in the midst of them. I looked furious and unhinged. I looked like someone who shouldn't be loose on the streets, a figure in a Surrealist painting.

The problem was endocrinal: an overactive thyroid gland rampaging into hyperthyroidism and thyroid eye disease. My resting heart rate was 127 beats per minute. The doctor put me on beta blockers and prescribed bed rest until radioactive iodine could be flown in to kill part of my thyroid. The pill was sealed in a special container that looked like an enormous lead Rolex box, and I wore special protective clothing to take it. For several days afterward, I had to avoid children and pregnant women, stay at arm's length from everyone else, use a bathroom no one else used, and flush twice.

Over time, my hands and thyroid levels stabilized and my eyes retrenched a bit, and I was left with my father's mother's stare almost exactly. It glares at me from photographs and subway windows; it captivates babies and antagonizes strangers. Regardless of my actual mood, it's a look eternally caught—until I glance down, soften the rest of my features, recalibrate—somewhere between surprise and anger. I'd grown accustomed to the things about myself I wished I could change: my pale skin, my freckles, my lack of coordination. I hadn't anticipated new ones, from Grandma, again.

Grandma never admitted to having had a thyroid disorder, and perhaps she'd never been diagnosed, but I'm sure at some point she had the same affliction I did. In childhood pictures, her eyes look as nondescript and narrow as mine once were. Apart from being dark brown rather than muddy hazel, they are precisely the same eyes I had as a girl.

BECAUSE OF MY FATHER'S LECTURES, I assumed Grandma was proud of her skin. Eventually, I learned it embarrassed her. She, too, weathered the late eighties by resorting to the orangey glow of self-tanner. As with the Confederate emblem on the state flag of Mississippi, she would have preferred something less distateful to U.S. culture at large. It surprised me that we agreed that the symbol should be removed, though it's safe to say that she did not share my vehemence.

Grandma's sister, Great-Aunt Pearl, was like a character in a Eudora Welty novel: full of cutting quips about everything other people were doing wrong. She often compared Grandma unfavorably to herself. Whereas Pearl was stylish, moneyed, and popular, Grandma was dowdy, boring, and clumsy, in Pearl's view. Pearl was nice to me when it suited her but not above mischief. During the era when my mom was trying and failing to transform toddler me into a tap dancer, Pearl gave me a baton and suggested I could be a majorette. "Let's see you twirl it!" she said, a gleam in her eye.

In an undated eight-page single-spaced recollection of life in the Delta that Pearl sent out to the family, maybe in the late 1990s, she recalled a party that she and Grandma attended as young girls in the 1920s. Afterward, Pearl remembered, "When we reached the steps to the house, Alice [Grandma] just fell on them and said, 'I am soooo tired!' Her dress had punch down the front of it and she had fallen several times and had a knot on her knee." More neutrally in the same letter, Pearl recounted, "There was no vaccine at that time, so Alice and I had all the children's diseases. We had chicken pox, measles, colds and coughs, mumps and other things. I remember once a friend saying to Mother, 'Mrs. Terry, do those little girls get enough to eat?' We had plenty, we just didn't have a large appetite."

Though I was required to finish every meal I was served as a child, people often thought I was too thin. I fantasized about not having a body at all. If only I could exist entirely in my mind, I wouldn't need to eat or sleep; I could escape sports and avoid being yelled at by my father. I so resented being tethered to earth by a physical self that I interacted with the world as if I were barely inside it, slouching in on myself, rushing from place to place, heedless of my surroundings, reading as I went whenever that was allowed, swallowing half my dinner without chewing and then asking to be excused. The backs of my feet were too narrow for most shoes, so my toes were always pinched up front while my heels slid out each time I lifted them off the ground.

At some point, for reasons unknown to me now, I adopted the habit of getting around on my tiptoes, or nearly, arches craning up like Barbie feet, so that only the tiniest possible part of me made contact with the ground. I remember a junior high classmate asking, with incredulous concern while we were doing laps around the parking lot, "Is that really how you run?" I tried reversing course, jamming my heels down instead, and a boy in the grade below us put it more bluntly. "That girl runs like shit," he said, pointing.

The lack of intelligence I had about my physical being and how to move it around was mortifyingly conspicuous. Whether this was primarily a result of genes, of anxiety, of spending my first weeks of life in an incubator, I don't know, but seeing Grandma knock around in the world, I trace at least some of it to her. I remember complaining about my terrible posture to Grandma once, when I was in my late twenties or early thirties. Though I didn't intend it, the rebuke to her own carriage would have been implied. Her curved upper spine was impossible to ignore. Grandma forced her shoulders back, raised her chin and her chest. Her hump persisted. She looked like a panicked animal in the glare of headlights. "I'm made this way," she said, her voice tinged with shame.

THE OLDER I GOT, the more aware I was that if my ambulation and posture didn't improve, I would end up with the same issue Grandma had—*the hunch,* my sister and I called it with dread, *the hunch.* Increasingly, I worried that I might even end up like the great-great-uncle my father described who was practically bent in half all the time, who slept on pillows that raised him almost to a sitting position. Still, it felt most comfortable to rush from place to place with my head sagging over a book (or, later, a phone) or just my own thoughts.

As I entered my forties, I had tried and failed at yoga and every other physical system I attempted. *The hunch* was beginning to set in. My neck and wrists ached and I was always turning my ankle. After many years of therapy, I knew that the way I moved through the world was also reinforcing my anxiety and distractedness. I decided to try the Alexander Technique, described to me as a method to improve posture. The Alexander Technique teaches students to reduce unnecessary tension in the body by becoming aware of their habits, of things that have come to seem inherent to an activity but aren't really. Thinking doesn't actually entail clenching your jaw or wrinkling your forehead, for example, even if you always do those things when you're concentrating. Sitting doesn't need to involve swinging your arms. Texting doesn't inherently involve hunching.

My teacher, Dan, approached the Alexander Technique through mindfulness meditation techniques that involve recognizing what's happening with your body, how your feelings manifest in your physical being, and accepting them, letting them be in the moment and then, in that acceptance, creating room for change. After my first lesson, as I walked to the subway, I found myself weeping. From my earliest years, I'd trained myself to operate my body as though I weren't really inside it. Showing up for the lessons week after week didn't allow me to keep doing that.

One thing I liked from the beginning was the emphasis on thinking. I'd always been told I needed to *think less* about softball or Frisbee or dancing to do them well, that I needed to just watch and then do them. For me, thinking less had resulted in the opposite of improvement. Dan showed me on a miniature skeleton what my bones looked like inside my body, how they were connected with one another, and how the—for lack of a better word—machinery was supposed to work. It was helpful for me to work more directly with what Dan called "that part of the body we call the mind."

I learned techniques that helped me see my habits more clearly and make room for the possibility of new, better habits. I could tell myself things like, *I am not sitting down,* even as I sat down, and see what happened. Sometimes I experimented with even stranger ideas Dan suggested, like telling myself, *I don't have a jaw.* After all, I couldn't clench it if it wasn't there.

I found that many aspects of my body and way of being that I saw as innate were at least partly the result of things I was doing to myself to avoid feeling pain. I'd permanently twisted myself after being kicked by a horse, for example, in an effort to walk normally, because my father was embarrassed by my limping. I'd done the same after slamming my jaw against the steering wheel in a car accident. And there were older and deeper habits, ways I'd learned to clench as my father shouted at me so that I wouldn't cry too soon. Before I could figure out new ways of being, I had to be willing to feel the pain that rushed in when I didn't clench and twist to avoid it.

I haven't eradicated those old tendencies, but I've reduced them, and some of the most remarkable changes have been to my feet. Both of my parents have high arches, and I always did, too, more like a Barbie doll's with each passing year. When I started lessons, my feet often ached in the middle and my toes were always cramped up, braced against the floor. Recalling this condition, Dan joked, "Rigor mortis would probably be too strong a phrase."

Now my feet are flatter and wider and, though still stiff, far more flexible. My arches are what you'd see on human feet rather than a doll's. When I'm standing, when I'm walking, I feel—well, I feel more grounded. "More aliveness" is what Dan observes, and that's true, not only of my feet. My breathing is less choppy, deeper, and more even. I'm less likely to get caught in feedback loops of panic as I try to calm myself. Several of my health problems, from an unhappy gallbladder to intense seasonal allergies, have partly resolved themselves. None of these were things I expected to be able to change, and the hunch is smaller now, too.

What surprised me most is that nearly everything I believed was involved in "good posture" turned out to be wrong. All the times my father tugged at my neck and shoulders and urged me to stand up straight, he was perpetuating our shared misunderstanding of what that meant.

When I think now of Grandma clutching her keys, fumbling with her coin purse, and tottering along on her little ankles, and when I imagine all the pictures in which she bravely smiled, trying and failing to "stand up straight," I have the sense of knowing, intimately, what it felt like to be her, and I'm flooded with sympathy. I realize that I can't know what her lived experience was really like. But as my body habits have become a little less like hers, as I've experienced other—less rigid and less frantic—ways of being, I realize how stressful it must have been to live that way.

I find myself thinking, too, of all the habits I share with my father: the choppy walk, the teeth grinding, the steely grip on a pen. Whether or not my father experiences himself as an anxious person, a person craving more connection than he's capable of, I believe he is one. I feel that I *know* he is one. It surprises me that my own body has come to seem like a doorway into how my father might feel when other, more usual forms of empathy have been a dead end.

THE LAST TIME MY grandmothers saw each other, one of two or three times I remember them being in one place with me, Granny came out on my mom's front porch to greet Grandma and Grandpa, who were in Miami on a rare visit to my dad. I believe I was eighteen, in my senior year of high school. My father had come to pick up my sister and me and take us out for dinner with his parents.

Granny, then in her mid-eighties, still lived in Dallas most of the time, but she spent longer periods of each year with us. Now recuperating from surgery, she stood with her cane. Just a few weeks before, her intestines had started leaking into her body. Scar tissue from a hysterectomy had ruptured, and as Granny had lain, wan and listless and in terrible pain, on a stretcher to be wheeled into emergency surgery, the surgeon had told my mom and stepdad that she might not make it. As I recalled the story, Granny had sat up on her stretcher and shouted at him, "Don't you tell them what I'm going to do, goddammit!" He stammered an apology.

In recent years, I checked with my mom, and she corrected me: "Granny looked the doctor straight in the eye and pointed her finger at him and said, 'I'll be right back!' Then she lay back and closed her eyes as if going to sleep." But my mom conceded, "What you said sounds just like something she could have said."

When Grandma saw Granny tottering toward us from the porch with a cane, she popped out of the car and rushed up the walk, her face evincing admiration but far more fear and pity. Granny was sixteen years older, from a different generation, a preview of what was to come. "Oh, Martha, you didn't have to come all the way *out heah*," Grandma said. Granny frowned and brandished her cane like something between a gavel and a scepter. "I'm a fighter, Alice," she said, "and you better learn to be, too, if you want to get to be my age." She turned to my grandfather, a fellow tenacious sort, now standing beside Grandma. "Tell her, Richard," she said, pointing the cane.

I WONDER WHETHER GRANDMA thought of Granny's stance as she began to contemplate her own end. Grandma often spoke of her horror of "becoming a burden." She wanted death to come easily, lightly, before some precipitous decline. She believed, with a low-key confidence, that she would end up in heaven, and she feared dying far less than lingering too long. Her great fear was that Grandpa would die first and she would be left alone, unable to care for herself. Several years before Grandpa's death, though, they called with news. Grandma, at age eighty-three, needed surgery.

She and I had gone through some rough times. It hurt her that

I wasn't close with my father and even more that I'd sworn I never would be. But we didn't discuss our disagreements on the phone that day. "The doctor found just a little spot of cancer on my uterus," Grandma said. She sounded cheerful, but putting a good face on a bad situation was perhaps Grandma's most singular talent.

The last time I'd visited my grandparents in Mississippi, Grandma had worn a catheter throughout my trip, but she never mentioned it or let on that she felt any discomfort at all. She'd taken my sister, Max, and me to the fanciest casino in Biloxi. She wore a silk blouse and silver shoes and walked the length of the resort. The news of the catheter had surfaced only when Grandma's kidney infection progressed so far that she wound up in the hospital. My aunt flew down from Tennessee and got the full story from the doctor. Seeing how dire the situation was, my aunt convinced my grandparents to sell their house and move to an assisted-living facility not far from her place.

And so, after talking with Grandma about the "spot of cancer," I called up my aunt and learned that Grandma's uterus had to come out entirely, that the cancer had spread beyond the uterine wall into her ovaries. The last time Grandma and I spoke before the procedure, I reminded her of Granny's exhortation to be a fighter. "I'm so glad you remembered that," Grandma said, again taking care to project optimism. "That's exactly what I'm going to think about on the operating table."

The cancer was more widespread than the doctors realized—widespread enough that it would eventually kill her. Almost immediately after the procedure, she had a stroke, then another. Half her body was paralyzed; she couldn't speak or see. The doctors didn't think she would recover. I got on a plane and rushed to her bedside. When my aunt told her I was there, Grandma made a noise, widened her already-wide eyes, opened her mouth, and closed it again. Tears ran from her eyes.

I sat with her and held her hand. I could feel her straining to stay, to connect. I told her I loved her, gave her water, and dabbed her lips with a warm washcloth. I'd been feeling guilty about urging her to fight if that wasn't what she wanted. It probably wasn't, I knew. After an hour or so, I told her that I wanted her to live if she wanted to live, but that if it was her time, she should go. We would be okay. We loved her and it was up to her.

I don't think I imagined the relief in her expression. Her brow unclenched; her hand rested in mine more lightly. She closed her eyes. As far as I know, she never stirred much after that, though she lived several days longer. Over the years since she died, I've mulled the grace and the strength in her readiness.

Chapter 14

THE FAMILY FACE

———

As NEWBORNS WE FOCUS ON FACES, THOSE REASSURING markers of our caregivers, before anything else. Soon we discover our own fingers, our mouths and toes. Around the age of two, we understand when we're seeing our reflection in the mirror, and then, sometime after this sense of me-ness takes hold, we start comparing ourselves with other children. Why is our hair black and our friend's blond? How come our ears stick out while our brother's lie flat? If we're short, we wonder what it's like to be tall. If we can roll our tongue or turn a cartwheel, we don't relate when other children can't do these things, and if we're hardy we can't imagine what it's like to spend a month sick with strep throat, then the flu, and then tonsillitis.

As a gawky kid, I was indignant that girls were judged on something as random and (I thought) insignificant as beauty, but I had little compassion for a tone-deaf friend who envied the way I could sing. Whatever the shade of our skin, the shape of our bodies, the extent of our abilities, some of the very first things we confront as children are the confines and triumphs of our physicality.

Our resemblance to grown-ups is difficult to fathom in childhood. It's hard to look past their wrinkles, breasts, and nose hair and their enormousness in comparison to us. No matter how many times we're told we look exactly like our great-uncle Benjamin, we aren't likely to see it. At some point, maybe we're presented with a photo of a relative said to have been practically identical to us at the age of six, and the similarities are striking enough to overcome all those things that make the pictorial past alien to children: the bee-hive hairdo, the thick goatee, the grainy mutedness of old film. There, beneath a newsboy cap, in front of a barn that was torn down fifty years ago, is a face that really could be our own. But for many of us it's only as we're getting older, watching our faces morph into our parents' and theirs into our grandparents', that we, too, find ourselves unable to stop marveling at how much little Olivia's scowl is like Aunt Matilda's.

The writer Sven Birkerts wrestles in an essay with the way his nephew's features are tangled up with a picture of his late father-in-law, Earl. "I knew this photo of Earl for some time before Matt leapt into it," he writes, "and now that he *is* there . . . I can't get Earl by himself anymore." "I'm the self-portrait of my father," says the speaker of Saeed Jones's poem "Hour Between Dog & Wolf," while standing before "the only unbroken mirror. . . . Even the rage is his." The poem was inspired in part by a family reunion where an older relative called him by his father's name. "For a brief moment," Jones told me, "she actually thought I was him." At times I nearly feel that way about my own face. Grandma's eyes look back at me as I glance into a store window, and I think, *Hi, Alice.*

Everyone who knows my husband exclaims how much my step-daughter favors him. She does: same nose, same lips, same cheek-bones and fingers. But people who know her mom are equally—and understandably—stunned at the resemblance between the two of them. I had a similar reaction to my young half-siblings, my dad's fraternal twins, whom I've never met. Their mom is Chinese Amer-ican, and in photos they look strikingly like her but also a lot like my sister and me, so much so that anyone who knew us as children would surely see us in them. I was unprepared for the protective feelings that welled up when I looked at their faces.

IF WE DON'T KNOW our biological relatives growing up, it can be surprising to encounter them later in life. In her memoir, *The Mistress's Daughter*, A. M. Homes writes of her search for the parents who gave her up for adoption. Finding them, she was astounded by how much she resembled her biological father and bemused that he would insist on a DNA test to establish paternity when her face and even her gestures were so similar to his own.

The writer Jennifer Teege, adopted at age nine, was horrified to discover as an adult that she's the granddaughter of Amon Goeth, the vicious commandant known as the "butcher of Plaszow," made famous by *Schindler's List*. Like her grandfather, Teege is tall and thin; unlike him, she's half-Nigerian. Goeth never would have been able to reconcile himself to Teege's existence, though she is his flesh and blood. And yet, she writes, in *My Grandfather Would Have Shot Me*, "When I look in the mirror, I see two faces, mine and his. And a third, my mother's. The three of us have the same determined chin, the same lines between the nose and the mouth."

Dani Shapiro recalls in her book *Inheritance: A Memoir of Genealogy, Paternity, and Love* the moment she, as a grown woman, first saw an image of the man who was her biological father. Her husband had pulled up a video. "I saw my jaw, my nose, my forehead and eyes," she writes. "I heard something familiar in the timbre of his voice. It wasn't merely a resemblance. It was a *quality*. The way he held himself. His pattern of speech . . . He held both his hands in front of him as if bracketing the air in parentheses—a gesture that I suddenly recognized as my own."

The genealogy site My Heritage has held competitions inviting users to submit photos showing an "uncanny resemblance" between themselves and an ancestor. Science writer Neal Ungerleider observed that many of the entries "looked as if they were of the same person." Over the course of our lives, in our own mirrors, we encounter many people who came before us. The past and present blur in our very being; the divide between living and dead becomes porous. "I am the family face," the poet Thomas Hardy wrote. "Flesh perishes, I live on."

Invisible resemblances of the flesh can be just as eerie. The first time I noticed Granny's scent coming from my own body, I froze for a minute, as if breathing might break the spell. The return of something I thought had died with her, something I couldn't imagine existing apart from her, seemed unreal, borderline supernatural. In truth, it's utterly ordinary. The genes we inherit from our ancestors have a lot to do with the odors we give off. It's even possible that newborns recognize their own biological mothers by scent and that mothers can identify their biological newborns the same way.

THE ANCIENTS GRAPPLED WITH questions of physicality in myth, religion, and philosophy. The Book of Genesis tells us that God created Adam in his own image, and later Adam became the father of "a son in his own likeness," carrying the resemblance to the second generation. Jesus's disciples connected physical disability with divine punishment, asking him, "Rabbi, who sinned, this man or his parents, that he was born blind?" Hesiod's didactic poem, "Works and Days," lauds a just, blessed, and peaceful society as one in which "wives give birth to children who resemble their parents."

Following the Hippocratics' fixation on transmission of traits like eye color from the parent with the strongest seed, Aristotle assigned deeper meaning to characteristics of the face. He argued in *Historia Animalium* that people with "a large forehead are sluggish; those who have a small one are fickle; those who have a broad one are excitable," and so on. By the eighteenth century, the mother's imagination was seen as the most powerful force in shaping a child's features.

As the twentieth-century view of genetics took hold, the genome was treated as an indelible code made up of simple dominant
and recessive genes that should be easy to identify and possible to
eradicate. Charles Darwin's cousin, Francis Galton, invented the
idea of improving humans through strategic breeding. The writer
Amram Scheinfeld's popular 1939 book, *You and Heredity*, provided
predictive "child forecast" tables for couples, offering a range of
likely skin tones and eye colors for their offspring. Scheinfeld surveyed musical ability, analyzing the families of Metropolitan Opera
musicians, and concluded it likely had a genetic component. He
debunked some of the most common, and most facile, legends
about "mental defectives" in families.

Scheinfeld was less enthusiastic than many of his contemporaries about the potential of forced sterilization to eradicate traits
like hemophilia and schizophrenia from the gene pool. He recognized that environment played a significant, elusive role. And he
observed that undesired traits seemingly eliminated through eugenics could resurface through mutation. As the Nazis consolidated
power, Scheinfeld rejected the ideas of racial purity and racial infe-
riority and highlighted the problems with the idea of "race" in general. Rebutting the Nazi ideal of an "Aryan race," he contended that
if a child of Adolf Hitler and the child of a rabbi were switched at
birth and "reared unwittingly by the wrong father, in all likelihood
Hitler's [biological] child would grow up to be 'Jewish' in temperament, behavior and social viewpoint," whereas "the rabbi's child
would be goose-stepping, storm-trooping and 'Heil-Hitlering' with
the most rabid of Aryans." Later in the book, though, Scheinfeld
toed the eugenics line, arguing that sterilization "can undoubtedly
eliminate many defectives" despite "serious limitations" and "inherent dangers."

After World War II, these kinds of eugenical practices began to
drop off, but the idea intermittently persisted that we needed only
to decipher our genes to crack open the secrets of everything: beauty,
disease, athletic prowess, creativity, and business acumen. By the

year 2000, scientists announced that they'd produced a working draft of the human genome, by which they meant a sort of map of human DNA, based on the genomes of several anonymous men and women. Former president Bill Clinton called it "the most important, most wondrous map ever produced by humankind." Francis Collins, one of the creators of the sequenced genome, called it "a history book—a narrative of the journey of our species through time" and a "shop manual: an incredibly detailed blueprint for building every human cell." Craig Venter, another creator, also heralded the making of "the human genetic blueprint." The blueprint was incomplete, though. "Some genetic influences lie beyond our DNA code," Venter conceded in his 2007 memoir, *A Life Decoded.* "Genes are not the whole story." In this he nodded to the influence of epigenetics, how our genes express themselves.

IT'S NATURAL TO WONDER why we look the way we do, why some people are more beautiful than we are and some less, some darker and some lighter, some more graceful and others clumsier. These kinds of differences are even more mysterious when we see them irregularly manifesting in our biological families. Like Montaigne, we want to understand how particular traits are selected to be passed down, why some manifest even when we're babies while others remain hidden until middle age and then burst into view.

Tim Spector, the genetic epidemiologist and physician who's spent decades closely studying identical twins, observes that, even when raised apart, twins not only look alike but "talk alike and have very similar mannerisms and facial expressions." And yet even conformity of facial characteristics among identical twins isn't ironclad.

His research has uncovered "major genetic influences" on many diseases, including some once thought to be the result of aging, such as cataracts, hemorrhoids, and varicose veins. But even diseases that "appear to be strongly genetic," such as rheumatoid arthritis, don't necessarily manifest in both twins. Of "identical women twins with the disease, 85 percent of the women never developed their sister's disease—even though they had the same genes and very similar lifestyles." For most diseases studied, "there was rarely more than a 50 percent chance of both twins getting the same disease, and usually the figure was much lower."

Sharon Moalem, the neurogeneticist, evolutionary biologist, and writer, also emphasizes that two people can be born with the same marker for disease but manifest that disease differently—or, seemingly, not at all. In *Inheritance: How Our Genes Change Our Lives and Our Lives Change Our Genes,* he tells the story of Ralph, a sperm-bank donor so popular that he became the biological father of at least forty-three children around the world. Unbeknownst to everyone, Ralph carried a genetic mutation that he had a 50–50 chance of passing along to each child. The gene was for neurofibromatosis type 1, which can cause disfigurations such as "enormous sacks of sagging skin, profound facial deformities, and growths that can resemble deep-red body-covering boils," along with "learning difficulties, blindness, and epilepsy." But in some cases it can manifest "so mildly that it's not recognizable." That's what happened in Ralph's case. Many of his kids weren't so lucky.

Underscoring the point, Moalem highlights a case of the neurofibromatosis type 1 gene in identical twins. One twin has a face so "bloated and disfigured" that a drunk club goer "once tried to rip it off, thinking it was a mask." Meanwhile, the other twin "could pass for Tom Cruise from a certain angle but suffers from memory loss and occasional seizures." This "variable genetic expressivity" is a truth Mendelian science failed to take into account.

Cultures have different standards of beauty, but research suggests that some aesthetic preferences are shared by most people. Humans tend to like symmetry. While Moalem emphasizes our power to influence our own gene expression, he also has a determinist streak, arguing that our faces and "the genetic workmanship that went into our fetal development" are closely linked. Humans evolved to find certain facial traits desirable, he argues, because they "provided the fastest way of assessing, ranking, and relating to the people around us" and they "divulge our developmental and genetic history. Your face can also tell us a lot about your brain."

People tend to be drawn to faces with eyes spaced so far apart that you could fit another eye between them. Modeling agencies seek out this trait (orbital hypertelorism), which, Moalem points out, both Jackie Kennedy Onassis and Michelle Pfeiffer possess. "Millimeters matter," and this makes sense because "the spacing between our eyes is a feature of more than four hundred genetic conditions." Very closely spaced eyes (orbital hypotelorism) are common in people with holoprosencephaly, "a condition in which the two hemispheres of the brain don't form properly," and in those with Fanconi anemia, which "often causes progressive bone marrow failure and an increased risk for malignancies." Much of the time, though, very closely spaced eyes seem to have no particular significance.

Patients often expect Moalem to begin an examination by analyzing their DNA. Instead, he starts with the body. He asks his patients to roll up their sleeves—not so he can draw blood but to "feel the texture of your skin and watch you flex," to "run my fingers along your wrist and stare deep into the crevices of your palm." Moalem mentions time and again that this or that characteristic—a bent pinky finger, for example, or a thumb as thick as your big toe— might mean you suffer from some terrible condition, or it might mean you just have a finger or toe that's a little out of the ordinary. So, too, with many genes.

In one troubling analogy, Moalem compares human faces to the Louis Vuitton logo and characterizes the face as "our most important biological trademark," a metric of "biological quality." Still, like Spector, he holds that tracing even our simplest physical traits through our DNA with any reliability is a tricky art. He once posted a photo of two infants to his Tumblr. One was a healthy sleeping baby in a blue onesie, with some kind of rash or blemish on their face. The other was tiny, less than half the size of the other, wearing a respirator covering half their face. Beneath the photo, the post said only, "monozygotic (identical) twins."

NOWADAYS WE CAN LEARN some things about our genetic markers through tests offered by companies like 23andMe. The site makes predictions as to eye color, hair texture, height, birth weight, and more. It attempts to project whether you are likely to tolerate lactose, to prefer bitter tastes, to flush when drinking alcohol. It purports to tell you your propensity toward disease, for yourself and your offspring—for example, whether you're a carrier for the more common strains of cystic fibrosis, whether you have increased risk for Alzheimer's or Parkinson's, how likely you are to respond to treatment for hepatitis B.

Some predictions are easy to evaluate by looking in the mirror. I do, as 23andMe suggests, freckle more than most people and have (to put it mildly) lighter skin than the average person. I'm also short, as my DNA would apparently tend to indicate, and I really *do* "hate the sound of chewing." My husband Max's test correctly suggests straight hair and brown eyes, and, given his hair at age forty-nine, "decreased odds of male pattern baldness" seems accurate.

But my results say, "likely no cheek dimple," when in fact the one on my right cheek was so pronounced in childhood, people liked to call me "Shirley Temple." "Likely no widow's peak" is also wrong. Looking a little more deeply into these predictions, even the stated odds of accuracy aren't great. While 69 percent of subscribers who share my nine markers don't have a cheek dimple, 31 percent do. In the case of the twelve markers considered significant for likelihood of widow's peak, 72 percent of subscribers don't have one, and 28 percent do. In each case, that's nearly a third who have the opposite characteristic from the one the result purports to show. Evidently, I also have the muscle-composition marker common to "elite power athletes," a miscasting I greatly enjoyed, particularly when the site used to frame the result as "likely sprinter." AncestryDNA (which offers fewer results but collects your genetic data all the same) correctly predicts that my ring finger is longer than my index finger based on two markers; this characteristic can indicate exposure to high levels of testosterone in the womb.

My eyes were "likely brown" in the initial 23andMe results but are actually a medium-to-dark hazel. The characterization was first changed to the much broader "likely dark" and more recently to 27 percent dark brown and 25 percent dark hazel. My mother's eyes—"likely blue" when 23andMe first put out this trait prediction—are also hazel but of such a pale variety that, in some light, they're as yellow as cats' eyes. Now her 23andMe prediction says "likely light."

In one sense, these predictions are a harmless novelty. We know what we look like, so it would be absurd to pick them apart, except that the idea that they are correct and worth relying on is fundamental to 23andMe, whose reason for being is genomic and medical research. AncestryDNA has also profited from lucrative genetic research partnerships but affords users even less transparency than 23andMe about its findings. The consequences of these predictions, however wrong, could be as far-reaching as Goddard's reductive eugenics.

Chapter 15

MUGSHOTS FROM DNA

———

I N 2014, I LEARNED OF EFFORTS TO MAP THE HUMAN FACE in 3D from DNA alone. The plan was to identify markers that create a jutting jaw or an underbite, an aquiline or a pug nose, eyes spaced near each other or far apart, and so on. This data would be used to create predictive mugshots. I found the prospect chilling even before I learned that the study was funded in part by the U.S. Department of Defense. The research was led by Mark Shriver, a population geneticist and anthropologist at Penn State University, whose bio notes that he "occasionally consults for law-enforcement agencies by helping officials to use science to further justice."

At a 2014 World Science Festival panel called "It's All Relatives: The Science of Your Family Tree," Shriver characterized his research into facial structure, skin color, hair texture, and more as an effort to unite rather than divide. These "superficial traits belie our interconnectedness," he argued, noting that his research to date had focused largely on people with mixed African and European ancestry. He displayed a graphic of a man's face—one he called the "consensus face" of his research—which he manipulated along a continuum, purporting to make the face "more European" or "more

African" based on the average in the database. "It's phrenology," whispered Shelley Salamensky, a writer and professor of global humanities at the University of Louisville, who'd gone to the lecture with me. Next, Shriver made the face "more feminine" and "more masculine." The transformation was eerily, dangerously transfixing. The young children next to us, otherwise fidgety and indifferent, sat spellbound as the face morphed.

Back then, when Shriver's research was published in *PLOS Genetics* and reported in *Nature,* his study had 592 fully genotyped participants, from which the researchers claimed to have identified twenty-four variants in twenty different genes that are predictive of facial characteristics. The idea was to systematically study facial variation stemming from "sex, ancestry, and genes" in order "to lay the foundation for predictive modeling of faces," including from DNA found at crime scenes. Other goals were to "predict the facial features of descendants, deceased ancestors, and even extinct human species." Participants agreed to take a complimentary 23andMe autosomal DNA spit test and allowed themselves to be photographed in 3D.

Once again, curiosity overrode my trepidation—and my disapproval. In July 2014, I took a trip to Penn State to participate in the study and to talk with Shriver and his co-author, Peter Claes.

SHRIVER IS AN ARTICULATE, fairly good-looking man, who was then in his forties, with a charm that's a barrier rather than a window—hard to see behind. Over the brief time I spent with him, I vacillated between viewing him as a character from the pages of *Brave New World* or a basically well-meaning guy who takes such a long evolutionary view of human beings that, despite knowing the risks of his "mugshots" being misused and the history of eugenics, still thinks the work might improve humanity as a whole.

Study participants signed a consent form acknowledging that while the research team would "take reasonable efforts to keep your participation in this research study confidential as required by law . . . other people may find out about your participation." Listed among the "people/groups" that could copy records of the research was the U.S. Department of Defense. The form plainly stated that genomic data uniquely identifies a person at least as precisely as their name or fingerprints do and that, consequently, "we do not believe that it is possible to guarantee the privacy, confidentiality, or anonymity" of an individual or their data. Participants thus assumed the risk of being identified, but the form did not disclose that participation has implications for volunteers' descendants, parents, siblings, nieces, nephews, and cousins—any close genetic relative. My half-siblings may never know me, but they share about 25 percent of my genome and could easily be identified if someone had their DNA and ran it through the database.

Someone at the World Science Festival asked Shriver why the military was funding the study. "To solve crimes," he said. At that time, Shriver's mugshots had already been used in at least two criminal cases, to try to identify repeat rapists. The panel's moderator, Randall Pinkston, noted that he himself had been a perpetrator of "the crime of WBB—walking by Black," and expressed concern about the potential for racial discrimination. Shriver countered that DNA evidence had frequently been used to exonerate persons of color. At his Penn State office, I raised the issue of the Department of Defense again, and he professed surprise. Only "a couple people" had been concerned about that, he said. Most participants were "really positive. People are interested in genetics these days."

Shriver had already been researching variations of skin tone and other traits across human populations when he discovered that he had a fairly large percentage of sub-Saharan African DNA—11 percent—which he told me he never knew about while growing up in southeastern Ohio. Both of his parents declined to participate in his research. His father, a computer scientist, cited privacy concerns, which perplexed Shriver, who said he doesn't understand "protectionist impulses." I asked if his parents were unhappy that he discovered Black DNA in their background. "I think probably unhappy," he said. "Their disbelief drove the disinterest."

Shriver is a libertarian who passionately believes in social freedom and opposes taxes. "You can't find examples of people who've been discriminated against based on their genes," he told me, whereas "knowing someone's genotype could protect them from disease." He lauded a federal law, the Genetic Information Nondiscrimination Act (GINA), which prevents health insurers and employers from discriminating based on genetic information. The late senator Ted Kennedy heralded GINA as "the first civil-rights bill of the new century of the life sciences." Maybe, but dangers remain.

In 2016, a couple of years after Shriver and I spoke, parents in Palo Alto, California, brought a suit alleging that the local school district discriminated against their son because he had markers for cystic fibrosis. In recent years, life-insurance companies have denied coverage to women with the BRCA1 breast-cancer gene. GINA doesn't protect people in either of these situations, because the discrimination doesn't involve a health insurer or an employer. A bill proposed by congressional Republicans in 2017 would have allowed employers to require their employees to undergo genetic testing or pay a fine if they refused.

IN 2015, SHRIVER'S DNA-MUGSHOTS technique was built upon by the private company mentioned earlier, Parabon NanoLabs, which sells the resulting images to law enforcement. A mugshot generated by Parabon that year reportedly helped identify a suspect in a double murder. First the suspect's DNA was matched to the crime scene using traditional DNA analysis. Then Parabon conducted a "face morphology analysis" that suggested "a wide facial structure" and "admixed ancestry, a roughly 50–50 combination of European and Latino ancestry," according to promotional materials. The suspect pled guilty.

It's hard to imagine this methodology bearing scrutiny in any rigorous scientific study. Even Parabon acknowledges that the pictures generated by its mugshot tool don't always look like the person they're purporting to depict. The company's director of bio-informatics, Ellen Greytak, emphasizes that they use data mining to give *probabilities*. One marker won't determine whether some-one has blue eyes, she admitted, even if it's "highly associative with blue eyes." Even five markers can't determine that. Parabon uses an "evolutionary algorithm" that "starts from a random population" and "scores" how well a particular marker associates with "pheno-type data." Learning of this, a friend of mine theorized that the MyHeritage contest I mentioned earlier, where users submitted look-alike photos of ancestors, was designed to harvest data for facial-recognition AI. A few months later, MyHeritage invited people to upload images of their ancestors and claimed to animate those images with its Deep Nostalgia™ "deep learning technol-ogy."

The databases Parabon draws on are only as good as the data in them, data highly unrepresentative of the population at large, so the company's algorithmic images have a high danger of racist uses and raise many ethical questions. Shriver initially helped Parabon se-cure a government grant, but according to a 2017 article in *Vice*, he soon stopped collaborating out of concern that they were "moving too quickly to market with unproven technology." He told *Philadel-phia* magazine in 2019 that Parabon seemed "'quite focused on sell-ing tests and not doing science quality tests.'"

Unlike Belgium and Germany, which prohibit DNA phenotyp-ing, the United States has no laws about DNA found at crime scenes. U.S. courts have ruled that bodily fluids no longer attached to their owner are abandoned, fair game for analysis, the equivalent of a fingerprint. Pondering the disturbing implications of this, the artist Heather Dewey-Hagborg spent a couple of years "obsessively collect[ing] shed hairs, smoked cigarette butts, chewed-up gum, and fingernails to research how much I could learn about people who have dropped them." She wrote in *The New Inquiry* that she discovered she could use "published research, bioinformatics, and machine learning tools" to "draw inferences or statistical predictions" about the individuals' appearance. For her art project "Stranger Visions," she created "life-size full-color 3D portraits" based on the projections, to increase awareness of genetic surveillance. Life imitated art a couple of years later, in 2015, when an NGO and an ad agency in Hong Kong used Parabon's Snapshot tool to produce what it presented as wanted posters of people who'd littered. Today's technology, Dewey-Hagborg argues, "masks a form of gender and racial stereotyping with the scientific authority of genetics."

In the end, perhaps because of the disconnect between stereotyping and reality, the mugshots have proven far less useful to crime-solving than autosomal DNA tests have. I've mentioned Parabon's lead forensic genealogist, CeCe Moore, who relies mostly on personal genomics databases as her starting point for crime-solving though she does feature related Snapshot images on *The Genetic Detective*.

In 2014, Ancestry released a customer's Y-chromosome data to Idaho police under a search warrant related to a decades-old rape and murder. The police identified a young New Orleans filmmaker as their prime suspect based on similar markers found at the scene. He had made a film about collectibles connected to violent crimes. He had connections to Idaho. The police interrogated him for six hours and took his blood for DNA testing. He remained under suspicion for a month until forensic DNA testing cleared him.

Later, the crime-scene sample was subjected to autosomal DNA testing, and CeCe Moore was able to identify the true culprit's great-grandparents. From there, she pinpointed suspects. Detectives collected DNA from discarded objects and eventually confirmed a match, who confessed, leading to exoneration of a man who'd falsely confessed to abetting the crime years earlier. Does this outcome excuse the methods or the errors along the way? I don't know.

In many ways, making predictions based on DNA analysis has as much risk as utility. I'm living proof that having the same muscle composition as an "elite power athlete" guarantees nothing.

Part Five

TEMPERAMENT

Chapter 16

GRUDGING KINSHIP

—

MY MOM ONCE DEVOTED HERSELF TO HER LOCAL CAT club so fully that, in 1968, *The Dallas Morning News* featured her as its president. The article didn't mention that she lived with more than thirty cats at the time, only that she had six of her own and that she cared for an unspecified number of rescues. When I asked my mom about the club a few years ago, she denounced it as "horseshit." The members were "ego-involved with their cats," only interested in purebreds, not in animals who needed them. Reading between the lines, I gathered that her efforts to transform the group into a rescue agency for cats had failed. In response, she rejected the whole venture, giving away all but three of the cats.

Later she became a preacher, a bird breeder, and a dog rescuer. To each of these endeavors she devoted the same intensity, until they palled. Her church congregation grew and then dwindled and disbanded. She attributed the decline to false prophets and gossip. Her avian holdings overflowed our house, but she rarely agreed to make a sale, judging potential customers flaky, undeserving, or possessed by demons. Eventually she moved to North Carolina and her flock wound up on a friend's farm south of Miami. Dogs have been a constant, though she's down to four from a high of sixteen or so.

While we were out of touch in the aughts (because of my anger over her refusal to acknowledge the harm of my stepdad molesting me), my mom turned to fruit trees. I learned of her orchard when I called on her seventieth birthday, in June 2010, after (notwithstanding our occasional email flare-ups) going seven years without hearing her voice. My joy at being reconnected was so extreme that I sat at my computer, quietly typing up much of what she said. While shopping the previous July, she'd "spied these wonderful dwarf trees that grow to be about six or seven feet tall." They were too expensive at first, but each time the price dropped, she bought a few. By the time we spoke, she had twenty apple, six peach, five nectarine, five pear, four apricot, three cherry, one mulberry, one plum, a dwarf lemon or two that overwintered in her greenhouse, and ten or fifteen assorted berry bushes. She was worried about the heat. Some leaves were looking "kind of brown and downcast," she said.

Downcast leaves! I thought fondly, tears welling up as I typed the words. I had missed her.

For years, much of her time went into tending the trees, securing their bounty from wildlife. But in recent years, unpredictable weather caused them not to bear fruit or to produce it too early. Squirrels bit into the apples. Deer ravaged the peaches. The remnants fell to the ground and rotted. My mom was getting older. Finally, by 2019, she'd had enough. She was going to ask her handyman to chop them all down.

I suggested keeping a few trees, maybe one of each kind, or two or three favorites.

"I just want to *set fire to them,*" she said.

I'd seen her between missions before, in the depressive lulls that preceded her Bible study, the church, the birds. I'd known what it felt like to be the core of a project of hers that revealed itself to be imperfect and for the whole endeavor to go sour. Like her, I knew the thrill of launching some new venture and the choke of defeat as I realized it was too big to wrangle, too slapdash to endure.

What I've longed for most in my life is to be like my mom: creative, original, joyfully intractable. What I've feared most, too, is being like her: impulsive, fervent, self-destructive, and rebellious, pouring myself into projects I later burn down.

I TRACE THESE SHARED propensities in large part to my mom's father, Robert Bruce. As a young woman, my sense of his life was spotty. What I carried forward was a sense of its merrily reckless, careening quality. Near the start of my family-history research, I emailed my mom to confirm exactly how many times he was said to have married. Thirteen, she replied. She added that one of Robert's wives might have shot him.

> Daddy was married thirteen times, I think: once before he married Granny, then two to three times to Christine. Next (I think) he married a woman named Evelyn, and, believe it or not, they lived on Daniels Avenue on SMU campus right down the street from my sorority house where I [much later] lived for three years. . . . She may be the one he was married to when he was shot in the gut and nearly died. I think she shot him but don't know for sure.

Was it really possible that my grandfather had wed more times than anyone else I'd heard of? And that one of the marriages culminated in a shooting? It seemed both objectively impossible and also, knowing my family, not unlikely. What would drive someone to live a life like this?

I asked my mom how she knew Robert had been shot but not who did it. She explained that a sorority sister's father had approached her at a college gala—in the early 1960s, when my mom hadn't spoken to her dad in years—to ask if she was Robert Bruce's daughter. The man had been the surgeon on duty after the shooting.

Realizing that my mom didn't know the story, he had to be the one to tell her that Robert nearly died of a bullet to the abdomen more than ten years before.

AFTER THE SPLIT FROM Granny when my mom was three years old, Robert occasionally picked my mom up to spend the weekend with him. At first these visits happened about every six months. By my mom's tenth birthday, she'd met two wives, but there were also years during this stretch when she didn't see her father at all.

And then, from the time my mom was about ten until her early twenties, Robert exited her life. Once or twice during the start of this long absence, he called from Hollywood to report on his marriages to aspiring starlets. After that, there was only silence until he rang up Granny one day, learned my mom was in college, and asked for her number. According to my mom, apart from the would-be movie stars, her father tended to court older women, "preferably ones with money, which he took and made tons more with." For most of his life, it appears, he lost any wealth he accrued as soon as he made it, owing to his other career as a high-roller alcoholic and ladies' man. (Not all of his wives capitulated to his financial schemes. He urged Granny to add him to the deed for her house, but she never did.)

My mom knew three specific women Robert married, beyond Granny. I had found a couple more. The others were a mystery. In 2015, I visited the Church of Latter-Day Saints' Family History Library in Salt Lake City, thinking that if anyone could help me, it would be the Mormons, with their history of sanctioned polygamy and vast research repository, which covers populations around the world, regardless of religious affiliation. But the helper I was assigned seemed to disapprove. "Why would you even *want* to find that?" they said. The searches they led me through there didn't turn up anything new. A trip to archives in Dallas proved more fruitful.

Between the courthouse and the library, I identified two additional spouses.

Robert was married at least three times before he and Granny wed, not just once, despite what my mom had said in her email. His alleged time in California and liaisons with would-be movie stars remain unsubstantiated. The ten marriages I've found to nine wives affirm the broad contours of my mom's recollection, though. And every few years, as more records have come online, I've discovered something new. It's highly possible that there are marriages I've missed.

Even as I probed my grandfather's history, my feelings toward him were slow to deepen. I had a sardonic fascination with his self-ishness and debauchery, as if he were a villain in a novel rather than my mom's father. He was backstory to my mom's odyssey, an unfortunate detour on Granny's, and a source of ill-defined dread for me. None of my other grandparents were chaotic and mercurial, and my fixation on policing those tendencies in myself made it hard for me to see exactly what I was afraid of in Robert and what might have survived of him in me.

A couple of years into my search, I discovered that Robert probably abandoned another daughter. This was news to my mom. "I was the only child he ever fathered," she'd told me in an email once, "except for an infant born to another wife besides Granny," who "was either stillborn or died as an infant." My feelings toward my grandfather tilted more explicitly toward disgust.

I have a photo of Robert holding my mom when she was about eighteen months old. His hair is slicked back. His shoulders are slumped. He has the most defeated look on his face. One arm wraps around my mom's torso; the other loops beneath her. His grip is tight, proprietary, desperate. My mom's face betrays confusion. One of her small hands rests on his. The other may be waving at the photographer, who was almost certainly Granny. Apart from their expressions, the scene could be a happy family afternoon. Robert stands in front of a car, eaves of a house visible behind him, wedding ring displayed. Ordinarily he photographed as a man of the world, but in this shot you can see the farm boy in him. Was his misery genuine or a performance?

Another photo, taken six to nine months before, shows Robert smiling and leaning against the same car, my mom a happy baby held against him on the hood, in an affectionate side embrace. He wears a tie, long-sleeved button-up shirt, handsome belt. His hair, glimpsed from the side rather than straight on, is artfully arranged in waves. A dog that could be part beagle sniffs at his feet. It's the happy family photo that the other is not. I suspect this shot was taken not long before my mom's first birthday, maybe even en route to the gala celebrating the garment workers' union Robert helped organize. This was the high point of my grandparents' marriage.

How did my grandfather feel as he churned through wives and livelihoods and opted out of parenting his children? Was he regretful? Optimistic? Indifferent? Photos, letters, certificates, and census data couldn't answer these questions, nor could my mom. I began to feel a sympathetic kinship with Robert only when I let my imagination and intuition become involved with what I knew of the evidence.

AS I PICTURE IT, Robert's early boyhood was happy. His parents were poor farming folks. Charley, a transplant from Georgia, was twenty-six when they wed, in May 1906. Rindia was sixteen, a Tennessee girl and ardent evangelical whose father had died young. She'd settled in Texas at around age ten with her mom, stepdad, and siblings, her grandfather and his second wife, and assorted aunts and uncles. Charley was far from home, the lone Bruce among his wife's people. He came from a religious family, too, revival-going Methodists.

Robert, their first child, was born in December 1907. In my

imaginings, he loved his mother but chafed at all the church and the praying. He tried Rindia's patience with his willfulness. And he idolized Charley, a tall, strong, charming man whom women were always swooning over, marveling at the likeness between father and son. The family lived outside Grand Prairie, a town at the edge of a prairie that extended into West Texas. By 1909, according to the official history online, the town, despite the "ever-present mud," had some amenities, everything from a cotton gin to a barbershop, post office, hardware store, millinery shop, and short-order stand. A trolley trip from the town into downtown Dallas ran a mere ninety minutes, but the trip by wagon for a farmer like Charley took a full day there and another back, a long haul in the Texas heat.

The Bruces' tiny rental shack sat next door to the (as I envision it) falling-down shotgun house where Rindia's mom, stepdad, and siblings lived, down the road from Rindia's granddad and his family. Up before dawn most days, Charley worked the fields. Rindia often toiled at his side, but she also cared for Robert, kept the house, milked the cow, fed the pigs and chickens, and took in sewing for extra money. Everywhere Robert looked, everywhere he went, he would have seen Rindia's people, praying and praising God. While Charley came from devout people, too, I imagine his relationship with God was less steady and all-consuming and that he started to drink too much after testifying in the trial that got his best friend, George, locked up. Maybe all the hallelujahs tried Charley's nerves and, in sympathy, exasperated young Robert, too.

Maybe when Rindia wasn't around, Charley told his son funny stories about George, pranks they'd pulled as bachelors new to Dallas, fishing trips they'd taken later, a night they'd tromped out onto the prairie after a goat of Charley's and found its carcass being devoured by a mountain lion. But Robert would have heard whisperings from Rindia's folks, too—how, when Robert was a baby, George tried to hurt his own stepdaughter. The girl, Bessie, had turned up at their family compound, trembling and bruised, after it happened.

She stayed the night with Rindia's grandpa and step-grandma, or so I infer from a court opinion on the assault-to-rape case, which mentions her seeking refuge with a Mrs. Haddock.

And then George got out of jail, swore revenge, and attacked Charley while he was unloading the wagon. Charley fended George off with the hay hook, catching him in the stomach by accident, he told his son. The small wound quietly festered into sepsis and death. As I picture it, Charley had been drinking and blaming himself for a couple of days before the police knocked on the door that night with a warrant for his arrest. "Take care of your mama and the girls, now, son," Charley might have told Robert, as the sheriff closed the cuffs around his wrists.

I IMAGINE THAT DAY as the worst of my grandfather's life. Then eight years old, Robert would have stood with Rindia and his little sisters, Mamie and May, crying but trying not to. May was five years old and Mamie was three. Maybe they hid in Rindia's skirts. Their mother's belly would have been starting to swell. Six months later, three days before Christmas, their baby brother would arrive. As the men rode off, Rindia fell to her knees and prayed, or something like that. Maybe it seemed to Robert, no fan of religion in his later life, that God was what got Charley into this mess.

Even in early-twentieth-century Texas, not exactly a bastion of law-abidingness, the case caused a stir. A blurb about the death by hay hook, one farmer killing another, appeared in newspapers around the state. But the neighbors came forward, and the grand jury declined to prosecute. Four days after his arrest, Charley was back home, freed of blame.

Not even a decade passed between the day the grand jury set him free and the day he was committed to the mental hospital, and while the exact form of his decline is lost to history, it's clear the accusation haunted him. Still, Charley and Rindia had three more sons during those years. In Robert's telling, this in-between time before his father succumbed to manic exhaustion didn't warrant mentioning. Nor did the near-rape of George's stepdaughter register as a major plot point. Robert drew a line from his father's grief over an ex-friend's death to Charley's own demise. Charley "lost his mind," my mom remembers Robert telling her, because he accidentally killed his best friend. I wondered if Robert's version of the story was a clue to his life. Did he come to see caring too much about someone as something to avoid?

IN THE SUMMER OF 1925, at the age of seventeen, Robert married Nettie Mae Mason, his neighbor. Nettie was also seventeen and a farmer's child. Like the Bruces, the Masons were poor. The families had lived near each other since at least 1920, when they appeared on the same page in the census.

Nettie was working by about age fourteen. She appears in the 1922 Dallas City Directory as a garment operator at Higginbotham-Bailey-Logan Co., a clothing manufacturer where Robert later worked. Was it just hormones and proximity that drew the two of them to each other, or something beyond that? I imagine Nettie was stylish and sophisticated by comparison to the other people Robert knew. Like all the women he married whom I've seen in photographs, she had dark hair and a pretty face. "Your grandfather had a type," a friend of mine said once, when I shared photos of Robert with various women, and it's true: chestnut hair, high cheekbones, intelligent eyes.

What else? Maybe Nettie inspired Robert's own transition into the garment trade; maybe she taught him what she knew. By 1930, one of Robert's sisters also worked as a seamstress. My mom recalls that his mom and other sister were also talented at sewing. Working with clothes may not have been a novelty for Robert, but industrial machines and a corporate employer would have been. Dallas clothing manufacturers depended on skilled garment workers but paid notoriously low wages to their mostly female employees, who toiled for long hours in poor conditions. Still, factory sweatshops probably paid better, and more reliably, than farming did. And a man working as a marker and cutter may have made more than the women and been treated with more respect.

Robert and Nettie might also have bonded over family troubles. When they wed, Nettie's mom was already sick with the tuberculosis that would take her life in 1929. Charley was struggling with bipolar disorder. I imagine that Robert hoped the marriage would somehow bolster his father, but Charley entered the mental institution two months after the wedding.

NETTIE GAVE BIRTH TO a daughter, Bonnie Katharine, in May 1926, nine months and three days after they married. The baby must have been named for Nettie's mom, Bonnie Bell, who was suffering from consumption. When I found Bonnie's birth listed in the official state index, a chill ran up my neck. A baby girl! Robert had lied about so many things, I didn't know what to think. What if my mom's half-sister was still alive? Within an hour or two, I'd learned that Bonnie really had died young and also that Robert's representation of her life was misleading. She didn't die as an infant but lived to be five years old.

In the years leading up to this discovery, I'd emailed my mom endless questions about Robert and his family. No, as a girl she'd never known anything about Charley, not even his name, she said. She hadn't seen much of Rindia growing up, especially not after Granny remarried. But she took pains to emphasize that "my daddy loved children":

He played with them everywhere he met them. He loved me, too, except I guess since he and Granny were divorced and I was not in his line of vision, so to speak, he didn't contact me often. Or, it could be that Granny made it difficult to see me. I really don't know. I don't remember ever missing him or asking to see him, but I did threaten Granny many times when I didn't get my way that I would go and live with my daddy if she didn't do what I wanted.

But then there was that line in the letter Robert sent Granny when she left him. "Tell Sandy Daddy loves her and will take her to the zoo if she comes home at once and if not she may never see me again."

The "come back now or else I'm going to abandon our child" approach doesn't suggest the most devoted of fathers. Now I'd found another child. How involved was Robert in her short life?

CHARLEY DIED OF MANIC exhaustion in the mental hospital not long after Bonnie's first birthday. Judging from Robert's grief when he told my mom the story more than four decades later, his father's demise hit him hard. If Robert wasn't a drinker before then, I suspect that's when he started. Maybe it's when he started smacking women around, too, if he didn't already.

Robert and Nettie seem to have stayed in Grand Prairie, close to family. In 1928, Robert was working for Nettie's former employer, Higginbotham-Bailey-Logan Co., as a garment cutter. In 1929, he was a garment cutter for a different company, Vaughan Hinckley Co. He divorced Nettie in a Dallas court that July, a couple of months after her mother died. Nettie didn't appear for the proceedings but was awarded custody of their daughter. In October, the stock market crashed, and the Great Depression began. By the 1930 census, three-year-old Bonnie was a "boarder," living without either parent or (seemingly) any relatives, in the Arcadia Park section of Oak Cliff, in Dallas. It's unclear who was caring for her or paying her room and board. Robert may have visited, but he didn't exactly live around the block. I can't find anything about Nettie's whereabouts that year.

How did Robert feel about all this? In 1930, he appears alone in the city directory, as a "marker" at Darling Dress Manufacturing Co. A marriage certificate attests that he married his second wife, a pattern designer, Clara Mae Brantley, in Oklahoma on April 19. It seems likely that Robert and his new bride met through work. Given his ambition, I suspect Robert wanted to advance in the clothing industry and was drawn to her at least partly because her knowledge and expertise surpassed his. I imagine the two of them debating the placement of seams, and how to economize on fabric, over drinks.

By 1931, Clara wasn't working, but Robert still had his job with Darling Dress as a marker. Their place was just south of what is now the Bishop Arts section of Oak Cliff, about a fifteen-minute drive to the place where Bonnie was living the year before. Bonnie died the following year, 1932, at five years and eight months old, in Roanoke, a small town northwest of Dallas. According to her death certificate, the cause was diphtheria, known then as "the deadly scourge of childhood." An aggressive vaccination campaign was under way, but maybe it took a while for word to spread, or traveling for the shot was too cumbersome or securing it too costly. If Bonnie was still a boarder, the people housing her may not have had the energy to care about someone else's little girl. The informant on Bonnie's death certificate wasn't a parent, grandparent, or known relative but a doctor.

Seventy-seven years after the fact, learning of my mom's half-sister's death hit me hard. Mindful of how rarely Robert was around for my mom after he and Granny divorced, I felt an elevator-sinking dread. Bonnie's fate could easily have been my mom's if she hadn't had Granny.

Chapter 17

CHASING THE DREAM

———

I N OCTOBER 2019, A DECADE AFTER I LEARNED ABOUT Bonnie, I was combing through databases and found a newly digitized obituary, DIPHTHERIA FATAL TO ROANOKE CHILD, which was published in the *Denton Record-Chronicle* on February 3, 1932. Coming upon the text without knowing more, you would believe Bonnie lived with her parents: "Bonnie Katherine Bruce, daughter of Mr. and Mrs. Robert Bruce of Roanoke, died of diphtheria in the home Wednesday morning at five o'clock. Funeral services were to be held Wednesday afternoon at four o'clock in the home, followed by burial in the Roanoke cemetery."

I probably rolled my eyes. *Of course* Robert wanted to put the best possible face on his abandoned child's death. But then I wondered: Could the obituary be a true representation of Bonnie's living situation? I hadn't found Robert and Clara in the 1932 city directory. Had they rescued Bonnie from the boardinghouse and moved north? Were they the "Mr. and Mrs. Robert Bruce" of the obituary? In marrying Clara, had Robert established a stable home for his daughter? My mom had said that Robert loved children, but, as with Charley and the hay-hook killing, I'd looked at the facts through the lens of blame and decided I knew better.

No sooner had I begun reimagining Robert's relationship with Bonnie at the end of her life than I checked the 1932 Dallas City Directory again and realized that Robert and Clara were listed under "C Robt Bruce" rather than the usual "Robt C Bruce." Clara's name was alongside his, in parentheses. No occupation was given for either. They lived far from the town where Bonnie died.

Still, having imagined an alternate reality, I found it difficult to return to my earlier mindset of utter condemnation. I couldn't fathom being a parent who left their child in a boardinghouse. Then again, I'd never had to support a family while working long hours for low wages. I had observed my mom's misery over the demands of mothering and, realizing I would feel the same way, resolved never to have a baby. Most divorced fathers working long hours during the Great Depression didn't take care of their children, who were often abandoned, apprenticed, or boarded as servants. When I knew her, Granny had the most finely tuned bullshit detector of anyone I've known, and (by my mom's account) she believed Robert was bereft over the death of his child. As an experiment, I decided to proceed as if I believed that, too.

SKILLED DRESS CUTTERS LIKE Robert made about ten to fifteen dollars per week in Dallas, compared to fifty dollars in other cities. Hours were long, typically fifty-four per week and often more; the factories were poorly ventilated and given to extreme temperatures. Black workers fared considerably worse than their white counterparts, toiling even longer for less.

As labor organized, newspapers like *The Dallas Morning News* caricatured the workers, depicting women who labored in the factories as coarse and unladylike. The major dailies "condoned brutal tactics" of the police and "frequently stirred racial antagonisms and anti-Semitism." As a white man, Robert was probably paid more than most but not fairly. The job required making precision cuts with heavy machinery for ten or more hours a day. Like Granny,

Robert had dropped out of high school. There was no family help if he fell on hard times. And given his father's history and Robert's erratic relationships and employment, I'm certain that he was bipolar. Sometimes he rode manic energy to glorious success, but more often he tried to self-regulate with alcohol. He lost jobs and destroyed marriages.

Robert was only twenty-five when Bonnie died in 1932. The city directory for that year suggests that neither he nor Clara was employed. Their marriage continued for a few years. In 1933, Robert worked as a superintendent for Darling Dress Manufacturing Co. I'm not sure what became of them for the next two years. In 1936, they were living together in an Oak Cliff apartment, with no occupation given for either. They divorced that June, six years and two months after they wed.

The following summer, July 1937, Robert married a younger woman, Rose Marie Camiani, in Rockwall, a town outside Dallas. Rose Marie was twenty-two years old to Robert's twenty-nine. She doesn't seem to have had a connection to the garment industry, and, as far as I can tell, neither she nor Robert was working in Dallas that year. Robert was again employed as a pattern drafter the following year. In March 1939, Rose Marie obtained an injunction against Robert, barring him from her premises, and an alimony award of ten dollars per week. They officially divorced in May, after less than two years.

BY THEN ROBERT HAD worked for more than a decade in the clothing industry. His third marriage had failed. He would soon be thirty-two years old. While he doesn't seem to have been prone to introspection, Robert must have taken stock and resolved to do things differently. By all accounts, he was a canny businessman. He was also an opportunist. Shortly before or after the split from Rose Marie, he started working for Justin McCarty, a Dallas designer. Granny was McCarty's office manager.

McCarty, a major player in the booming Dallas garment industry, considered Robert a natural talent, his best designer and pattern
drafter, whose future was dulled only by his drinking. My mom remembers Robert bringing home chic blouses and dresses for
Granny, who didn't like to wear them. "He always dressed well," my
mom said, "and wanted his women dressed well, too." Decades later,
my mom experienced his expert eye in action. She made her own
clothes sometimes, beautifully, just as she would later make dresses
and ball gowns for my friends and me. Because my mom was a
small, short young woman, she could buy fabric remnants cheaply
and convert them into stylish outfits that other people admired.
Robert noticed her shortcuts. "That skirt would be prettier if you'd
cut it with the grain instead of across it," he said once.

My guess is that Robert courted Granny more as a strategic
move than a romantic one. She was his boss's trusted assistant. She
may also have been, and I use the term with no small irony, the
wealthiest woman Robert had managed to woo by that point. Having squirreled away most of her wages from nearly two decades of
stenography and bookkeeping, she owned the house where her parents lived. She cared for her mother and father, and she paid her
own way. Granny was smart, self-made, and, for a working-class
woman, successful. She was thirty-four, older than Robert by two
years, and she was pretty. And then she got pregnant.

I imagine Robert moved toward marriage with excitement over
being a father again, with some optimism that he and Granny
would be a good match, and most of all with the expectation that
he would be able to dominate her and her savings. I picture Granny
proceeding with some mixture of hope, embarrassment, and sour
trepidation. I've already been over the ultimately dismal trajectory
of their marriage, but they wed in October 1939 and my mom was
born the following June.

No doubt Robert was quick to accept McCarty's assessment of
his talents. He must have wanted to build his own business rather

than being paid an hourly wage. And while he and Zone, Granny's father, ultimately loathed each other, I suspect Zone influenced Robert at the start of the marriage. Granny always said, with a roll of the eyes, that her father was a communist. My mom recalls Zone holding forth on *Das Kapital.* He was a card-carrying socialist as far back as 1913, when he co-signed a letter, published in *The Dallas Morning News,* to recall the mayor and city commissioners because of monopoly electric pricing. Socialist fervor had gripped parts of Texas at the start of the twentieth century, waned in influence, and had a brief revival in the 1930s, a few years before Robert met Zone. Zone's arguments against plutocrat bosses may have persuaded a son-in-law also possessed of talent, unconventional intelligence, and similar bad habits. I suspect it was some combination of Zone's influence, the residual New Deal spirit of the day, and exasperation with his own continued financial struggles that jolted Robert, who had no prior or subsequent history of organizing or known humanitarian impulses, into spearheading a union.

The month my mother turned a year old, Robert and other garment cutters announced their union, Dallas Cutters Local. Robert became the first president. On June 11, 1941, *The Dallas Morning News* ran a puff piece on the group: GARMENT CUTTERS WILL CELEBRATE ORGANIZING UNION. In the accompanying picture, Robert looked handsome, feeding fabric to a motorized knife alongside his union deputy. The photo caption noted that they and other union volunteers were cutting and assembling 20,850 garments to donate to aid "the British victims of disaster" during the Blitz.

Granny pasted the article and photo in a scrapbook along with another clip of unknown provenance, dated July 1, 1941, which touted Robert and the union celebration. But Robert's attempt at organizing came at least a few years too late. Wealthy manufacturers had been successful in turning the public against unions, and anti-communist fervor reigned. Organized labor, to the extent it remained, was typically in the pocket of Dallas business leaders.

GRANNY DIVORCED ROBERT OVER his affair in February 1944. He doesn't seem to have spent much time mourning the breakup. Eleven days later, he and Christine applied for a marriage license in nearby Rockwall County. They must have married soon after.

On September 6, Christine filed the first of many divorce actions that punctuated their marriage. By October, they had evidently resolved their differences, and that case was closed. Still, they did somehow obtain a divorce, because the following January, they secured another marriage license, this time for the marriage of Robert C. Bruce to "Mrs. Christine Bruce," and married again. And then, on June 29, it was Robert who filed for divorce against Christine. By August, he had dropped the suit.

Over the years, Christine idly petitioned for divorce three more times that I know of, in August 1946, in May 1949, and in October 1949. "They were just playing around," a Dallas County district clerk official said as he handed me the records.

During his marriage to Christine, Robert left the clothing business. He became, according to my mom, "the best auto mechanic with a full-repair location in Dallas": Bruce Motor Service. In 1947, a photo of Robert and Christine sitting in front of the company truck with another couple and two long rows of fish appeared in a newsy Oak Cliff shopping circular. They look happy, Christine far more at ease with Robert than I imagine Granny ever was. "Robert C. Bruce, Sole Owner," it said on the side of the truck. The caption is titled "Fishing Party Brings Back Proof." Anyone with "fish tales to swap" is invited to "drop around and have a tale-telling bee with Mr. Bruce. True to tradition the party reports that the biggest one got away."

Three years later, on May 24, 1950, Christine divorced Robert for good. The auto-repair business was no longer. The decree recounts that they'd already sold their community property—income and as-

sets each had acquired during the marriage—and divided it between themselves.

EIGHT DAYS AFTER THE final divorce from Christine, Robert
married Olgie Evelyn York, a forty-five-year-old beautician and
widow who went by Evelyn. She owned three beauty salons and
was three years older than Robert. When they got married, Robert
was running a grocery store in Oak Cliff. It may originally have
belonged to Evelyn's first husband, or maybe Robert bought it with
proceeds from the sale of Bruce Motor Service or with financial
assistance from Evelyn in the lead-up to their wedding.

My mom hadn't seen her father in a couple of years when, at age
nine or so, she heard people praising him as a "true master grocer."
I can easily picture people recommending the store to Granny, and
Granny trying not to roll her eyes while mulling whether to reveal
that he was her ex.

My mom biked over to see the place for herself. It was a long
ride. Robert proudly introduced her and then drove her home. Not
long after this, my mom met Evelyn, and then Evelyn picked up my
mom for the day to perm and style her hair. She accidentally left the
developer on too long and, as my mom put it, "burned off" all her
hair, but my mom liked Evelyn anyway.

Less than a month after Robert and Evelyn's marriage, my mom
celebrated her tenth birthday by spending a night at their new
home. It was just down the street from what would later be her
sorority house, along the SMU campus, in the quietly posh University Park neighborhood. They took my mom to Neiman Marcus
and let her pick out a pool toy, though she really wanted a swing set.
That was the last my mom saw of her father's sixth wife.

A month later, on July 23, Evelyn shot Robert in the stomach at
two o'clock in the morning. A brief in the *Daily Times Herald* noted
the short duration of the marriage. The shooting, it said, "apparently

followed an argument." I'm guessing Robert was drunk. And not blameless. I imagine Evelyn standing, in their last moments together, on their porch in a silk robe late at night, her hair pinned up, a gun trembling in her hands.

According to the surgeon's account a decade later, Robert's wounds were so severe, it wasn't clear he would live. Granny, who must have been disgusted and mortified, and maybe also a little concerned, didn't tell my mom anything. My mom learned about it only by chance. If her friend's father hadn't deduced years after the shooting that my mom was Robert's daughter, she might never have known.

Soon after Robert was out of the hospital, my mom's stepfather, Smith, told Robert to stay away. Smith promised to care for her as a father, and Robert agreed. This arrangement sounds cold to me, but I asked my mom how she felt about this when it happened. She insisted that, while she didn't feel any love for Smith, Robert had been around so rarely, she doesn't recall feeling much at all. I asked how she thought Robert would have felt. Relieved, she imagined, not to be expected to pay for her upkeep. Not sad? I asked. No, she didn't think so.

By the end of August, a little more than a month after the gunfire, Robert was well enough to file for divorce. The dissolution of marriage was granted on October 26, 1950. Evelyn was awarded the house, which she'd bought. He got the grocery store.

MY MOM ONCE JOKED, as we were contemplating the trajectory of Robert's life, that her dad "probably decided to trim his sails and settle down" after the shooting. This seems to have been true eventually but not right away. On January 29, 1951, five months after his divorce from Evelyn, Robert, then forty-three, married Vera Fern Sebastian, who was twenty-five years old; the dark-haired beauty went by Fern. It was her second marriage.

As a girl, Fern had ambitions to perform. At age twelve, she and her sister won the chance to perform a "harmony duo" in a competition for a "Future Stars" radio contest. Other clippings from Fern's teenage years suggested her interest in show business persisted. I wonder if Robert and Fern made their way to Hollywood, where, my mom maintains, Robert married aspiring actresses. Maybe he designed dresses for Fern. Regardless, the union didn't last long. Fern divorced Robert in Dallas on August 21, 1951, less than eight months after their wedding. He did not appear in court.

My mom seems to recall that, during his Los Angeles period, "Daddy did more dress designing. One of his [wives'] names out there was Hevelyn (I think)—sounds pretty Hollywood, doesn't it?"

At some point after this, Robert relocated to Phoenix, Arizona. His obituary claims he settled there in 1948, but that can't be true, or if it is, the stint was a short-lived trial that was later revisited. Whatever year he arrived, I think he was definitely living in Phoenix by 1952, because in January of that year, a man with his name married a woman named Delores Lillian Preston in Phoenix. The document doesn't provide birth dates or birthplaces or other concrete data to prove this was my grandfather, but he's the only Robert Bruce with a "C" initial I've found in the directories from the years I know he lived there and the years surrounding them. Knowing Robert's ways, I count Delores as a confirmed spouse, though no proper genealogist would make that sort of leap and I can't find a divorce.

In 1954, mentions of leases negotiated by a "Robert Bruce of Grace and Grace" realtors began appearing in the real estate section of *The Arizona Republic*. This was my grandfather. Later, as Robert's prominence grew, the newspaper would include his middle initial. By 1955, Robert was evidently married for the tenth and final time, to his ninth wife, Eleanore D. Havel Lussier, a comfortably middle-class widow with horn-rimmed glasses and, according to my mom, a low-key knack for keeping him in line. She was one year younger than Robert and, my mom says, deferential to him. With Eleanore's help, Robert quit drinking. He became a stepfather and a step-grandfather, and around 1963, after his life had stabilized, he got back in touch with my mom. They met up at the Dallas airport briefly. Over the years that followed, they visited each other a few times.

Eleanore may have helped fund Robert's most successful enterprise, Bob Bruce Realty. *The Arizona Republic* announcement of the opening on June 19, 1955, referred to "Robert C. Bruce, widely known in local real estate circles." I found this documentation many years after my mom's original email outlining all of Robert's jobs. "My dad was the FIRST industrial realtor in Phoenix," she'd told me. "He did this without any real estate training. He just began appraising industrial real estate and it went on from there—the same way he did the grocery business, service-station business, dress-designing, etc."

Robert's success in real estate is a source of pride for my mom, but it depresses me to see his transformation from a union leader to a booster of an enormous city built in a desert, a seller of land in a county that bears the name of the Maricopa people but does not acknowledge their claim.

A 1965 *ARIZONA REPUBLIC* article establishes that Robert was the third rather than the first realtor from the area to "be installed as a member of the Society of Industrial Realtors," an "exclusive group," but the seat-of-the-pants approach my mom describes is one I'm intimately familiar with, through years of being raised by my mom and even more years of being me. Until his death in 1970, Robert's real estate career advanced. One year, he was named Phoenix Realtor of the Year. By 1968, he was president of the Phoenix Real Estate Board and on the board of the Industrial Development Committee of the Society of Industrial and Office Realtors. *The Arizona Republic* relied on him as a source of real estate insight and occasionally published his boosterism in op-eds. By the time he died in 1970, he was well known enough that his obituary was itself news: ROBERT C. BRUCE, 62, LEADING CITY REALTOR.

The last time my mom saw her father, she and my dad visited around Christmas 1969, a few months before their wedding. Robert's health was poor. For the first time, he confided in her about his father's death. Robert had sent my mom a dress that didn't fit properly, and he took her to Neiman Marcus to return it. He picked out an expensive pale-yellow suit for her instead. ("Little blondes" like my mom, he always said, should wear creams and pastels.) Eleanore's sister was visiting from Wisconsin and disapproved, perhaps getting the misimpression that Robert often lavished gifts on my mother this way.

Robert privately warned my mom against marrying my father, whose awkward personality and lack of charisma must have amazed him. He urged my mom to meet his lawyer, but my parents decided to leave early, ostensibly because Eleanore's sister kept all the doors and windows open, so my parents were freezing. I'm sure my mom was cold. Knowing my father, I suspect he wanted to prevent my mom from being advised to insist on a prenup.

Robert had agreed to walk my mom down the aisle at her wedding the following April, so she told herself it wasn't a big deal to cut the visit short. But when my mom glimpsed Robert's sad face from the plane window, she had a premonition that she would never see him again. She was right. As mid-April approached, Robert was too sick to travel. His death came in the hospital five days after the wedding, on Granny's sixty-fifth birthday.

When I asked as a child about the cause of his death, Granny implied it was a result of complications from alcoholism. My mom ascribed it to aftereffects of being shot. The reported obituary in *The Arizona Republic* attributed his death to a "heart ailment." What I learned when I tracked down his death certificate is that, at least according to the coroner, he died of a coronary occlusion after being treated for two weeks.

I wonder how much Robert thought of my mom as he lay in the hospital bed. Did he know she'd tried to kill herself less than a year before her wedding day, a week before meeting my father? Robert had known and disliked her first husband—"buy her the god-damned cigarettes," Robert shouted at him once—and he'd witnessed that marriage fail spectacularly. Did Robert recognize the kinship between her bad choices and the poor judgment of the women who'd married him? I imagine my mom would have been on his mind at a time when he was supposed to be, as she puts it, giving her away. The newspaper announcement of my parents' marriage makes no mention of Robert, though it was published on the day he died.

Someone once said that my grandfather must have been a hopeful man to embark on so many marriages. I thought they were being sarcastic, and laughed. Their interpretation struck me as an attempt to put a kindly spin on the indefensible. Eventually, though, I wondered if they were right. Many of Robert's choices were mercenary, abusive, erratic, and narcissistic, but did he believe in each of his relationships, his careers? Did the marriages hold the same kind of hope and allure for Robert that the cats and the church and birds and trees each did at times for my mom? I asked my mom what she thought. "He *was* hopeful," she said. "He was never depressed. He was always ready to go to the next business or whatever." We agreed that the "whatever" often seemed to come in the form of a woman.

From *The Atlanta Constitution* I learned that Robert's great-grandfather, Elias Bruce, met and married a woman at a Methodist tent revival in September 1886, when he was seventy-four. Elias's wife had died the year before. According to the article, he and his bride met and "professed to attain perfect love" at the campground.

AT TIMES IT FEELS like an overreach to compare myself to my grandfather and my mom. I haven't gone on benders and gotten married ten times, or started a union, then a service station, and then a grocery store. I haven't founded a church in my living room or taken in thirty cats. But I am also vigilant against excess. I set rules for myself. I no longer stay out drinking, talking, and playing poker until four o'clock in the morning. I quit smoking cigarettes years ago. I can't claim to be a teetotaler, but I opt for herbal tea more often than whiskey for a nightcap.

Still, I do have a history of starting projects, pouring time and energy into them, and then, when they don't turn out exactly as I want, tiring of them, rethinking them, sometimes abandoning them. I see grand connections between things, connections that I've learned to be cautious about. In speech, I often interrupt myself to clarify or moderate a point I'm making before I've actually made the point. In my blogging years, I went through phases of feeling like I needed to be posting things constantly because an audience might show up at any moment. When I wrote something I felt unsure about, which was almost everything, I put up something else as soon as possible in case the original thing wasn't good.

"It seems as though you feel that you start each day without any credit or goodwill," said my late therapist, Dan Cohen, "as though you feel you have to prove yourself from scratch every day." Yes, of course, I agreed. How else would one approach life? Maybe, in a less self-flagellating way, Robert felt this, too.

Once or twice a week in the early aughts, I'd stay up all night blogging (a pastime unique to weirdos then) and go to my job. The less rest I got, the more I told myself I didn't need as much sleep as normal people, that my brain worked just as well without it. I'd always had periods like this, of racing thoughts and sleepless nights that compounded one another. Dan pointed out that going without sleep can make people feel anxious, depressed, and more than a little unhinged. He must have told me this many times, but I didn't hear it until I was ready to make the change. I started treating sleep as a necessity, and I did feel better. Later I learned that Charley had died from manic exhaustion, and I remembered my own sleepless nights and scrabbling brain.

Seven or eight years after I started blogging, Charles McGrath, a onetime editor of *The New York Times Book Review,* kindly invited me to lunch. By then I'd written some reviews for the newspaper, although not during his tenure. Over our meal, he asked why I had "decided" to blog rather than work for the *Times.* I was confused. Blogging was free. I'd had no credentials for a newspaper job and had never seen one as a possibility. I had student loans and other bills to pay, I explained, so had always had a "real" job and written on the side. McGrath looked skeptical, as if he thought that I'd considered becoming a newspaper reporter or critic but decided against it out of some outsider perversity. Maybe he thought I was independently wealthy, or that I made money from my website, which I didn't.

I liked McGrath, but the conversation hearkened back to a time when I sat on endless panels about whether bloggers were "killing book reviews" in professional publications. Eventually I realized I could just say no to the panels, and I pronounced myself retired from them. The blog I wrote had become known as a book blog, a label I didn't seek or endorse, though I did often write about books and writers. Early on, as people began to expect book chatter, I felt increasingly obliged to provide it, even to pander, but every time I felt overwhelmed by the project and exhausted by my own tap dancing, I reminded myself that I could write whatever I wanted. Sometimes I had these reckonings publicly. In a post called "A dictatorship, not a democracy," I wrote that if someday I decided to devote the blog to speculations about the inner lives of snails, there wasn't anything readers could do.

It took me a long time to realize that some people are wired for operating within existing systems and don't see another way. Others don't see an obvious place for themselves in a system and look for a different route. I don't mean to discount the advantages my education gave me, the privileges of being a white person who grew up middle-class with a lawyer father and an English-major mother, or the extent to which these factors fed into the acceptance my writing has received. But all my life, when I've felt excluded from something I wanted to do, I've tried to create a path to doing that thing.

Nowadays my blog archives feel like a testament to wasted time; to critical opinions, many of which didn't need airing; to a younger, angrier self who makes me cringe. I imagine the blog's defects strike me like the disappointing fruit trees did my mom when she decided she wanted to set fire to them, like the empty seats in her church must have hit her before she let the ministry go.

For all the frantic pointless posting that went into the site, though, there were good impulses behind it, too. The blog was where I first found readers who cared about the things I cared about. It was where I first wrote regularly about the preoccupations that would coalesce into this book. It was through the blog that I realized my strongest writing would be the highest and best manifestation of my own perspective and strangeness. This book would not exist if I hadn't written the blog. And this book would not exist if I were not Robert's granddaughter.

Chapter 18

EMOTIONAL
RECURRENCES

——

WHEN THE WRITER KURT VONNEGUT ARRIVED HOME
on leave from the army for Mother's Day in 1944, he
learned that his mother had overdosed on sleeping pills the night
before. Decades later, he took medication for his own depression. In
a 1972 letter to friends, he traced his "formless anger" and need for
solitude to "bad chemicals in my bloodstream" and his mother's suicide. The same year, in a letter to his daughter Nanette, he shared a
realization that he was prone to "terrific depressions" regardless of
what was happening in his life. "We inherited those regular dips,"
he wrote. "I scarcely know which ancestor to thank." He cautioned
her against taking pride in "the family disease," to lean away from it
rather than in. Still, he emphasized that their legacy had its gifts,
too: The women could draw. He closed with a request for one of her
drawings.

Nanette Vonnegut was about eighteen at the time. She was already an artist, and still is. Her work, some of which is reproduced
online, is full of rich color and dreamy figures that to me evoke
mythology and the primal figures of Chagall. The images also suggest dollhouses and fairy tales. In recent years, Nanette Vonnegut

has admitted that she writes, too. She used to be secretive about her prose because of the weight of being "a Great Writer's child," she says on her website, but now that she's older, writing feels "pleasantly urgent," less like something to hide.

She is preoccupied with her dad's mother, who killed herself, and with her mom's mother, who was institutionalized. The order committing her granny to the state hospital "allowed for sexual sterilization, citing 'the best interest of society.'" The medical records classified her as "'Manic Depressive Reaction, Manic Type,'" and said she was "high school Valedictorian, unusually able in literary matters, particularly writing . . . Lesbian tendencies.'"

"I weep," Nanette Vonnegut writes. "She got out and went on to be the most boring, sweet-smelling Granny ever.

"At the root of a lot of art," she maintains, is an "injury that needs addressing." In an interview, she described her work as "all about family."

Mark Vonnegut, brother of Nanette and son of Kurt, has written about his own experiences with bipolar disorder. In his memoir, *Just Like Someone Without Mental Illness Only More So*, he writes of generations of "manic depression," of "episodes of hearing voices, delusions, hyper-religiosity, and periods of not being able to eat or sleep. These episodes are remarkably similar across generations and between individuals. It's like an apocalyptic disintegration sequence." He posits that "creativity and craziness go together," because "if you're just plain crazy without being able to sing or dance or write good poems, no one is going to want to have babies with you. Your genes will fall by the wayside."

EMOTIONAL RECURRENCES IN FAMILIES have consumed me for as long as I can remember. The more I feed my fixations, the sooner they tend to wither, but this one tends to permeate my perception of humanity. I often think family patterns are the primary existential conundrum we all have in common, apart from death and basic needs like food and shelter—but, then, questions of sustenance and longevity are intensely tangled up with our ancestors, too.

In my early thirties, I discovered Kay Redfield Jamison's *Touched with Fire: Manic-Depressive Illness and the Artistic Temperament*. It was the first book I read that posited a sweeping connection between mental illness—bipolar disorder in particular—and what she calls the artistic temperament. The book is filled with quotes and anecdotes tracing mental illness through the families of writers, including Mary Shelley and Mary Wollstonecraft; Henry, William, and Alice James; Herman Melville; Lord Byron; Virginia Woolf; and Alfred Lord Tennyson.

Anyone who's read Mary Shelley's *Frankenstein* is familiar with the sadness and alienation of both the monster and his creator. Jamison draws from letters in which Mary Shelley spoke of her own depression, an "'illness—driving me to the verge of insanity. Often I felt the cord would snap.'" Her mother, Mary Wollstonecraft, author of *A Vindication of the Rights of Woman*, attempted suicide twice. Wollstonecraft's father was an alcoholic, her sister suffered from depression, and her eldest daughter, Fanny, killed herself.

Charlotte Gordon's *Romantic Outlaws: The Extraordinary Lives of Mary Wollstonecraft & Mary Shelley* considers the resonances and differences between mother and daughter, noting that while "Wollstonecraft, like many Enlightenment figures, had believed that suicide was an honorable option," Mary Shelley disagreed, and her half-sister's fate, Gordon suggests, may have made her feel more vulnerable. "Their mother had struggled with depression. [Mary Shelley's father] had acknowledged this legacy by teaching the two girls that they should guard against their dark moods and stamp out the tendency to brood. Fanny had lost a battle that Mary continued to fight." Jamison highlights one of Mary Shelley's last journal entries: "'My mind slumbers & my heart is dull—Is life quite over?

Have the storms and wrecks of the last years destroyed my intellect, my imagination, my capacity of invention—What am I become?'"

Jamison herself has bipolar disorder and a wonderful aptitude for metaphor—a talent that, the book implies, goes hand in hand with mania. Brilliantly, she evokes the racing mind, the associative and grandiose thinking, the bursts of high creativity and then plummeting into depression, that an artist with bipolar tendencies can experience. Her natural fascination with the subject and the quotes she includes give the book a thrilling intensity.

"'For no reason,'" Theodore Roethke wrote, "'I started to feel very good.'" "Suddenly I knew how to enter into the life of everything around me. I knew how it felt to be a tree, a blade of grass, even a rabbit." On little sleep, he moved through life intoxicated by a sense of unity with all things. One day, imagining how it was to be a lion, he ordered a raw steak at a diner. But when he started eating, the other customers were aghast. "And I began to see that maybe it *was* a little strange."

When I first read *Touched with Fire*, I could see that Jamison was doing some creative, slippery, usually posthumous diagnosing of writers, artists, and their ancestors with bipolar disorder, but I didn't mind, because I related to much of what she described and I enjoyed feeling special. The particular type of family tree that populates Jamison's book is called a genogram (or sometimes a genosociogram). These graphs can be useful for mapping traits through families but are similar to those used for pedigrees generated by the Eugenics Record Office, a research institute established at the Carnegie Institution of Washington's "Station for Experimental Evolution" in 1910. The graphs were connected to the idea that mental illness "could be attributed to a heredity disposition," Staffan Müller-Wille and Hans-Jörg Rheinberger observe in *A Cultural History of Heredity*, and that "unimpeded spread of these conditions would cause sweeping degeneration" in the population. Patients' case histories charted "the incidence of mental diseases, mental retardation, suicides, and alcoholism" among their relatives. The Eugenics Record Office sought "evidence of Mendelian inheritance patterns in particular families," to create "an 'inventory of the blood' of entire nations."

Genograms have troubling applications even now. In his memoir, *Boy Erased,* Garrard Conley describes their use in the "ex-gay" movement. His pastor father and devout mother enrolled him, when he was a college student, in a camp that promised God would cure him of his attraction to men. Among many horrible things, including watching his writings be destroyed in front of him, Conley was required to create a genogram that according to the program leaders would show how various tendencies in earlier generations were antecedents to his queerness.

Jamison argues that bipolar disorder is largely hereditary—she doesn't examine environmental factors to any significant degree—and that we as individuals and as a society should not be afraid of this truth, because the condition also bestows enormous creativity. *Touched with Fire* is, in a sense, a love letter to bipolar disorder. As someone who's on the lower end of that spectrum, the book seduced me.

WE MAY BELIEVE WE have more answers about temperamental and emotional inheritance than the ancients did, but we still have little predictive ability. Current science tells us that depression, bipolar disorder, and schizophrenia are at least partly hereditary, and we know all three can and often do surface multigenerationally in families. In twins, they're more likely to correlate than in the general population, even when the twins are raised apart. But there are also plenty of twin pairs for whom this isn't the case. One twin struggles with manic episodes; the other doesn't. Even the most comprehensive efforts to pinpoint a gene that dictates mental-health characteristics haven't been successful in a predictive sense.

From time to time, a discovery is announced—the "empathy gene," for example—but the results are disputed and difficult to replicate.

Complicating things further, natural selection doesn't always select against genes associated with mental illness. Sometimes it's the opposite. Esmé Weijun Wang's *The Collected Schizophrenias*—an intimate and intricate rendering of her own mental-health history, which becomes the compassionate lens through which she considers schizophrenia more broadly—highlights research suggesting that "twenty-eight of seventy-six gene variations connected to schizophrenia" appear to be evolutionarily preferred.

In a 2007 article in the journal *Proceedings of the Royal Society B: Biological Sciences* to this effect, the evolutionary biologist Bernard Crespi and his co-authors discuss the "evolutionary-genetic paradox" of schizophrenia: It has "strongly negative" effects on longevity and reproductive potential but also "high heritability," persisting "at a prevalence of approximately 1 percent across all human cultures." Complicating matters further, the line between schizophrenia and bipolar disorder is indistinct. The conditions "exhibit substantial overlap in cognitive symptoms as well as their genetic basis." Both have been repeatedly linked "with creativity and imagination."

Wang summarizes three common theories about why the markers associated with schizophrenia not only persist but may be positively selected for. The first is that "the evolutionary development of speech, language, and creativity, while bestowing significant gifts, has 'dragged' along less desirable genetic tendencies with it." The second is that "schizophrenics are, evolutionarily, meant to be ad hoc 'cult leaders' whose bizarre ideas split off chunks of the human population." The third is that "schizophrenia *itself* has evolutionary advantages," that it "persists because it promotes creativity." Wang, who has reckoned with the symptoms and diagnosis of schizoaffective disorder for most of her adult life, finds this last explanation both tempting and, in its romanticizing of a serious condition, dangerous. Had Socrates been privy to the science of our era, he might have subscribed to this schizophrenia-positive view. In *Phaedrus,* he called madness "'the channel by which we receive the greatest blessings.'" Madness "comes from God," he said, "whereas sober sense is merely human."

SCIENCE CAN'T TELL US with certainty if particular genes cause schizophrenia. It can't tell us when having genetic markers frequently associated with schizophrenia will actually cause a person to develop schizophrenia. Nor can science tell us why the condition persists. The same is true for bipolar disorder and depression—and for sunny dispositions. One study purported to find correlations between optimism and a GG marker on the oxytocin gene, but mental-health findings of this kind are often criticized for small sample size and dubious methodology, and the optimism study is no exception.

Although science can't nail down causation between DNA markers and mental health, research has shown that environment can influence emotional wellness, in part by changing the way our DNA encoding is expressed. Children exposed to neglect, abuse, and other forms of trauma often fail to develop the ability to self-soothe. Their levels of cortisol—an adrenal hormone associated with metabolism, mood, and responses to stress—become aberrational. Their endocrine systems have trouble ramping down. Even if circumstances improve as the child matures, their system may continue to generate anxiety when none is needed. Everything feels like an emergency.

The genes themselves don't change in this process, but their manifestation does, through epigenetic responses and instructions. People whose bodies undergo these changes in response to trauma as kids are more likely to suffer from depression and other psychiatric disorders as adults. Their immune systems tend to work less well, leaving them more vulnerable to inflammation and disease.

Positive epigenetic changes can occur, too. Exercise can lead to a decrease in modifications associated with aging by slowing the loss of DNA methylation, for example. Physical activity may also improve cognition, particularly the memory loss often associated with age. Meditation and other contemplative practices tend to result in a decrease in perceived stress, among other reported benefits. Despite a rush of enthusiasm following one study several years ago, though, so far efforts to pinpoint associated epigenetic changes have been inconsistent and thus inconclusive.

Although the science of epigenetics is still in its infancy, and scientists don't always understand what triggers these kinds of changes, we do know that modulation of gene expression occurs throughout our lives. As we've seen, some studies suggest that epigenetic changes could potentially be passed down from parent to child, or even grandparent to grandchild. One study of worms reportedly showed transmission across fourteen generations, but of course worms and humans are very different sorts of beings.

Our science is only as good as the questions we ask, as the participants in any individual study, as the ways of seeing open to us. But we know that our behavior has the potential to change our own epigenetics, for good or ill. So while the language used by laypeople is often imprecise, I'm puzzled by the derision and contempt that flow from some corners of the scientific community toward psychological and spiritual practices designed to promote positive changes in gene expression that may have ancestral origins.

EVOLUTIONARY PSYCHOLOGISTS CONTEND THAT some of our actions are decided at a neurological level that we justify after the fact. Early support for this idea came from the so-called "split brain" experiments of the 1960s and '70s, which focused on patients whose connections between the left and right hemispheres of the brain had been severed (usually in an effort to prevent recurring epileptic seizures). In the studies, the researchers showed a word to a patient's left eye and visual field that was not visible to the right eye and visual field. The word presented to the left eye was processed by the right hemisphere of the brain, but it's the left side of the brain that (in common parlance) usually processes language. The patients didn't seem to realize they'd seen the word but would draw a picture associated with the word or choose an object to match it.

The professor of science and religion Robert Wright discusses these experiments in his book *Why Buddhism Is True*. As he puts it, "when the left hemisphere is asked to explain behavior initiated by the right hemisphere, it tries to generate a plausible story. If you send the command 'Walk' to the right hemisphere of these patients, they will get up and walk. But if you ask them where they're going, the answer will come from the left hemisphere, which wasn't privy to the command. . . . One man replied, plausibly enough, that he was going to get a soda. And the person who comes up with the improvised explanation—or, at least, the person's left hemisphere, the part of the person that's doing the talking—seems to believe the story."

Recent studies of patients with separated brain hemispheres have cast doubt on aspects of the earlier findings. Participants in a study led by the Dutch cognitive scientist Yaïr Pinto "showed full awareness of presence and location of stimuli throughout the entire visual field—right and left, both," Pinto wrote in *Aeon*. It was as though each participant experienced "two streams of visual information, one for each visual field," and couldn't fully "integrate the two streams," as if they watched "an out-of-sync movie, but not with the audio and video out of sync. Rather, the two unsynced streams are both video."

Whereas earlier studies "provided strong evidence for materialism (split the brain, split the person)," he argues, "the current understanding seems to only deepen the mystery of consciousness. You split the brain into two halves, and yet you still have only one person."

The earlier studies were relied upon in evolutionary psychology and cognitive neuroscience to formulate the idea that, to put it roughly, some of what we think of as decisions are actually set in motion by (to use a disputed but widespread term) brain modules formed from the experiences of our ancestors, a set of tools developed from the way the ancient humans who made us learned to survive and solve problems. As I understand it, these internal psychological mechanisms are thought to be like computer programs running in the background, beneath our conscious experience, programs that sometimes motivate us more powerfully than our reasoning does.

The idea is that the modules arose from natural selection, as an adaptation to the environments our ancestors navigated. Two prominent evolutionary psychologists, Douglas Kenrick and Vladas Griskevicius, authors of *The Rational Animal: How Evolution Made Us Smarter Than We Think,* argue that we have seven sub-selves, each tied to one of the following motives honed by our ancestors' evolutionary needs: evading physical harm, avoiding disease, making and keeping friends, attaining status, acquiring a mate, keeping a mate, and caring for family.

As Wright observes, these objectives overlap. And the modules idea is far from universally accepted. Some evolutionary psychologists prefer the term "networks," which conveys the interconnectivity of these goals far more than the word "modules" does. Whatever the terminology, I'm by nature averse to viewing human behavior in the mechanistic and reductive way some evolutionary psychologists do. But I became interested in these studies because of Wright's book, an argument for meditation through a (highly simplified for the layperson) scientific lens. Some of the studies he cites on the modules theory of mind aren't especially surprising. For example, marketing researchers found that people shown two ads for a museum were more likely to respond favorably to the "Visited by Over a Million People Each Year" pitch if they'd just watched a scary movie, because they felt safer in a crowd, but more likely to respond favorably to the "Stand Out from the Crowd" pitch if they'd just seen a romantic film.

But in another study, participants were offered a reward if they squeezed a hand grip hard enough. Before each squeezing session, the amount of the reward flashed in front of the subjects. Even when the amount was communicated subliminally—a single frame on the screen for a split second, not long enough to reach conscious awareness—the subjects squeezed harder when the reward was higher. Simultaneous brain scans showed that a region "associated with motivation and emotion" and "thought to encode information about rewards" was reliably more active when the reward was higher, a pound rather than a penny, and this was true whether the information was presented long enough to enter consciousness or only subliminally.

Wright details many other studies that suggest our decisions are often based on factors other than rational decision-making, and I especially relate to Wright's description of how mindfulness meditation exposes sudden unexpected feelings and strains of thought to the meditator, who ideally will sit there noticing what's coming up and then turn their attention back to the breath rather than riding away on the feeling or stampeding into a discursive series of avoidant thoughts. As my meditation teacher Ethan Nichtern once said in his Buddhist studies class, the conscious mind is not the originator of our experience but the recipient of our experience. In his book *The Dharma of the Princess Bride,* Ethan observed, "Your habitual tendencies get knotted up with those of your family like a ball of rubber bands," an insight I connect to these networks or modules and my ponderings on their potential interplay with epigenetics. If the modules exist, if intergenerational transmission of epigenetic changes do happen in humans and affect this kind of programming, how quickly could modules adapt in any individual family? In trying to leap from a moving car just as my mom had leapt into the dumpster, was I enacting some epigenetic programming?

As you might imagine, given the uproar surrounding transgenerational epigenetics research in humans, the difficulty of control groups, the problems with sample size, the stripping away that happens in methylation, the issue of the womb environment, and so much more, questions about the possible impact of any given person's epigenetic changes on their descendants remain in the theoretical realm. Scholars are pondering these questions, though. Karola Stotz, a philosopher of biology and cognitive science, argues in the journal *Frontiers in Psychology* that developmental environments "do not just select for variation, they also create new variation by influencing development through the reliable transmission of non-genetic but heritable information." She advocates studying the relationship between cognition and "those aspects of extended inheritance that lie between genetic and cultural inheritance, the still gray area of epigenetic and behavioral inheritance systems."

My interest in emotional recurrences in families isn't limited to what (current) science shows. The box of materialism is too tight for me. Speculations can be worth considering whether or not they're backed by millions of dollars in research funding and a PhD in one of the hard sciences. Most of us have had visceral reactions to something"—a bug or a food or a place or a person—that can't be explained by our direct experiences, that feel rooted in a kind of instinct.

TO UNDERSTAND OURSELVES, CARL JUNG argued, we need to understand our ancestors. "Our souls as well as our bodies are composed of individual elements which were all already present in the ranks of our ancestors," he wrote, in *Memories, Dreams, Reflections.* "The 'newness' in the individual psyche is an endlessly varied recombination of age-old components. . . . The less we understand of what our fathers and forefathers sought, the less we understand ourselves.

"I feel very strongly," he wrote elsewhere in the book, "that I am under the influence of things or questions which were left incomplete and unanswered by my parents and grandparents and more distant ancestors. It often seems as if there were an impersonal karma within a family, which is passed on from parents to children. It has always seemed to me that I had to . . . complete, or perhaps continue, things which previous ages had left unfinished."

Jung wrote of the dead and his ancestors in this way in his published writings, but in *The Red Book*—a journal of his that wasn't published until 2009—he recorded what he believed to be his communications with spirits or beings of his subconscious. Decades later, he said of the book that to an outsider it would look merely like madness, but also that all the works for which he's best known originated with "those initial fantasies and dreams." In 1913, as he began to have visions and hear voices that led to the book, he worried that he might end up "doing a schizophrenia." In *The Red Book* itself, he wrote that madness "is not to be despised and not to be feared" but to be given life.

He came to believe in the importance of the dead and that, in ignoring them, in separating ourselves from them, we have done ourselves and the whole of the world a grave disservice. "Turn to the dead," he wrote, "listen to their lament and accept them with love."

I'd been put off by Jung in the past because of what I saw as his insistence on particular symbolic interpretations that didn't resonate for me. His binary approach to sexuality was a particularly bitter pill. But the historian Sonu Shamdasani, translator of *The Red Book,* contends that Jung wanted individuals to discover their own language and cosmologies, rather than being bound by his insights. At the same time, in *Lament of the Dead: Psychology after Jung's Red Book* (a conversation between Shamdasani and the late psychologist and writer James Hillman), Shamdasani acknowledges Jung's attempt to extract "general principles from his fantasies," to "indicate that his fantasies didn't concern himself alone." Hillman agrees, observing that the fantasies for Jung connected with voices of the dead. They represented "collective strength, and collective message, a collective importance" in what comes up for each of us.

This tension between the individual and the "collective un-conscious" obsessed Jung. While I don't accept the whole of his framework, I, too, have become consumed with my—with our—connections to the humans whose bodies and spirits led to ours. I, too, am limited by my own language and cosmology. And I, too, believe that our family dead, and our relationships to them, are im-portant, to me as an individual and to humanity as a collective.

Part Six

INHERITANCE

Chapter 19

HEIRLOOMS AND
DISINHERITANCE

———

G RANNY GAVE ME A RING THAT I WORE FOR YEARS AND then lost. It was white gold, with Art Deco filigree scaffolding that rose to a diamond in a hexagonal setting flanked by two marquise sapphires turned on their sides. The diamond was large, with blue-grayish glints—a blue diamond, Granny said.

I loved that ring. From the time I plucked it from Granny's belongings at age nineteen, with one sapphire missing, and she allowed me to wear it back to college, I rarely took it off. I wore it in the shower; I wore it swimming daily. Soon it was understood that the ring had become mine. Seven or so years later, when Max and I decided to get married, I had the missing sapphire replaced instead of getting an engagement ring that would have cost far more and I would have liked far less. The new stone cost maybe a hundred fifty dollars. It was darker and duller than the intense royal blue of the remaining original, but the symmetry was an improvement. I gathered from the jeweler's blasé reaction that the ring wasn't as valuable as I'd believed it to be, which was a relief. It was a fancy ring of its era, with a large diamond cut in an unfortunate, old-fashioned way that muted its appeal. Knowing this only endeared the ring to me more.

One day, when I was thirty or so, a co-worker pointed out the fragility of the setting, that the diamond might fall out just as the sapphire had. A jeweler she recommended said there was no way to secure the stones. I should be more careful with the ring, he said, take it off before doing dishes or bathing, never sleep in it. At first I was diligent about putting the ring in the same spot each time, but I grew careless. It only took once. I have a dim memory of rolling it into the pocket of my jeans one afternoon so I could wash the dishes. I never saw it again.

Granny's ring isn't the only family heirloom I've mismanaged. Far from it. I used to have a habit of sliding rings on and off, and in that way I lost my great-grandmother Mama T.'s wedding band. It was thick yellow gold, set with a pretty, pale-pink princess-cut topaz. At a football game with my high school boyfriend, I slid it off and dropped it beneath the bleachers.

It seems magnificent and dreadful to me now that I was entrusted with Mama T.'s ring at the age of sixteen. It was Grandma's sister, my extravagant, funny, overbearing, and frequently unbearable great-aunt Pearl, who gave it to me, as Mama T.'s eldest granddaughter. The gift was a rare and opulent token of belonging to that line of my father's family—a token I didn't deserve, and one, I am tempted to say, that in some cosmic sense wasn't meant for me, though I don't have that feeling about Granny's ring, which I still consider, wherever it is, to be mine forever.

I HAVE BEAUTIFUL THINGS Granny made: an intricate bedspread she crocheted from twine, probably during the Great Depression, that won first prize in the Texas State Fair and later was chewed on at one corner by mice in my mother's basement; five or six quilts with gorgeous floral patterns constructed from pieces of men's pajamas found at the Goodwill; a black wool afghan with brightly colored patterns; and some elaborately sequined Christmas stockings. I also have her coral cameo ring; a gold cat pin with a jade belly and amethyst eyes; a delicate glass bottle in an etched sterling-silver casing; a blown-glass pitcher of pink swirls from her rarely used parlor; and two glass vanity jars with ornamental lids. I have Granny's cookbook and many of her photos and documents.

Over the years, my mom has passed along more of Granny's possessions: a rocking chair built by her father, Zone; a satin-covered footstool used by her mother, Alma; another footstool of unknown provenance, decorated with Granny's needlework and re-inforced underneath with the side of an old whiskey crate, no doubt also Granny's doing. I have some of Alma's correspondence, and I have Zone's wallet and Social Security card, and a Captain of Port ID with his fingerprint on it. Granny and her family are all over in my home.

The three or four houses Granny amassed across Dallas in her lifetime by hard work and then marrying a rich man are long gone, as is her money, both what she earned on her own—before her union with Smith and after he died—and what she inherited from him. As a child, I was confused about my family's status. Some-times, as a young girl, I thought we were rich, because my father was a lawyer and kids at my school seemed to think so. Later, after my parents divorced, when our car door broke and we didn't fix it, and my mom went a summer in the Miami heat without running the air-conditioning to save money, and rats were allowed to build a nest under the garbage disposal, I knew we weren't.

Or were we? Even as all that was happening, I learned that I had stock from a Texas insurance company where Granny's husband Smith worked for many years. She herself had something like $600,000 in company shares by 1988; my mom had about $350,000 worth, given to her by Granny over the years; my sister and I had maybe $35,000 each. This was revealed to me as the Texas legislature contemplated changes to state insurance laws and Granny was warned to sell. She declined, Smith having advised her to keep it forever. The law took effect and the stock value started to plummet. Still, Granny held fast. The company had never let her down, she

said, and she would not let them down now. Eventually a representative from the company itself called my stepfather to enlist him to
persuade Granny to sell. She refused. My stepdad sold the stock
that belonged to my mom, sister, and me, salvaging a tenth of its
value. Soon the stock was worthless.

Granny had intended her resources to see her to her death,
which they did, and then to pass to my mom and ultimately to my
sister and me and our children. Despite Granny's thrift in her lifetime, all her money, her assets, are gone. She helped my sister and
me out with college, with high school trips and buying our first
(used) cars. She helped my mom out with things, too. What was
left when Granny died—a couple of houses, some money (I don't
know how much)—went to my mom's monthly bills. Leaving aside
her preacher years, my mom was last employed when pregnant with
me, so her monthly Social Security payments don't cover much.

AS FOR MY DAD'S PARENTS, Grandma gave me a cross when I
graduated from high school. It's a pretty piece of jewelry, with tiny
but dazzling diamonds and a small, bright marquise ruby, the Platonic ideal of a ruby, the color of blood from a prick test. It came on
a thin gold chain. I wore the necklace a couple of times in my youth,
but as I grew into a committed unbeliever, putting it around my
neck would have felt like a violation of my own beliefs and a mock-
ery of my grandmother's.

For nearly three decades, it sat in a drawer, behind less costly
jewelry that I actually wore. I'd happen upon the cross when looking for something else, an earring back or an old rhinestone brace-
let, and its dormancy disturbed me. Seeing it conjured up Grandma's
and my fraught relationship, underscored how since her death my
life had tracked ever further from the path she would have chosen
for me. Her judgment seemed to inhabit the necklace, to glint out
at me from the jewels. A friend urged me to melt it down, to create

something beautiful I'd like to wear, but it felt wrong to destroy an object Grandma intended me to treasure.

I considered passing it along to my sister, but I knew she wouldn't wear it. Nor would my stepdaughter, nor my niece. But then one of my cousins had a daughter, Grandma's great-granddaughter, who I knew would be christened and raised in the church. The cross finally had a destination. Grandma would have wanted it to go to her, and so it did.

MATERIAL OBJECTS CAN BE moved around. A ring can be worn or given away, a quilt folded at the foot of a bed, a stocking hung from a mantel. But they also conjure deeper connections, deeper questions. I have photos of Grandma, a birth certificate, a death certificate, some letters she wrote me. I have her skin, her tiny wrists and ankles, her fidgety way of moving. The bulge of my eyes is like hers. Every day I use a pretty set of inexpensive cutlery that she gave Max and me when we got married. Apart from a red lipstick she deemed too bright for herself, though, the necklace was the one physical object she gave me that she herself had once worn. And aside from scans of some things he wrote, I don't have anything of Grandpa's.

That's not exactly what my grandparents intended. When they moved into an assisted-living facility in 2003, they shipped most of their furniture and many other belongings to my father. Down to Miami went their mahogany desks, their cherry dining set and china cabinet, their sofas and cut glass, and Mamma's silver. Ultimately, they intended my father to pass these things along to my sister and me, but this was wishful thinking on their part. We were both already estranged from him. As the schism deepened over the years that followed, our grandparents died, and our father started another family. The hand-me-downs will naturally pass to our half-siblings, who will have grown up with them close at hand.

Long before any of this, in my junior year of college, I wrote my grandparents a letter asking if they'd be willing to help me buy a car. As it happened, just as I was mailing the letter, they were trading in their car for a newer one. When my request arrived, my grandfather went back to the dealership and renegotiated, gave them more money so that I could have the old car, some American sedan, make and model now long forgotten. I was amazed and moved that Grandpa had gone so far out of his way for me.

My father was angry. He didn't want me to have a car, especially not from his parents. He promised that if I didn't take it, he would give me his car, an older Cadillac Eldorado, when I graduated. He would cover costs, including insurance, which was the wrinkle in my existing plan. I capitulated, turned down my grandparents' car. When I graduated a year and a half later, my father pretended not to remember our agreement. I tried to enlist support from my grandparents, but by then they were as exasperated with me over the car as they were with him, and I can't say I blame them. In the end, Granny gave me some money, and I bought an old Toyota hatchback.

WOMEN IN MY MOM'S line have a perverse nostalgia for terrible memories. We hang on to documents most people would find too painful to revisit. Granny kept correspondence about my grandfather's affair. She kept documentation of her sister's death in the mental institution. She preserved the newspaper announcement showing that she and my grandfather got their marriage license less than eight months before my mom was born. A few years ago, my mom shipped me a card I'd made in a rush and tucked under her pillow when I was nine years old. I remembered the day well, but I'd forgotten the note until I saw it again. That afternoon, my parents had fought, more ferociously than usual, about my mom's church. After she screeched off in the car, my father phoned his parents in

Mississippi. Then he told my sister and me that we would be flying out that night to stay with them. He told us to pack.

I staged a rare revolt. I sat on my bed, arms folded, and refused. Instead of spanking me, my father filled our suitcases himself. Before we left for the airport, while he was engrossed in last-minute planning, I made the card. "MOMMY," I wrote with blue crayon on the outside of a purple envelope, "pray for me!" The sheet tucked inside reads, "I didn't want to go, but Daddy made me. I protested as much as I could. I took the dresses for church out of my suitcase. Don't get mad at me, it wasn't my fault, please call me." I sealed the card with five pink pig stickers and hid it on my mom's side of the bed, where she would find it and my father would not. When she got home and discovered the card late that night, my father refused to say where we were. Desperate, my mom called our friends' parents. She called people we hadn't talked to in years. Finally, my father admitted that we were with his parents. She rang them up and (though I didn't know this until much later) threatened prosecution for kidnapping.

Within a couple of days, we were headed to Granny in Dallas. Grandpa and Grandma stood in the airport, tears streaming down their faces, as we waited to board. "I just hope we'll be able to see y'all again," Grandpa said. I hoped so, too. I didn't see why we wouldn't. Mostly I felt relieved to be getting away.

NOT LONG AFTER SENDING the card, my mom offered me her file documenting the aftermath of my parents' divorce. If I didn't want it, she was going to throw it away. Curiosity overrode my trepidation, and I knew it would be helpful for verifying my memories as I was writing this book.

"You will remember," my mom wrote to my father in 1989, in a letter cc'ing his parents and others, "at the time YOU DIVORCED ME, I did not secure an attorney because I trusted you. You told me to save attorney's fees and that you would take care of the whole thing. And you really did! You shortchanged me from the beginning, and you know it. The divorce papers were set up entirely by you and solely to your advantage. I was so glad to get out of the marriage that I did nothing but acquiesce to your terms just to keep from having to deal with you and your arbitrary, argumentative harangues—still believing that you would be fair." This continues for five single-spaced pages, and the file is hundreds of pages thick. In notes to her attorney, my mom recounts my father's efforts to control us, his cruelty, and his racism. I'd forgotten he used to kick our animals, until I came upon her mention of it. The scenes flashed back with painful clarity.

My mom sued my father to increase child support and to force him, several years after the divorce, to finally pay her for her half of the house where he still lived. Granny sued him for never repaying her loan to him and my mom, years before, to fix up the house. My father threatened to file an ethics complaint against their lawyer, who in his final letter wrote to my father that "all of your many suspicions and fears about me" were "entirely unfounded" and "must be motivated by factors that are exclusively internal to you." The lawyer was eager to settle the case, "with the knowledge that I shall hopefully not have to deal with you again any time in the future."

Granny kept a will handwritten by my mom's father, Robert, on October 13, 1944, eight months after their divorce was final. In it, he grandly bequeaths my mom, then four years old, "all propertys that I may own at the time of my death as her property absalutly and for ever" (the spelling is his). As far as I know, he had no property(s) at the time. My guess is that Robert drafted the will as a dramatic display of his devotion to my mother after having consistently failed to pay Granny the five-dollar weekly child support she was owed under the divorce agreement. She always said he didn't help support my mom.

When Robert died in 1970, he left everything to his last wife, Eleanore, under a will executed in 1961. My mom and Eleanore's two children were to split his estate equally if Robert and Eleanore died simultaneously or if Eleanore, as the lawyers say, predeceased him. At the time that he signed the will, Robert and my mom hadn't been in touch for about a decade. A couple years later, he reestablished contact. The last time my mom saw her dad, when Robert warned her against marrying my father, Robert predicted that my father would use her to support him through law school and then divorce her. He urged my mom to meet his lawyer. As I've said, I suspect he wanted the lawyer to persuade her to insist on a prenuptial agreement, but she didn't.

My mom has always speculated that there was another, secret will that Robert planned to unveil in the meeting with the attorney. "He told me he was leaving me land in Dallas," she wrote in an email once, "and a sizeable money inheritance in his will. His wife and her sister stole it from me." Historically, I discounted the idea that Robert meant my mom to have more of his wealth than she ended up with. But in recent years, I started to wonder. The will that went through probate was signed by Robert while he was still estranged from my mom. Later, he wanted my mom to meet his lawyer, and she didn't. Had Robert drafted a codicil that his wife didn't know of, that my mom didn't find out about because she skipped the appointment? It's possible. On the other hand, Robert's lawyer never reached out to my mom. Maybe Robert considered a revision to his estate plan and, when my mom left early, decided not to implement it.

IN A TWIST THAT is so very *my family*, I came to have Robert's probated will not through Granny's papers, not through my mom's file, but from my father. In 2003, I interrupted our estrangement by emailing him and asking for a collection of letters my mother wrote and carbon-copied to our family when I was a small child. Everything else I'd left in his house I could easily part with, but not those.

I tried to phrase the request casually, so as not to underscore that

I still didn't intend to be in contact going forward. I knew he would wonder if the request was an opening. I felt a little guilty about that, but I desperately wanted the letters.

To my relief, my father did send them. "Also enclosed," he wrote, in a note accompanying the parcel, "is certain probate court information regarding Robert Bruce." Beyond the will, he included a photocopied summary of some disinheritance provisions of Arizona law, with the following sentence highlighted: "Children living when the will is executed and not mentioned therein have no rights in the estate."

It was a message to me about the future as much as about the past. The surprise wasn't that my father was threatening to disinherit me but that he thought I didn't expect him to do so. I'd gone to law school at his urging. Then I'd capitulated by taking a basic income-tax class, which I loathed until realizing my classmates were there to learn how to help rich people game the system. I forced myself to pay attention, and then I took more tax classes. In the end, I received the "book award"—the highest grade—in estate planning. I knew the law, and my father knew that I knew it. I was well aware that in cutting ties with him I was also cutting myself off from his money.

I GREW UP THINKING of wills and inheritance as the purview of my father and people like him. He emphasized saving and the idea of family land and family assets. His practice focused on estates. He helped clients structure wills and trusts so that their money passed to their heirs rather than to taxes and, to the greatest of his ability, so that the money passed to their children only if the children did what they wanted. For one client who feared his daughter would not marry a white man, my father added a clause that the daughter would inherit only if she returned to live in her country of origin, where, in my father's and the client's view, she was less likely to meet a Black person. Both the client and my father would have preferred a more direct proscription in the will, but it would have been unenforceable.

I remember him recounting all this to my sister and me with pride. He often discussed his estate-planning strategies while we were in the car. Sometimes my sister or I, whichever of us was sitting up front, would try to make the other laugh by putting a hand around back to give him the middle finger as we feigned interest in what he was saying.

When I was getting married, in 1997, before my father and I were estranged, I told him by letter that Max had a daughter from a previous relationship. My father had opposed my relationship with Max from the start. He'd urged me to date someone with lucrative career prospects rather than an artist. Instead, I'd made clear that Max would be part of my life and my father's participation was optional. Unable to deter me from this course, my father pushed me to insist on a prenuptial agreement. If I didn't, he said, I'd forfeit my right to inherit any of his money outright. He intimated that he had amassed—or eventually would amass—several million dollars, and if I had a prenup in place, I might be given the power to withdraw a percentage of trust assets each year.

Max didn't want to enter into our marriage under this kind of constraint, and neither did I. I loved my stepdaughter, who was four when Max and I married. I knew I would want anything I had to pass to her and Max if I died. I didn't plan to have biological children or to adopt. But I was torn about a prenup. I was reluctant to irrevocably part ways with the possibility of a future windfall. Maybe even then some part of me still wanted to please my father, too.

My sister, who was already estranged from our father, counseled against any sort of agreement he proposed. First there would be the prenup, she said, and then other conditions. If I did have a child, I'd have to send them to a certain school, take them to a certain church. If I didn't have a child, I'd be disinherited for failing to produce an heir.

I knew my sister was right. Our father had a habit of extending offers that later he denied having made, once I'd fulfilled my part of the bargain. In 1993, a couple of years after I fell for the false promise of his car, he said that if I went to law school at a state university instead of an expensive private one, he'd pay the full tuition and all my living expenses rather than the half my parents' divorce agreement obligated him to pay. I asked for the promise in writing. When he refused, I made sure to repeat the conversation with him over the phone while my then-boyfriend and other members of his family were in the room. I wanted witnesses. Predictably, I went to the University of Florida and my father denied having made the agreement. I took out loans to finance the education I'd embarked on to please him. I considered suing him, but who wants to sue their father?

A few years after I graduated from law school, Max was finishing film school in Tallahassee and we were deciding where to go next. My father exhorted us to move back to Miami so I could fulfill his dream of a family law firm: Newton & Newton. By then I'd worked for a law firm, which I didn't like, and as an attorney for the Florida Department of Revenue, which I did. I enjoyed making corporations pay taxes they owed to the state.

Max also grew up in Miami. We hadn't planned to return. Nor did I want to work for my father or help wealthy people evade taxes. But I wondered if I should do it anyway. Maybe my father would pay me a big-firm salary. He could, if he wanted to. Luckily, he didn't offer. He wouldn't specify what he'd pay. He wouldn't put anything in writing. I found a job in New York City, where Max wanted to work in TV and film. For the first six months, I worked at a big accounting firm, advising corporations. I didn't feel good about the work as a matter of policy or politics. And I wanted to be a writer. So I took a legal-publishing job, writing about tax. It paid the bills and allowed me to write on the side.

What's explicitly handed down to us is only part of our inheritance. I've benefitted from the privileges I had, the education my parents had, the means my ancestors had, their struggles in and contributions to the world, and the wrongs they perpetrated. I grew up with a tax lawyer for a father. Grudgingly, out of fear of him and of my own failure, I wound up with a law degree and tax expertise myself.

Ultimately, I'm glad that my father was withholding rather than generous, unreliable rather than a safety net, so I didn't have to find out exactly how many compromises I was willing to make. It frightens me to wonder what I might have chosen to overlook, what I might have chosen not to say, if my father had doted on me.

Chapter 20

MONSTROUS
BEQUESTS

———

S A YOUNG GIRL, I KNEW MY FATHER BELIEVED THAT every Black person, everywhere, should be out in fields picking cotton, following a white man's commands. Luckily, no one else I knew in Miami defended slavery or mourned the end of it. So I knew early on that my father was wrong.

His vague descriptions of benevolent masters and grateful "negroes" aside, my father didn't offer details of our ancestors' involvement in slavery. In my twenties, I realized that my great-grandfather, Daddy Joe, had become an overseer on a plantation starting only in the mid-1930s, seventy years after the Civil War ended, and I began to hope my father had inflated our family's role, that he'd invented (what he saw as) a lofty antebellum past to bolster his pedigree.

Once I started digging, I found so much enslaving that I kept losing track: twelve people bound by this fourth great-grandfather, nineteen by another, six by this fourth great-grandmother and two by that one. To this day, whenever I try to add up all the human beings my ancestors subjugated on this continent, I realize how incomplete my research still is. Then I dig deeper and find more. In total, the number is in the hundreds, if not thousands.

The older I get, the more recent this history seems. I was born in

1971. The Civil War ended in 1865. A hundred and fifty years is nothing. It's the blink of an eye.

IN MY ANCESTORS' WILLS, human beings are bequeathed to wives and children alongside money, land, tools, and beds. The first document I turned up along these lines was signed in Georgia in 1816, by a fifth great-grandfather, Davis McGee, my ancestor through Grandma, who left to "my beloved wife Nelly McGee my land Household and kitchen furniture, and also my Negroes, to wit: Grace, Sall, Mary, Pat, Stephen, and Nemrod, and all my stock and plantation tools, that is to say my estate both real and personal during her natural life or widowhood."

Davis's third son, Joseph, was my fourth great-grandfather. By the 1840s, Joseph had migrated to the Mississippi Delta, not far from where my father was born a century later. Joseph's will, probated in Holmes County in 1855, provides that all his "land, stock, and property of every description except my negroes be sold." His youngest daughter, my third great-grandmother, Sarah Ann McGee, then sixteen, was to receive "a bed stead and all necessary furniture in addition to her distributive share of my estate." Perhaps in reaction to the lone dollar Joseph's own father bequeathed him, Joseph's will directs that the twelve people he enslaved be "divided into seven lots" by "five disinterested men" and distributed equally among his seven children.

> . . . the residue of my property consisting of the following ne-
> groes and their increase viz Burwell and Joan, Bob, Martha,
> Esther, Buddy, Ralph, Alfred, Randle, Kat, Burwell and Jim
> be divided into seven lots, Burwell and Joan constitute one
> lot so they not be separated and divided by lot among my
> seven children. . . . the division to be made by five disinter-
> ested men in such manner as for all to be made equal. In the
> event that my daughter, Sarah Ann McGee, shall be single at

the time of such division, I will that she have the choice of the lots so made.

Was this what my father meant when he extolled the kindness and generosity of our ancestors?

In the end, Sarah married two months before Joseph died, so rather than choosing which human beings to call her property, she would have inherited whatever "lot" she was assigned by "the five disinterested men." Five years later, by the 1860 census, she and her husband, John William Bailey, my third great-grandfather, enslaved a total of ten people. John's father, Jordan, appears on the same page of the slave schedules, with nineteen people listed alongside his name.

In true Mississippi Delta fashion, I'm descended from John William Bailey's grandfather, Jeremiah, in two different ways. Grandma's parents were second cousins once removed—this would happen if, say, the child of your first cousin married your own grandchild—and the relationships get confusing. Here's a visual representation:

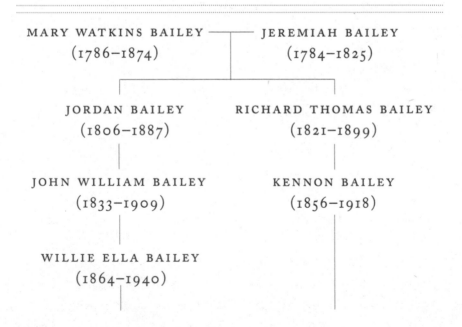

MARY WATKINS BAILEY —— JEREMIAH BAILEY
(1786–1874)   (1784–1825)

JORDAN BAILEY   RICHARD THOMAS BAILEY
(1806–1887)   (1821–1899)

JOHN WILLIAM BAILEY   KENNON BAILEY
(1833–1909)   (1856–1918)

WILLIE ELLA BAILEY
(1864–1940)

LAURA FRANCES BAILEY ── JOSEPH EVERET TERRY
(1889–1985)   (1889–1970)

GRANDMA
(1921–2005)

My father took especial pride in the Baileys. The family tree he showed me with tears in his eyes traced back to Jeremiah's father, Benjamin Bailey, who was born in Virginia in 1755 and fought in the Revolutionary War. It was through this lineage that my great-grandmother, Mama T., the one whose pink-topaz wedding ring I lost, joined the Daughters of the American Revolution.

The Baileys, said to be English and Scottish by background, wound up in Virginia because an unnamed ancestor was given a land grant by the king, a common tactic for offloading evangelicals to the colonies. Another of Jeremiah's lines included John Easter, a preacher that a historian of Methodism called "one of the most zealous, powerful, and successful" Methodist preachers ever, "an uncommonly faithful and holy man." The compiler of the official Bailey family tree wrote in the introduction that Jeremiah and his children "inherited a religious fervor" from Easter.

From their earliest days on these shores, European colonizers and settlers cloaked themselves in religion, bound together in congregations they told themselves were chosen by God, while justifying slavery as part of God's plan. In his autobiography, Frederick Douglass invokes the biblical Book of Matthew in condemnation. "Never was there a clearer case of 'stealing the livery of the court of heaven to serve the devil in.'"

We have men-stealers for ministers, women-whippers for missionaries, and cradle-plunderers for church members. The man who wields the blood-clotted cowskin during the week fills the pulpit on Sunday, and claims to be a minister of the meek and lowly Jesus. The man who robs me of my earnings at the end of each week meets me as a class-leader on Sunday morning, to show me the way of life, and the path of salvation. . . . The slave auctioneer's bell and the church-going bell chime in with each other, and the bitter cries of the heartbroken slave are drowned in the religious shouts of his pious master. Revivals of religion and revivals in the slave-trade go hand in hand together.

GRANDMA DIDN'T SEEM ZEALOUS compared to my mom, or even in comparison with my father's Presbyterian church or my fundamentalist schools, but she was a churchgoing Methodist, and I remember her horror when my parents briefly tried to compromise on a Baptist church.

One night, contemplating my Bailey ancestors, trying and failing to imagine how they justified enslaving fellow human beings, I realized that both of Grandma's Bailey great-grandfathers died on my birthday, May 21, one in 1899 and the other a decade later. The date brought a reckoning before I even existed. To me, it feels fated—and so spiritually Southern—that I've ended up being the descendant of theirs who can't stop pondering responsibility for the harm they did.

APART FROM WILLS AND census data, I don't have direct insight into these great-grandfathers' lives. As for their descendants in the Jim Crow South, my own great-grandparents, Mama T. and Daddy Joe, only indirect accounts survive. Mama T. kept daily house diaries of life on the plantation that Daddy Joe managed, but Grandma threw them out. I imagine she wasn't eager for them to see the light of day ("Those old things?" she said, when I asked why she'd tossed them), but as an immaculate housekeeper, and in contrast to my mother's side of the family, she was also an enthusiastic purger in general. She donated my father's comic books while he was away in grad school. Each day's newspaper was in the bin by 8 A.M.

In the mid-1990s, Grandma's sister, Pearl, and Pearl's husband, John, wrote their memories of life on Four Fifths Plantation as it was in Daddy Joe's time. Aunt Pearl and Uncle John have since passed on, but they mailed these recollections to the broader family. I believe they intended their accounts as a record for posterity, a corrective to the prevailing view that plantations were exploitative and unjust, and that they would have been glad for the accounts to be shared. To me, their memories underscore precisely what Pearl and John hoped to refute. They lay bare the mechanisms of white supremacy and its connection to the economy of the South.

"The size of those mules!" John wrote of his first visit to the place, to meet Pearl's family. "I had only seen the smaller mules that were used on the Tennessee farms. I never knew about those mules that worked the Delta land. There was no comparison. These mules were about twice the size. . . . And then the black men that drove them! They were so big and strong. I had to admire these powerful men. Mr. Joe knew their language and everything that they were doing. He had a saying that I will always remember 'always leave the blacks with something to laugh about.' He could do that in such a wonderful way." Uncle John described Daddy Joe as:

> an example for me and others in his integrity and proud honesty. He was a great one to observe the humanity that surrounded him in his managing such a large plantation. The responsibilities to the owners of the property and his understanding of the needs of the black people who did the work there. No one I have ever known was held in higher respect than he was among the black people of the Mississippi Delta. He had a reputation among them of being able to afford them good living conditions and ending up the year with

money in their pockets. He was completely fair and considerate in all his dealings.

Reading this part of Uncle John's reminiscences felt a little bit
like being at the dinner table with my father again. In fifth grade I'd
learned in school that, before the Civil War, enslavers frequently cut
off the toes of enslaved people who escaped and were recaptured.
When I told my father this at dinner, he was so angry, he seemed to
levitate. He canceled our weekend plans and spent that time sketch-
ing Civil War battlegrounds, lecturing me about the benevolence of
my ancestors and the importance of cotton.

A few years ago, someone whose grandparents had been sharecroppers on Four Fifths Plantation during the time Daddy Joe
managed it emailed me because of a blog post I'd written. They were
trying to figure out whether their grandparents had been born
there. I wasn't able to answer that question but invited them to
share their family's experience, explaining that I felt responsible for
reckoning with that history in whatever way I can. They regretted
not remembering more of their grandparents' stories but replied
diplomatically, saying, "I do remember my mother telling me that
of the sharecroppers in the area, our family were relatively 'comfortable,' as my grandfather was able to supplement his income by
hunting and my grandmother would babysit the owner's children
and take in laundry. Other families would often come to them for
food or help." According to Isabel Wilkerson's *The Warmth of Other
Suns*, "Fewer than one out of five sharecroppers ever saw a profit at
the end of the year," so in that sense Daddy Joe was comparatively
equitable, but the extra jobs the family had to take on just to be
"comfortable" are telling.

By way of example of what he considered to be Daddy Joe's
good sense and fairness, Uncle John recalled that:

Once, one of the blacks had been put into the jail in Greenwood because he had been threatening his wife and family.

Of course, he was drunk. The Sheriff picked him up because his family was afraid of him. Mr. Joe had called the Sheriff to go get him. On Monday, Mr. Joe went to get him out. Evidently, Mr. Joe wanted to get him off the place. So when they got back on Four Fifths on highway #49, Mr. Joe stopped the car and got out along with the black man. Mr. Joe said to him "Four Fifths Plantation runs north and south of this highway. Highway #49 runs east and west. Now you go this way on #49. Do not go north or south from here." "Oh Mr. Joe you don't want to run me off this place. Why you put my first pair of pants on me on this place." Mr. Joe with his quick wit replied "Yes, and don't let me tear the last pair off you on this place." That was an example of what I was talking about. He handled that with humor and got the desired result.

No judge, no jury—my great-grandfather deprived a man who'd served his time of his home, his family, and all of his belongings without due process of law.

When I was growing up, Grandma, Aunt Pearl, and the rest of the family often reminisced about Daddy Joe's poor hearing. As early as middle age, he began turning up the radio as far as it would go. He sought to dispel everyone's concern and feelings of responsibility for all the missed conversations and anecdotes by joking, "I didn't want to hear that anyhow." (I sympathize. My own hearing is deteriorating so rapidly, I've considered having a disclaimer tattooed on my wrist to display in crowded bars.) To compensate, Daddy Joe was said to have developed minute observation skills and an uncanny intuition about people's needs and why they might be approaching him. Uncle John writes that he first witnessed this when one of the sharecroppers came to see Daddy Joe, who had the sense that the man had come to ask for help for his sick family.

I remember clearly Mr. Joe walking up to this big black man and putting his body so close to the man's that they touched.

This was so he could hear what was said. They talked like that for some minutes. There was such a genuine feeling of one human being for another of deep concern. One had troubles and the other could help. I was so impressed.

I'm glad Daddy Joe was willing to coordinate medical care for people who worked on the place, but I'm considerably less surprised than Uncle John that Daddy Joe could sense when something was seriously wrong. Most people, Black or white, tend to have an urgent way of presenting themselves in a health emergency.

Uncle John also remembered that workers often knocked on the exterior door to Daddy Joe's and Mama T.'s bedroom at night. Mama T. usually answered to see what they needed, and then, if necessary, Daddy Joe got involved. In Uncle John's telling, people usually sought help because someone (i.e., a Black worker) was "drunk and threatening others." In that case, Daddy Joe called in the sheriff and went back to bed. If someone needed medical help, Daddy Joe and Mama T. assured them the doctor would arrive in the morning. And then Uncle John recounted:

> Once, Viola, cook maid or whatever, came to the back door at two o'clock in the morning and announced she had killed Lon and for Mr. Terry to call the Sheriff. As she said, "He was breaking up my furniture so I slapped him up the side of his head with an ax. He is out in the cotton dead." The Sheriff came and could not find the body and so he left. [Lon] showed up a few days later and was received in Viola's home as though nothing had happened. So it went on Saturday nights.

I must have been about twenty-five years old when this letter arrived. I called my sister, and we marveled at the blithe language: "cook maid or whatever." Could Uncle John genuinely not remember Viola's role, or was this a way of underscoring her role as comic relief in his story? Maybe a bit of both. "He handled that with humor and got the desired result." "He was completely fair and considerate in all his dealings." I felt disgusted but also impotent, not avoidant exactly—I showed it to Max, called up a friend or two, sparred with my father—but unsure how best to atone for or work against this history. Close friends and loved ones aside, I often found that when I tried to discuss my family's past with other white people, they were eager to change the subject. Some seemed to view my preoccupation with that past as a defect in me. Occasionally I wondered if they were right. Then a letter like this would arrive, or my father and I would argue about the Confederate flag, or a Black person would be killed in police custody, and I'd be filled again with the frantic urge to *do something*, still with little concrete sense of what that something might be.

WHITE WOMEN IN THE Jim Crow era enforced segregation and class boundaries as zealously as the men did, and sometimes more so, in an extension of their earlier role as enslavers. Historian Stephanie E. Jones-Rogers contends in *They Were Her Property* that before the Civil War, white women may even have been more invested in slavery in some ways than white men were. While most of the woman's property came under her husband's control at marriage, she could use legal loopholes to maintain control over the people she enslaved. By taking someone else's freedom, the woman secured more for herself.

So running a plantation behind the scenes was something a Southern belle was expected to be able to do. And in memories of my great-grandmother, sent in the same mailer, Pearl called Mama T. "'the power behind the wheel' of all that she and Daddy Joe did during those years." Pearl remembered her parents meeting in the hallway each night at the plantation, where they moved around 1937, to plan for the next day. Her father always sought her mother's advice on how to solve problems.

Everyone, the sharecroppers included, knew "that to get Mr.
Terry to do something you first had to get to speak to Mrs. Terry,"
my great-aunt wrote. Twice a month, Mama T. joined Daddy Joe to
pay wages from the back office in the plantation's general store.

> The blacks would line up to receive wages at the door of the
> office. . . . Not a cent was paid out without Mother by Dad-
> dy's side. . . . Daddy always knew who the blacks were and
> what was going on in their family. You know, there were
> ninety families of blacks on Four Fifths. He was dear to them
> because he cared for them and he could speak their lan-
> guage. . . .

Aunt Pearl had fond memories of life on the plantation, and also
recalled all the things requiring Mama T.'s oversight: care of the
garden, chickens, a cow, and hogs.

> Then Mother had to see about the housework and look after
> the children. Daddy had the farming, cotton gin and the
> stores to look after. Then there were many black families that
> always needed something, sickness, child birth, housing, set-
> tling disputes among family members, getting some of the
> men out of jail over the weekend. It never stopped. The cot-
> ton crop had to be raised along with worry about the threat
> of weather. There was no end to it. It took two strong people
> like Mother and Daddy to do all this.
>   Daddy was a strong person and he held up well under all
> this. But it took Mother to watch and handle all the details.
> This was done in such a quiet and efficient manner. Daddy
> would turn so many things over to her because he knew that
> she would do it so well. The planning of the garden was hers.
> When it came hog killing time the plans for this was [sic]
> handled by her. Daddy would say "Baby, you see about that."
> Mother would put on some warm clothes and direct the work

of the blacks who had brought their sharp knives and did the work. Daddy would make himself scarce and let "Baby" do it. Then we had plenty of sausage and hams and other good things. Word would be passed around their friends and family and all would come and feast at the Terry's [*sic*]. Henry was our cook and he prepared such good things.

"It took two strong people like Mother and Daddy to do all this," I said to my sister. "Yep, *alllll* this," she said. I couldn't attribute Aunt Pearl's near-erasure of the workers and their labor to my great-grandparents, who weren't alive to answer my questions and hear my concerns. But still, as I read and reread the letter and mulled my family's participation in the plantation system of the Jim Crow era, I felt angry, revolted, implicated, and stuck.

Chapter 21

NOT RACIST

———

R EADING THOSE MEMORIES REINFORCED MY SENSE OF distance from my father's family and my sense of alignment with Granny's. Unlike Grandma and her people, Granny came from poverty. She drove a musty old Buick. She loved playing solitaire against "old Sol" on her deck of Budweiser playing cards. She chewed toothpicks, bought her clothes secondhand, hung them on a line out back to dry. *She* didn't come from plantation types. Except, I learned when I started researching our family history, she did.

I'd imagined Granny's mother's ancestors as poor Appalachian folk, Scots-Irish settlers. Maybe some were, but Alma's father's father's people, the Kinchens, were more likely English, early arrivals to Virginia who migrated into North Carolina. A William Kinchen to whom some trees trace the line executed a will probated in 1735, through which he bequeathed nineteen enslaved people to his family. Whether or not my Kinchens originated with this man, they ended up in St. Helena Parish, Louisiana. There my ancestors not only enslaved people but sued one another over who had the right to enslave them.

Granny's great-grandfather John Kinchen was born in Louisiana in 1822. His mother, Nancy Kinchen, died soon after the French-man she married ran off. John, a baby, was raised by Kinchens. A few decades later, he and some of Nancy's siblings sued his grand-father, Nancy's dad. In the complaint, John and his aunts "respect-fully state" that:

In the said estate are the following slaves:

RACHEL, age about 45 years, light complexion;

JINNY, age about 17 years, dark complexion;

MINERVA, age about 14 years, dark complexion;

PHREM, a man, age about 26 years, light complexion;

SHERRED, a man, age about __ [left blank]

and also a considerable quantity of land. Petitioners state they never have received anything from the succession of their deceased mother [John's grandmother], that there has as yet been no partition, either legal or otherwise, and that all property has remained in the possession of William. . . .

Petitioners pray for legal relief as the heirs of Mary Gol-son.

The outcome is lost to time and a courthouse fire.

IT CHILLED ME THAT Granny, so benevolent toward me, so hu-mane toward strangers, so valiant in her childhood poverty and te-nacious in rising from it, came from this history. Granny always said that the Great Depression taught people that anyone might wind up poor, anyone could need a helping hand. During my childhood, she rented a house to an elderly blind woman who also relied on Granny to take her shopping and to forgive what she couldn't pay.

Looking back, though, there were clues. I remember her disgust at my father's racism, but I'd nearly repressed the times that, after hours spent outside pulling weeds or doing some other chore, Granny characterized what she'd been doing as "n—— work." She said it in a lighthearted tone, as if to particularly congratulate herself for having done labor so onerous. I notice, too, that I've found occasion to mention that Mama T.'s cook and housekeeper, Geneva, was Black but not until now that Granny's housekeeper, Carrie, who began working for Granny late in her second marriage, was also Black.

Sometimes Granny berated my father in front of my sister and me. Once, she told him, "You treat these children like n——s, and when they grow up they won't have anything to do with you." Usually I liked it when she stood up for us, but I flinched at this, knowing that word was the worst possible epithet and that the way he treated us was not remotely comparable to enslaving someone. I knew that word was wrong from everyone around me, but I first learned it was wrong from my father. Like his ancestors in their wills before him, he preferred what he considered to be the more genteel "negroes." My father explicitly advocated slavery, but I guess he wanted it to sound high-class.

Into my adulthood, I assigned one side of my family the role of "racist" and the other the role of "not racist," or "not *fundamentally* racist." But culpability is everywhere, going back generations, down to me, from all the times I stayed silent when I should have spoken up, to my participation in the systemic racism that my ancestors helped create. When I was fifteen, I told a racist joke to impress someone who had told it to me. I knew it was wrong. I did it anyway. I don't remember the joke but can easily summon the shame and disgust with myself I felt afterward.

Omitting unwanted recollections of Granny—from my memory

or from this book—would foreclose the true, deep reckoning I know is needed. It's one thing to acknowledge bigotry and inhumanity where we expect it, where we've always judged it, in people we already view critically. It's another thing to face and acknowledge it in the people we love most.

MY ANCESTORS THROUGH GRANNY perpetrated other large-scale wrongs, too. I'd never imagined my own forebears interacting with Indigenous people of this land. That history, like the *Mayflower*, felt remote, like something that couldn't have involved my family directly, even though I knew that they—and I—had benefited from systemic injustices against Native people.

When I first discovered that my ninth great-grandfather, Cornet Joseph Parsons, was, as many sources put it, a "founder" of Northampton and Springfield, Massachusetts, I was excited to find an ancestor outside the South and amazed that he'd been involved in establishing the town where my sister lived. I hadn't expected to find New England in my family background, especially not through my mom, whose ancestors I'd pictured as poor rural Southerners going back centuries.

I soon read in an account published by one of Parsons's descendants in 1912 that the first record of him, in 1636, "was as witness to a deed given by the Indians to William Pynchon and others of lands at and about Springfield, Mass." I felt vague unease on encountering this, knowing that the Puritans slaughtered many Indigenous people and drove many survivors from ancestral lands. Over the years, I've learned that Parsons was instrumental in decimating the Norwottuck, Nonotuck, and Agawam villages in what is now known as Western Massachusetts, first by trade and bargaining, with the deals becoming increasingly unfair, and then by military force. There's reason to believe that the lofty Pynchons enlisted Parsons, a trader, in their land deals because, unlike the other settlers, he could communicate with the Native people.

In an 1898 book on Parsons, Henry Martyn Burt and Albert Ross Parsons write that "Trading with the Indians brought the subject of this sketch into friendly relations with them and he appears to have been consulted when important transactions were to be concluded. . . . It is probable," they contend, "that Joseph Parsons had a more intimate acquaintance with the Indians than any other inhabitant of Northampton, or Hadley, as his trading with them must have taken them to their villages up and down the valley." My ancestor's ability to talk with the Pocumtuck and Nonotuck ("his dusky friends") in their own language is what "made him so valuable," according to the authors. "It also gave him a much more extended acquaintance with the country and of the most desirable lands."

Documents maintained by the English settlers of the day establish, the professor of anthropology Margaret Bruchac argues, that the settlers "regarded the Pocumtuck as shrewd traders, desirable allies, and powerful enemies," as the "Nonotuck Indians began bargaining away their independence in land transactions with the English." In 1668, after negotiating a transfer of land to John Pynchon, Parsons held a "mortgage" on fifty or sixty acres in Hockanum, according to the 1898 history of my ancestor. "Wequagon and his wife Awnusk, and Squomp, their son . . . owed [Parsons] 80 beaver skins for coats, wampum and goods, and if it was not paid before the first of September, he was to have the land." Later he took and sold the land "to the inhabitants of Hadley, for a considerable sum." He also participated in negotiating a 1664 agreement with the "Nowatugue [a phonetic rendering of Nonotuck] Indians that were the Inhabitants of the place," authorizing them to build a fort in Northampton, subject to various Puritanical rules, and promising them protection, which he and the other colonizers failed to provide.

Parsons became known as Cornet only in 1678, because of his military role in what was called in his time King Philip's War. The chief of the Wampanoag led many peoples of the Connecticut River Valley, including the Pocumtuck, in a war to drive out the settlers. Many of the Native people were murdered or fled elsewhere, but others stayed on their ancestral homelands, moving to the periphery of colonial settlements. A headstone in Northampton's Bridge Street Cemetery falsely declares Sally Maminash, who died in 1853, "the last of the Indians here."

When I visit Northampton now, walking with my sister and her family and our dogs along the river, driving on the highway or coming in on the train, I think of the violence my ancestors did to the people who communed with and cared for the land of the Connecticut River Valley for at least 12,000 years before the Europeans arrived. Their descendants live on, cellular and spiritual repositories of this history. What is my responsibility to them?

MY GREAT-GREAT-GRANDFATHER SYLVESTER GARFIELD Kinchen descended from both Joseph Parsons and John Kinchen (of the slavery lawsuit). Sylvester was Granny's maternal grandfather. In surviving photos, he's a tall skinny man with a long white beard. In one shot, taken about 1915, he drives Granny, age ten or so, and her younger sister somewhere in a covered wagon pulled by an emaciated horse.

Sylvester and my great-great-grandmother Martha Caroline were poor. In his late forties, Sylvester worked as a laborer. In his fifties and sixties, he worked as a peddler (as the city directory said some years) and traveling salesman (as it said in others). I have a photo of Martha Caroline scowling in front of a barn, Granny and Louise young girls glowering by her side with filthy bare feet. A friend compared it to Depression-era photographs of people starving in shacks. Sylvester's and Martha Caroline's poverty was real, and in her youth so was Granny's. But the fact that they were not visibly, actively benefiting from our ancestors' wrongs during those years doesn't erase what our people did or my responsibility for reckoning with that history. Nor does it mitigate the systemic racism that enabled Granny and her descendants to prosper while oppressing descendants of people our ancestors enslaved, killed, and displaced. Granny was able to pass along wealth to her descendants. Her housekeeper, Carrie, who died while living with Granny a couple of years after I was born, was not.

Here in my house on the land of the Lenape people, far from the places where my ancestors did all this harm and profited, I'm only beginning—and still pondering how—to make amends. Unlike my ancestors, who stayed silent or who used their words to manipulate and maintain power over others, I can acknowledge and own this history. I can dedicate time and money to dismantling white supremacy, advocate for reparations and apologies, urge other people with this history to do the same. And I can listen. But what, concretely, day to day, can I do?

An Indigenous organization I support, the Manna-hatta Fund, urges settlers to acknowledge and honor that we are on Native land; deed land to Native peoples directly if possible; and, when this isn't possible, give at least 2.4 percent of any land sale to Indigenous people. They advise regular donations to the Native people of the land where we live, work, and hold events; support of land-reclamation efforts and Indigenous-led environmental work; return of stolen objects; and removal of colonial monuments. Know from whence you came, they also say, where your own people are from.

Not long after reading this, in December 2020, I visited the original home lot of my ninth great-grandparents, Joseph and Mary Bliss Parsons, on Nonotuck land. Now a Northampton museum commemorating the Parsons family but closed to the public for repairs even before the pandemic, the place felt somber and misguided, a dubious monument that should be rethought. The day was gray. The plants were brown and dry, at rest for the winter. No one was in sight.

I asked forgiveness of the land and its Native people, living and dead. On the worn dirt at the foot of a bench, I emptied a bottle of wine as an offering.

Chapter 22

DISCONNECTION

———

A PERSON'S FATE ISN'T NECESSARILY SEALED BY THEIR belongings or status, but how we grow up sets us on a course. Circumstances frame our sense of who we are and can become. What we eat in our youngest years affects our future health and potentially our children's and grandchildren's. The air we breathe, the objects we treasure, the places we inhabit, and the resources we have shape us in intricate and unpredictable ways. My mother's belief in demons predisposed me from a young age to see repetitions of trauma, poverty, and displacement as a kind of multigenerational haunting.

The writer Sarah Smarsh was born to parents who came from generations of poor Kansas farmers. She imprinted on prairie farmland, on common sense and hard work, and became hell-bent on ending the generational pattern of being a young mother trapped in poverty. "Though I wouldn't know for years that I'd been an accident," she writes in *Heartland: A Memoir of Working Hard and Being Broke in the Richest Country on Earth*, "I felt the knowledge at an atomic level."

In her memoir, *Searching for Zion: The Quest for Home in the African Diaspora*, Emily Raboteau traces her own search for belonging to her father, who fled Mississippi as a child with his mother after his father was murdered in 1943. Raboteau took on her dad's feelings of homelessness like "a gene for being left handed." There's a spiritual tenacity to these books, a way of seeking backward, forward, and in the present all at once. In his essay "Inheritance," Alexander Chee reckons with a trust he inherited when his father died far too young, a large sum of money that, while it lasted, made Chee feel both "invulnerable and doomed," and conjured complex associations with his father's father's wealth back in Korea. As the eldest son, Chee was expected to keep the family records, perform the *jesa*—an annual ceremony to honor the ancestors—and look after "the entire family, the living and the dead." Decades after his father's death, Chee performed his first *jesa*, of his own design. He created an altar, made an elaborate Korean meal, poured soju. He wrote a letter to his ancestors, "telling them how angry I was with them, asking them to tell me what they wanted from me. Then I burned the letter, to send it to them."

As time passed, Chee began to contemplate his grandparents' lives under Japanese occupation in a new way. He'd grown up knowing that, when they met in elementary school, Chee's grandmother admired his grandfather's vocal insistence on the importance of ancestor worship for Koreans. What Chee didn't realize, he wrote in a later essay, was that his grandfather's evangelism "could have sent him to jail or cost him his life." However grudging Chee's *jesa*, it was the fulfillment of a dream a grandfather had long before his grandson existed. To me this echo is almost unbearably touching, because so many of us spend our lives struggling with or against our ancestors' dreams without knowing precisely how or why.

MY MOST TENDER ANIMAL self developed on drives to nursery school, my mom's cigarette smoke clouding around us, her keychain jingling as we talked. It developed as I sat on Granny's lap, twisting the rings on her fingers while she reminisced about growing up hungry, as I ate cut peaches at her kitchen table and the attic fan dragged hot air through the room. It developed as my grandfather introduced me to pralines, molasses on biscuits, and fishing from his little boat. It developed nights sitting across from my father in his study, the pendulum of his wall clock ticking, while he shouted and I dug my fingernails into my palms. And it developed as I sat under a tree in our backyard, watching manatees drift along the canal, from a particular spot on earth I doubt I will set foot on again. These experiences, these memories, are part of my inheritance.

Humans throughout time have believed objects and places to have mystical significance, but in the rational, capitalist West, many of us are taught to think of these relationships in terms of rights of possession, what is codified, so that what is left behind no longer belongs to us. As a girl in Miami, I felt especially alive sneaking into an enormous cemetery near a friend's house, where we'd been forbidden by our demon-obsessed mothers to go. The bright bouquets of flowers, set against rows of somber headstones and our awareness of the bones beneath, lured us there again and again until our mothers had a falling-out. My friend told me that your hair and fingernails continue to grow after you die, and we stood in horrified respectful silence, imagining all the skeletons.

I don't recall visiting a grave any other time during my childhood. In my mom's view, cemeteries are pointless and morbid. After death, only the spirit matters, the spirit up in heaven with God. Any inclination to the contrary fills her with rage. When my step-grandmother died in 2016 following a long decline, my mom was increasingly furious every time we spoke before I flew down for the funeral. "I'm *not sad*," she shouted at me that first day. "I'm *glad!* She's *with Jesus now.*" In the next call, she was even more livid, recounting the indignities of the day. *So many people were coming for the funeral.* My stepdad had *bathed his mother's body,* of all things, and was *still sitting in the room with it.* Later came the crowning outrage. "And then the *neighbors came by*"—she paused for emphasis—*"with their long faces"*—another indignant pause—"to *tell me how sorry they are!*" She was literally screaming by the end of this sentence. She had adored my step-grandmother but did not attend her funeral.

My mom enjoys recounting my request, at age three, to stay home from school the day after one of our cats was killed by a car. Apparently I wanted to sit with the body until the city came to pick it up. "She's just going to decay and rot," my mom told me. "But I want to watch her decay and rot," I said. My mom likes this story because I couldn't have known what "decay and rot" meant, and so she sees the request as hilariously outlandish, whereas I relate to my young self's desire to sit with our cat and bear witness rather than putting her out on the porch in a bag. In the way of daughters, I eventually reacted to my mom's insistence that burial and bones don't matter by becoming convinced that they do. Then I set about immersing myself in research to confirm I was right.

MANY OF MY PEOPLE came to these shores from England, an island invaded and conquered so early and often, it's impossible to speak with certainty of traditions indigenous to the place. Whatever practices existed there in antiquity were at least partly overlaid by those of the Vikings and the Romans. A later resurgence of paganism that accompanied the invasion (or, as some see it, triumphant return) of the Anglo-Saxons after the Romans withdrew was plainly influenced by the previous successions of occupying forces and the Saxons themselves. By the seventh century, Christianity dominated once again, and whatever pagan traditions remained in England were largely overwritten or driven underground. Records embedded in Roman writings and Christianized grimoires (medieval and later books of spells, demonology, and ritual magic) are so syncretized that their value as history is questionable.

Prehistoric monuments like Stonehenge, whose stones are aligned with astronomical phenomena, reveal that the earth and heavens figured into ancient spiritual practices of people on that land. Cremated remains establish Stonehenge as a cemetery, but the erasure of ancient religious practices and the destruction and reinterpretation of religious texts obscure how ancestors figured into all of this, if they did. Like many people newly interested in these histories, I feel sure ancestors were revered, but I can't prove it. And while I am inclined to resent the Christian church's role in this erasure, some scholars are quick to point out that the record doesn't quite support the idea that the church curtailed clear, established practices of this kind. My suspicions percolate along anyhow.

Beyond England, my ancestors came from Scotland, Ireland, France, the Netherlands, and no doubt many places I don't know about. As of this writing in early 2021, 23andMe has amended my ancestry assignments again, to 91.4 percent British and Irish ancestry (up from 53.5), 5.3 percent French and German (down from 29.3), 2.9 percent broadly Northwestern European (down from 14.4), zero Southern European (down from 2), 0.3 percent Levantine, and 0.1 percent unassigned. I don't lend much credence to these assignments, which according to the site look back only about two hundred years.

By then, every ancestor of mine I know of had already migrated to this continent. In all my years of searching, the most "recent" arrival I've found to these shores was a Frenchman who had settled in Louisiana by 1821, when he married and impregnated my fourth great-grandmother and then ran off, probably back to France. Even that large chunk of "British and Irish" only tells me so much. Like us, people in the past moved around; populations were not static. The Celts entered Ireland only around 500 B.C.

By the time my people began to arrive in the American colonies, the idea of a spiritual connection to ancestral land would have been, to most if not all of them, ungodly, pagan, and forbidden. Many of my ancestors were fervent Protestants. Some were Puritans who left England before feudalism was abolished. Whatever connection they may have felt to the places where our ancestors were buried, my people turned their attention to taking this land from the people who already lived on and cared for it. They viewed the earth as a commodity they had the God-given right to exploit. By this reasoning, they sanctified their subjugation of the land and its people.

By the late 1800s, bodies of people indigenous to the area of Western Massachusetts my ancestors had colonized were being unceremoniously dug up and the skeletons displayed "in libraries, museums, and physical anthropology laboratories," as evidence of the false claim that "the Indians" were extinct. In reality, despite the genocide of many Nonotuck people and the displacement of many others, some moved to the periphery of the colonial settlement and continued to live on their traditional lands, near the sacred bones of their ancestors.

MANY PREHISTORIC HUMANS BURIED their dead with care. Even some Neanderthal burials suggest intentionality. But the exact content and meaning of these practices is impossible to trace more than 40,000 years later. Scholars disagree about composition and meaning of still-ancient but considerably more-recent practices, too.

As I began researching funeral rituals and reverence for family dead in the West, I discovered the Victorian historian Fustel de Coulanges's 1864 book, *The Ancient City*, which posits that in ancient Greece and Rome, "the ancestor remained in the midst of his relatives; invisible, but always present, he continued to make a part of the family, and to be its father." Relying on ancient writings from classical Greece and beyond, de Coulanges argued that patriarchs were buried steps from the front door of the family home or even beneath the hearth. A character from Euripides's *Helena* greets his father in his tomb. "I buried you, Proteus, in this passageway so that I could address you," he says, "and always, as I enter and leave the house . . . call on you, father." A dialogue attributed to Plato speaks of a time when people buried their dead in the home.

Contemporary archaeologists haven't found evidence of these

burials near the home, and many modern scholars reject ancient literary references as primary evidence of funeral practices. Instead,
scholars tend to insist on physical evidence. In a different context, the
historian Charles W. King pushes back against this demand, asking
in his 2020 study, *The Ancient Roman Afterlife,* whether, given the
small number of surviving graves compared to actual deaths, ancient
graves are really more representative or "statistically valid" than literary sources. So I concede that the evidence doesn't show burials of
the kind Euripides or Plato describe. Perhaps those descriptions
were fanciful or mistaken or home-burial practices weren't widespread. But many scholars altogether rebuff the assertion that ancient Greeks and Romans venerated ancestors in any significant way,
and I side with recent works that survey the evidence and come to
the opposite conclusion.

In both Greece and Rome, funeral rites were often connected to
inheritance of land and wealth but had spiritual significance, too. In
The Restless Dead, Sarah Iles Johnston writes that ancient Greeks
believed funeral practices "to benefit the dead," whereas withholding rites resulted in "an unhappy afterlife for the disembodied soul,"
who might become angry and vindictive. Familial dead usually pro-
tected the living family, but neglected ancestors could transform
into *elasteros,* who persecuted the living family with curses like
madness and infertility. The dead could also "suffer the consequences of transgressions that they committed while alive," but rites
performed by the living could remove this burden.

Funeral offerings included food and drinks and sometimes also
everyday objects like jewelry, flowers, swords, and mirrors. As Johnston says, it's "hard to avoid the conclusion" that some of these "were
expected to be useful in the afterlife," particularly given stories of
the "dead demanding objects that were forgotten or omitted at the
time of burial." In the days, weeks, and years following the funeral,
rites continued to be performed at intervals at the grave, and some
also seem to have been performed at home. Johnston posits that
purification rituals probably helped the recent family dead join the

more distant *tritopatores*, ancestral spirits—"thrice-fathers" or great-grandfathers—that had "passed into a new, pure state of existence," thanks to their descendants' offerings and acts, which likely included anointing of statues or altars.

Charles W. King rebuts scholarship that insists *manes*—ancient Roman deities—were always collective, arguing that Roman families worshipped dead individual humans, too. Some, but not all, *manes* worshipped were ancestors of the body. As in ancient Greece, rites in Rome were a family religious duty. Death extended reciprocity of family obligation into a new form. With proper rites, the family member became a deity who could extend life, but neglecting the dead would "remove their protection and thus hasten death." Without funeral rites, a spirit "was trapped in the vicinity of its physical remains." Cicero "presents the heaping of earth" on the grave as "the minimum necessary element" for a grave to become sacred, and in King's reading, the burial and accompanying sacrifice of a pig seems to have commenced "worship of the new *manes*."

Where ancestor veneration survives today, rituals are often practiced collectively in cemeteries—as with the Day of the Dead in Mexico, Tomb-Sweeping Day in China, and All Souls' Day in New Orleans—and also sometimes at ancestral altars. Burials near the home do persist in places. Some Christians in Cameroon bury their dead in front of their homes, as their Fang ancestors once did. Even in the United States, some families maintain cemeteries on family land. But so many of us in the Christianized West have lost a sense of ongoing connection to family dead. After shunting them into cemeteries, we walk away. We believe our relationship to them dies when they do. What if we decided otherwise?

IN THE BIBLICAL BOOK of Genesis, Rachel steals her father's teraphim, household gods, the existence of which are mentioned without censure. There's substantial evidence that family religion was practiced alongside devotion to Yahweh in ancient Israel, in private at least and possibly even in public, until it became seen as a threat to the dominant religion and kings and prophets tried to stamp it out. Even those efforts were inconsistent—and, possibly as late as the first century A.D., seemingly ineffective.

As the story of Rachel and the household gods goes, Rachel's husband, Jacob, has spent twenty years working for her father, Laban. Jacob feels he's received little in return, apart from two wives, the one he chose (Rachel) and the one he was tricked into marrying (Rachel's sister, Leah). While Jacob stews about the unfairness of his lot, the Lord appears and instructs him to "Return to the land of your fathers and to your kindred." Rachel and Leah agree that they should go.

Before they flee, Rachel takes the teraphim while Laban is away shearing his sheep. A week or so later, Laban catches up with the caravan and denounces his son-in-law, asking why Jacob absconded with his daughters. Laban also expresses some compassion for Jacob, suggesting his son-in-law has "longed greatly for your father's house." He seems chastened, too, telling Jacob that "the God of your father spoke to me last night." But why, he asks Jacob, "did you steal my gods?" Unaware that Rachel was the thief, Jacob tells Laban to search the caravan. Perhaps in a nod to how serious the theft of teraphim is considered to be, Jacob promises his father-in-law that "Any one with whom you find your gods shall not live." Laban goes from tent to tent, searching, but Rachel has stowed the gods in her camel's saddle and tells her father that she can't dismount because she has her period. In the end, he and Jacob make peace, and Laban leaves without the gods.

Many argumentative gymnastics have been performed over time in trying to reconcile the passage with Judeo–Christian monotheism, but the scholar Susannah Rutherglen makes a strong argument that Rachel took the gods for the most logical reason: They represent a connection to her ancestors, to her father and his forebears, blood relatives she's leaving behind. Rutherglen detects meaning in the fact that Rachel's deception "involves her own blood—the one link to Laban that Jacob cannot sever."

> The objects and symbolism of family lineage are too strong here to be fortuitous: a man speaking to his blood daughter, who is about to go far away from him; the daughter, fertile because she is menstruating, the mother of the twelve tribes of Israel; her blood, which is half her father's, concealing objects of reverence for one's ancestors. It is difficult to imagine a more potent convergence of images centering on Rachel's inextricable bond to the hearth and lineage of Laban.

The spiritual practices of women in Rachel's time were treated as secondary, as the spiritual practices of women still are today, and because women were less likely to know how to write, those practices were more rarely recorded.

The Book of Judges mentions that a man named Micah had teraphim and in the next verse suggests that, because Israel had no king at the time, "every man did what was right in his own eyes." In another Old Testament story, in the Book of Samuel, King David's first wife, Michal, places a teraphim in the bed to trick her father, Saul, as David flees through a window. Teraphim were prohibited three Old Testament books later, in Second Kings, by King Josiah, but reappeared in Hosea, where the absence of teraphim and king are connected to the exile of the people of Israel. Much later, in the first century A.D., Josephus mentioned the custom of Jews taking household gods on their wanderings into new lands. Biblical condemnation of veneration practices surrounding the dead may have been a strategy to shore up the centrality and exclusive role of Yahweh.

SOME YEARS AFTER RACHEL stole the household gods, she died at Bethel, and Jacob marked her tomb with a standing stone. According to the historian Francesca Stavrakopoulou, author of *Land of Our Fathers: The Roles of Ancestor Veneration in Biblical Land Claims*, while these stones were typically placed at temples rather than graves in Israel, they were common to "many death cultures throughout ancient West Asia and the eastern Mediterranean." Monuments inscribed in Egyptian, Mesopotamian, and Phoenicio–Punic explicitly allude to the stones' "cultic, mortuary associations." For example, an Ugaritic tale describes "duties of the ideal son" in what is now Syria to include setting up a stone "for a divine ancestor." Ugarit ancestors remained part of the family in death and were often buried beneath the house and referred to as "the god of the father."

Ancient standing stones survive in Africa, Asia, and Europe, although their original significance is often uncertain. Stavrakopoulou acknowledges ambiguity surrounding the extent to which Middle Eastern standing stones were considered to "manifest, deify, or merely symbolize or represent the dead." But while many scholars have been puzzled by Jacob's decision "to bury Rachel at the roadside rather than transport her corpse to the patriarchal tomb," Stavrakopoulou argues that he did so to render Rachel's burial place "a monumental cult site." The "territorial potency of the dead" is often invoked, Stavrakopoulou contends, to imbue Yahweh with an ownership claim similar to that of family dead.

Of course, sacred ancestral gods and relics, such as the teraphim, *manes,* or *Tritopatores,* were by no means unique to ancient Israel, Rome, or Greece. I'm focusing on these traditions because of my own background and historical ignorance and because so many of us Protestants who descend from European Christians have been taught to view ancestor reverence as something exotic, foreign, and inaccessible. Given what we know of humans across the earth and across time, we in the contemporary West who do not venerate ancestors or minister to them in the afterlife are the aberration, not the other way around. Ancestor reverence of one kind or another was practiced in ancient Babylon, ancient Egypt, ancient India, ancient China, and ancient Mesopotamia, as well as among the Bantu and in many other places and cultures. Ancestor veneration survives now in many parts of the world, sometimes merged with monotheistic religions.

Relics of the Fang, Kota, and Mahongwe peoples, among others of Central Africa, are the unacknowledged underpinnings of the most celebrated works of Western modernism. Picasso, Matisse, and their contemporaries marveled over and were deeply influenced by African carvings of human figures that contained (or were attached to a platform containing) sacred relics: an ancestor's skull and other physical remains. By some accounts, the sculptures were meant to guard the bones; by others, they were intended to evoke the ancestor's spirit. Picasso acknowledged his debt to the original artisans more than the other well-known modernist artists did. His "'greatest artistic emotions,'" he said in 1917, "'were aroused when the sublime beauty of the sculptures created by the anonymous artists of Africa was suddenly revealed to me. These works of religious art, which are both impassioned and rigorously logical, are the most beautiful of all the products of the human imagination.'" Yet curator Alisa LaGamma observes in *Eternal Ancestors: The Art of the Central African Reliquary*, a collection of essays published by the Metropolitan Museum of Art for an exhibition by the same name, that "there is virtually no record of any curiosity" from Picasso and his contemporaries "concerning the original significance and function of these objects." And, in fact, the objects were not art; they were sacred-ritual objects.

Many of the carved reliquary figures remain in the possession of museums and collectors, rather than in the hands of the descendants whose ancestors they were created to honor. A common justification, concisely articulated on the website of the Stanley Museum of Art, is that because the bones and not the figures were sacred, there was "no apparent contradiction to individuals in selling what in effect was the tombstone of their ancestors for considerable profit to art dealers." Perhaps. But most of the Fang and others selling the carvings didn't know how valuable the works already were to Western artists. Missionaries insisted to Fang elders that the artifacts "were worthless and were to be destroyed," even as the missionaries collected the objects, according to LaGamma. In 2020, a century after Picasso's praise, Sotheby's sold a single "Fang–Betsi ancestor head" for $3.5 million and heralded the price as a "testament to the sculpture's aesthetic legacy in shaping the style of Western modernism."

Only the sculptures had value to "the late-nineteenth-century European colonialists who first collected many of the works," as a 2007 *New York Times* article puts it. The remains were usually "tossed away." But the Metropolitan Museum of Art collection includes three figures that still include the sacred bones of ancestors. This strikes me as an apt metaphor for the spiritual vacuum at the center of the dominant white culture in the West. Drawn to the beauty of someone else's ancestral relics, we have taken the objects without respect for their spiritual significance, and in so doing we deprive other people of the connection with ancestors that we ourselves lack. Judging by some popular Disney movies of the last few decades—*Coco, Moana,* and *Mulan*—many of us yearn for this connection but view it as some exotic fairy tale for children.

Chapter 23

UNACKNOWLEDGED
REMAINS

———

THE CLOSEST I CAME TO GRANNY'S BODY AT HER FUNERAL was an enormous closed casket. Though I'd known she was dying, I had trouble processing the loss. After the memorial, I moved a short distance from the grave and watched as men lowered the casket into the ground and shoveled earth on top of it. From the parking lot, my mom watched me watching them, her arms crossed, her mouth a grim line of disapproval. The workers also seemed perplexed by my presence, maybe even offended by it. "Do most people not stay?" I asked. "You're the only one," one man said.

Granny was buried in Western North Carolina, in a Baptist cemetery down the street from my mom's house, but very far from Dallas, where Granny lived nearly all her life and had made arrangements for a cemetery plot decades before. The decision made me sad, though the spot is beautiful, with mountain views she would have liked. Every time I visit Granny's grave now, I wonder how my distance from her remains and the rest of my family dead affects my sense of myself and my relationship to the world. I think about all of us in the West in a similar predicament.

My preoccupation with unacknowledged remains extends to Max's ancestors. Luckily, I married into a family that, like me, loves cemeteries. Some of Max's forebears migrated to New York City from Switzerland in the mid-to-late 1800s and are buried in a cemetery not too far by car from our house in Queens, though the actual location of their graves has proven elusive. Several years ago, we went looking for the parents of these ancestors in the old country.

On a warm summer day, Max, my stepdaughter, and I visited the town cemetery in Bubendorf, with my mother-in-law and her partner, and one of my brothers-in-law and his partner. Driving over from Basel, we arrived at a hill covered with orderly graves alongside a modern-looking church. Cattle grazed above us, bells clanging, as we climbed into the rows to find the headstones.

The first graves we passed were entombments from the 1970s and later, so we split up to start from different places, hoping to locate the older section. No matter how far in we got, we found more of the same. A couple exited the church, and I approached them with questions. Was there an older cemetery in town? There was not. Was there another section farther off where we might find eighteenth-century graves? Again, no. The graves were only *leased* at a person's death, they explained. The deceased was entombed until the lease ran out. Then the spot was rented to the relatives of a more recent corpse.

What happened, I asked, to the bodies when the lease was up?

The couple shook their heads. They didn't know, they said, and hurried away.

Later, I learned that twenty-five-year leases on cemetery plots are the norm nowadays in tiny Switzerland, apart from families who own or have long-term leases on graves that usually house the remains of generations of dead. When the time on the short-term sites runs out, according to the Swiss Center of North America, the remains are typically placed in a communal site, usually at the cemetery. The headstone is returned to the family or, if they don't want it, crushed as road aggregate.

Too many bodies in too little space is a problem throughout Western Europe. Many countries have instituted grave term limits, and Greece's three years may be the shortest repose allowed to a corpse. The writer Alex Mar has written about the tension between Greek law and the prevailing religion. The Greek Orthodox Church holds that cremation is pagan, that "the body, as the 'temple of the spirit,' must be buried whole to make resurrection possible." A permanent plot cost more than $200,000 in 2011. When no one was able to attend the exhumation of Mar's grandparents after their three-year term was up, their remains "were placed in a mass grave and dissolved with chemicals."

HISTORICALLY, THE CONNECTION BETWEEN humans and the land was obvious. People were of the land, nourished by it and buried in it, and thus nourished it in return. The earth was kin. The last couple of decades in the West have seen a growing desire to embrace the inevitability of rejoining the land when our time comes. This death-positivity movement brings hope that we can find a better way of returning to the earth. But so far, even in some green cemeteries, human bodies are a problem. Modern corpses don't decay as quickly as they would have historically. Decades pass, and when new bodies are added, the old ones are as preserved as if they were mummified. No one is entirely sure why. Is it the preservatives in our food? The depletion and degradation of the land over centuries?

The conundrum strikes me as emblematic of the ways many of us in the West have separated ourselves not only from the humans who came before us but from the earth as a whole. The earth doesn't know how to take us back the way it once did. All these generations since Europeans first set foot on this land, writes the biologist Robin Wall Kimmerer, a member of the Citizen Potawatomi Nation, in *Braiding Sweetgrass,* and "some of the wisest of Native elders still puzzle over the people who came to our shores. They look at the toll on the land and say, 'The problem with these new people is that they don't have both feet on the shore. One is still on the boat. They don't seem to know whether they're staying or not.'"

Many in this country, like my mom, won't commit to the land because they're waiting to be raptured up. Some of these evangelicals implicitly celebrate the degradation of what they see as their earthly home because they believe its destruction will hasten their liberation from this lowly sphere and resurrection to heaven. But the problem is much more far-reaching. Most of us in the West have been taught to see trees and birds and flowers and mountains as "nature" and ourselves and the habitations we build as something apart from nature, but we are also nature. We are all of the land. Our ancestors back through time have already returned to the earth. We have disavowed that kinship, too.

Part Seven

SPIRITUALITY

Chapter 24

THE WITCH

——

TWENTY YEARS AGO, I SEARCHED MY GREAT-GRANDMOTHER Alma's name online. Up came a tree tracing her line to a notorious accused witch in Puritan-era Massachusetts: Mary Bliss Parsons, my ninth great-grandmother. I soon found a University of Massachusetts website devoted to Mary, featuring a portrait of a woman in late middle age wearing a black pointy hat. She held a bouquet and small book, perhaps a Bible. Eventually, I learned that the painting wasn't really of Mary, but that day I searched the face for similarities to Granny's, my mom's, my sister's, and mine. She didn't look like us, exactly, but, with her large face and high cheekbones, she didn't look unlike us, either.

Mary was accused of consorting with spirits. This history fascinated and disturbed me because, when I was eight years old, my mom reported seeing angels and demons. God's messengers appeared rarely, but Satan's minions were everywhere. She described desiccated gray "Antichrist devils" that she said possessed my father and, through him, also me. "I bind you, Satan, in Jesus's name," she screamed. She insisted that she really saw these spirits. If only I shed my doubting demon, she said, I would see them, too.

I berated myself for my lack of spiritual certainty and discernment. I longed for proof that my mom was right and that the people at my father's church who told me that she would go to hell for interacting with the spirit world were mistaken. As I grew up, I started to fear I might have a conversion one day, too. Would I have visions? Start a church in my living room? Roam the streets, preaching salvation?

By coincidence, in the mid-nineties, my sister and her spouse moved to Northampton, down the street from the cemetery where many of our Parsons ancestors are buried. On a late November day a few months after I learned of our connection to the place, we walked there to wander among the graves and found a Parsons family monument commemorating Mary, her husband, and their descendants. Many old family headstones were no longer legible, but a marker for Mary's eldest son, Joseph, Jr., my eighth great-grandfather, was perfectly clear, etched with a winged skull. Later we learned that my sister-in-law has ancestors in the cemetery, too.

Our connection to the place felt uncanny in part because my sister and her spouse had moved to Northampton spontaneously, after other plans had fallen through. It was the only move either of them ever made like this: to a place they'd never been, with enormous optimism and no planning. They'd packed up a moving van and headed north, not knowing where they'd live or what they'd do for work but confident they'd be happy, and they were. They settled a short walk from where Joseph once lived.

In recent decades, the old house on the Parsons's original home lot has become a museum commemorating Joseph and Mary and the early history of the town. Known as the "Historic Parsons House," thought to have been built by one of their grandsons, it's the place where I poured the wine as an offering of prayer and apology.

THAT THE FAMILY IS celebrated in Northampton nowadays is ironic, given the infamy of Mary Bliss Parsons in her own time. The historical documents agree that she was beautiful and talented but, as a genealogy compiled by one of her descendants puts it, "not very amiable." In *Entertaining Satan: Witchcraft and the Culture of Early New England,* the historian John Putnam Demos assembles Puritan-era testimony of her "harsh, or openly accusatory" manner.

In this, Mary may have taken after her mother, Margaret Bliss, also a formidable person. A Bliss family genealogy disputed on other grounds describes Margaret as a "good-looking woman, with a square oblong face," a person of "superior abilities, great resolution, and uncommon enterprise," and "vigor of mind and constitution." Demos reports that Margaret more than tripled the "relatively meagre" resources left by her husband at his death, despite also being left with seven minor children. She was litigious, frequently prevailing in the many lawsuits she filed concerning property, contracts, and the interests of two grandsons. "It made an unusual record by any standards," Demos says, "and, for a widow, perhaps a unique one."

Margaret and Thomas Bliss set sail from England for the Puritan colonies in 1635. Mary, their third child, was probably between eight and ten years old when her family arrived in Boston that year. Ultimately, they settled in Hartford. Little is known about Mary's life before she married Joseph Parsons of Springfield, Massachusetts, in 1646, and moved to join him. Joseph, as I've mentioned, was a trader and businessman, canny and useful to the prominent Pynchon family but not in himself a posh guy.

A year after Mary moved to Springfield, she gave birth to Joseph, Jr., their first child. Despite the new baby, her adjustment to the place was rough. In 1649, she had another child, or possibly twins, who died. Her father passed the following winter. A different Mary Parsons of the town, no relation, was accused of being a witch. My Mary, Demos says, "was herself deeply affected by these proceedings. She suffered fits (though beyond the usual age for such experiences); she roamed about in a distracted manner; she talked of encounters with evil 'spirits.'"

Her husband doesn't seem to have been a source of comfort. On the contrary, as Demos recounts, Mary and Joseph were "frequently and notoriously at odds with one another." One public episode in the town "amounted to a family free-for-all. Joseph was 'beating one of his little children, for losing its shoe,' when Mary came running 'to save it, because she had beaten it before as she said.' Whereupon Joseph thrust her away, and the two of them continued to struggle until he 'had in a sort beaten [her].'" At another point, Joseph "sought to confine her to their house."

Later, a barrel-maker who'd visited their home in this era testified that Joseph accused Mary of being "led by an evil spirit," to which she replied that "he was the cause of it by locking her in the cellar" with the spirits and leaving her there. Mary allegedly told the barrel-maker that she "threw the bedstaff" at the spirits, followed by "the bedclothes and her pillow, and yet they would not be gone." Later, while she was doing chores, the spirits "appeared to her like poppets."

LIKE MY MOTHER AMONG Miami evangelicals many years later, Mary was an infamous character in Springfield, fodder for eerie stories and legends. Imagining Mary's dynamic with Joseph, I can easily substitute my parents for the two of them.

According to a neighbor, Joseph confided that he would hide the key from Mary but she could always find it and that Mary "'would go out in the night and that when she went out a woman [i.e., a spirit] went out with her and came in with her.'" The neighbor said Joseph tried to spin this by offering it as evidence that "God preserves his [children] with his Angels." Another neighbor testified of a man who claimed to have followed Mary "in her fit" and seen her walk on water. While he "was up to the knees," Mary "was not wet."

Given the spectacle Mary and Joseph made in Springfield, it's not surprising that they moved to the new settlement of Northampton around 1654. They must have hoped to start again and leave the gossip and spirits behind. Despite Mary's notoriety, her husband Joseph's fortunes continued to rise. In *Entertaining Satan*, Demos details Joseph's many successful business enterprises, including as a fur trader, retailer, "part owner of the first gristmill in Northampton and also owner of its first sawmill." He was granted a license to run an ordinary, where customers could eat prepared meals and drink liquor. Later in life he "bought a warehouse and ships' wharf in Boston," and by the time of his death in 1683 he owned land and other properties in several towns, was worth more than £2,000, and had given some of his older children "handsome 'settlements' of their own." Much of his wealth and land came from cheating, displacing, and murdering many Nonotuck, Pocumtuck, and other Native people of the area and helping others do so.

Demos theorizes that the Parsons family was disliked in Northampton for Joseph's success, for flourishing above their station. The Bliss genealogy also suggests that jealousy motivated the gossip and charges that came. Joseph ultimately evolved a spotty reputation of his own. He was in and out of court, frequently in actions involving business issues but also on personal matters. Though often the plaintiff, he appeared "occasionally as a defendant." According to court documents Demos cites, in 1664, three years after obtaining the license to run the ordinary, Joseph was "admonished" for "lascivious carriage to some women of Northampton." In the months that followed he was fined for his "high contempt of authority," his "contemptuous behavior toward the Northampton commissioners and toward the selectmen," and his "disorderly carriage."

But the family settled in Northampton about a decade before these rebukes of Joseph, and witchcraft accusations against Mary surfaced practically upon their arrival. She gave birth to a healthy baby boy, Ebenezer—"the first English child born in the town"—on May 1, 1655. Later the same month, her neighbor, Sarah Bridgman, a fellow transplant from Springfield who'd known the Parsonses there, had a baby who died. The grieving mother told townsfolk that Mary had cursed the baby.

Mary's mother, Margaret, confronted Sarah. Rather than backing down, Sarah insisted that she had been told Mary was a witch, recounting a story that after Mary had argued with a blind man in Springfield, "'the child of the blind man had a sounding [?] fit.'"

Joseph sought to protect the family's name by filing a slander suit. This approach was tricky and fraught. While the "immediate outcome of [slander] actions was usually favorable to the plaintiff," Demos writes, the "long-range effects were mixed."

At trial, Sarah testified that while in bed, with her baby on her lap, she heard "a great blow on the door, and that very instant . . . my child changed." She "told my girl I was afraid my child would die." Peering through a hole in the door, Sarah "saw to my apprehension two women pass by the door with white cloths on their heads, then I concluded my child would die indeed. . . . They made me think there is wickedness in the place." Sarah and her husband sought to tie the baby's demise to Mary. As proof, they claimed that when their elder son suffered an injury and "'was in grievous torture about a month,'" the son feared that "'Goody Parsons would pull off his knee'" and that he insisted, "'there she sits on the shelf.'" Another neighbor testified that several suspicious deaths of animals followed altercations he and his wife had with Mary. His cow died after a dispute between Mary and his wife over yarn that became mysteriously knotted as the wife spun it for Mary; his sow died after Mary confronted him for mocking a public altercation she'd had with her husband in Springfield; and his ox died from a rattlesnake bite after Mary chided him for mistreating oxen sold to him by her brother. "She said you put them in the middle where they are always under the whip," he recalled. "I told her they were not any way wronged," but "she went away in anger."

On the other hand, three women contended that Sarah's baby was "sick as soon as it was born." Sarah herself was said by the women to have thought that the infant "'had taken cold,'" that from the start he manifested an unusual "'looseness.'" And while Sarah had invoked the magistrate John Pynchon, Joseph's business partner, as suggesting that Mary "'could not be right,'" Pynchon rebutted Sarah's memory. "'I accordingly declare to my remembrance that I never said any such word,'" he testified. "'Neither do I remember any reports that I have heard which have given me occasion to speak any such words of Goodwife Parsons.'" At first more neighbors had taken Bridgman's side at the 1956 trial, but several changed sides, joining Joseph, Mary, and their powerful allies. Demos suggests that, because of the Pynchons, the social "rank and prestige" was on Mary's side from the beginning and "may have tipped the balance." Whatever the reason, the Parsonses ultimately prevailed in the slander case. Still, the verdict was far from the conclusive exculpation they sought.

SUSPICION AND ILL-FEELING ROILED until new witchcraft claims landed Mary in court again eighteen years later. The rumblings began in Northampton, in 1674, when a daughter of Sarah Bridgman (of the erstwhile slander lawsuit) died unexpectedly at age twenty-two. The young woman's husband and father contended that she "came to her end by some unlawful and unnatural means"—through "some evil instrument."

The court opened a criminal inquiry into the matter. The husband testified; the father offered a statement. Mary herself chose to appear, according to records, "'she having intimation that such things were bruited abroad, and that she should be called in question . . . she voluntarily made her appearance in court, desiring to clear herself of such an execrable crime.'" The following January, the county magistrates took additional testimony. Again Mary asserted, as they put it, "'her own innocency . . . how clear she was of such a crime, and that the righteous God knew her innocency—with whom she had left her cause.'" The bereft widower, Sarah's son-in-law, again offered accounts, "many and various, some of them being demonstrations of witchcraft, and others sorely reflecting upon Mary Parsons as being guilty that way."

The magistrates concluded that a Boston court had jurisdiction in the matter and ordered that Mary's body be inspected for "'any marks of witchcraft.'" The resulting report was not disclosed in Northampton but forwarded to the Boston court along with the other records. In Boston, Mary was imprisoned during the 1675 trial. The indictment reads: "Mary Parsons, the wife of Joseph Parsons, . . . being instigated by the Devil, hath . . . entered into familiarity with the Devil, and committed several acts of witchcraft on the person or persons of one or more." The record reflects that she appeared in the courtroom, "holding up her hand and pleading not guilty." The jury consisted of strangers, "twelve men, of no particular distinction, from Boston and the surrounding towns." No record of their thinking or of evidence from the trial survives, only the verdict: not guilty.

Later that year, Mary's son Ebenezer was killed at age twenty in an uprising led by the Wampanoag chief Metacom, often called King Philip's War. According to the Bliss family genealogy, Mary's accusers back in Northampton saw divine judgment at work in Ebenezer's death: "'Behold, though human judges may be bought off, God's vengeance neither turns aside nor slumbers,'" they said. (Given the way Ebenezer's father, Joseph, swindled, displaced, and butchered the Pocumtuck and other people native to the area, justice may have been meted out that day, but probably not by God.)

Ebenezer's death was considered particularly significant because he was Mary's child who'd lived when Sarah Bridgman's baby had died, a living symbol of the original accusations.

MARY AND JOSEPH LEFT Northampton and returned to Springfield a few years before Joseph's death in 1683, but local suspicion that Mary was a witch held strong.

In 1702, an enslaved woman preserved in historical memory as "Betty Negro" apparently told one of Mary's grandsons that "'his grandmother had killed two persons over the river and half-killed the Colonel, and that his mother was half a witch.'" The boy's father, Mary's son-in-law, sought an indictment against Betty for "foul language striking his son." The proceedings were a family operation. Mary's son Joseph (my eighth great-grandfather) was one of the two justices. John Pynchon (Joseph Parsons's erstwhile business partner) was the other. According to the brief record, Betty confessed. The judges found her "very culpable for her base tongue and words as aforesaid" and sentenced her "to be well whipped on the naked body by the constable with ten lashes well laid on: which was performed accordingly by constable Thomas Bliss," Mary's brother.

I didn't realize how prevalent slavery was in colonial Massachusetts until I learned that my own relations orchestrated this appalling pageant, a warning by the Parsons family and its allies. They brutalized a Black woman to silence the white townspeople who'd originated the gossip. To exalt Mary, they served up a woman with far less power.

To some degree, this ploy seems to have worked. Nearly a decade later, Mary's granddaughter, also named Mary, married Ebenezer Bridgman, the grandson of Sarah Bridgman. The elder Mary died three years later, in 1712. Her granddaughter's children were named Joseph, Ebenezer, and Mary. I wonder how many of Mary's descendants have shared her blunt ways, her visions of spirits, her empathy toward animals, her poor choice in men and reliance on those men, and her willingness to inflict violence to preserve herself. The echoes in my own life, centuries later, still astound me. What would Mary make of them?

Chapter 25

GENERATIONAL
CURSES

———

IN MY EARLIEST MEMORIES, MY FAMILY DIDN'T GO TO CHURCH. God was a focus in our house only at meals, when my father thanked "the heavenly father" for our food, and at bedtime, when I had to say my prayers. Soon I began to ask questions. Why did God have so many names? How was he connected with the meal we were eating? What was my soul and why should I want him to take it?

My parents' vague answers raised more questions, I suspect for my mom as well as for me. It wasn't in her nature to go through ceremony she didn't fundamentally believe in, and saying grace was a legacy of my father's family, not hers. If her heart wasn't in it, how could mine be, I imagine her thinking. I don't remember for certain how old I was at this time, but judging by the letters she wrote, probably three.

At the Presbyterian church, my mom got "saved" and "born again." She initiated my father, who'd been raised Methodist but enthusiastically embraced the Presbyterians' idea of the "elect." He liked the idea that he was predestined for salvation, that the Lord had chosen him and his family, that we had only to accept the Lord and reap the full benefits of being the highly select sort of people

my father had always known himself and the rest of us (being affiliated with him) to be. And so, when I was not yet four, my newly
born-again parents sat me down to impart the good news about
Jesus, the son of God, who was born in a manger surrounded by
sheep and donkeys and ended up being nailed to a cross on a hill
and dying there. On the third day, he rose from the grave (you could
tell it really was Jesus from the nail holes), and he did all of this to
pay for my sins. If I accepted him into my heart, I would be re-
warded with everlasting life in heaven. Otherwise, I would burn
eternally with the devil in hell. So we needed, urgently, to pray.

"Right now?" I said, or something like that. I remember not feeling 100 percent ready to ask this undead man, with his holey ex-
tremities, to dwell inside me.

"Well, yes," I recall my mother saying. "Unless you'd like to spend
eternity in the lake of fire, crying out for a drink of water."

My father laid his hand on my shoulder. "We don't want that, do
we?"

"Daddy and I would hear you from our mansion up in heaven,"
my mother said. "But we wouldn't be able to help."

So I repeated after them, inviting Jesus into my bosom. And
then, for years afterward, I lay awake half the night, fearful of my
own heartbeat, worried about what the savior might be doing in
there. I was filled with doubt, which was a sin, but I was also anxious enough about eternal damnation to endlessly beg the Lord's
forgiveness for doubting.

THE VERY THING THAT drew my father to the Presbyterians—
the idea of being chosen for salvation that wasn't available to all—
was what sent my mother searching for a deeper, more personal
relationship with her savior. She read the Bible, cover to cover, and
then she read it again. Soon she'd accepted the Holy Spirit. She
spoke in tongues and laid hands on people to heal them by faith.
She heard directly from God. She saw demons. Yes, she said, sigh-

ing theatrically, she *literally* saw them. Satan's minions were *right there:* possessing news anchors, the Presbyterian minister, the man in the drive-through line at the bank teller, and the woman filling up her car at the gas station.

She said everyone was born with demons because our ancestors' sins created generational curses that attached to a family line for seven generations. Our own sins also brought on demons that would be passed down. There seemed to be yet another type of demon possession that was like catching a cold, if your spiritual hygiene wasn't good enough. You should never let anyone touch your head, for example, because demons were easily transmitted that way.

I wasn't sure how to protect myself the many times I sat on a church lady's sofa while my mom led exorcisms in the next room. I often knew the people being delivered, but through the wall their voices sounded low and raspy, or furious and shrieking. Occasionally there would be a scuffle, the sound of punching or shouting or things being thrown, or the person would weep or vomit. I was supposed to be doing my math homework, but it was hard to concentrate when I knew the demons could easily slip under the door or my mom might get hurt. My father didn't know about these sessions, but my mom's fervor alarmed him all the same. He commanded her to shut the church down. She ignored him. He'd come home during the closing songs on Wednesday nights, to the sound of fifty tambourines clanking out across the canal, and order everyone out of the living room. "Do I have to put up big, blinking lights?" he shouted once. "You're not welcome here." The congregation cleared out in a hurry.

Meanwhile, my mom believed that the Lord had called my father to co-pastor her church and that he was failing to heed God's plan. Often, we'd stand in our front yard during Sunday-morning shouting matches as my mom hollered at my father's demons. Afterward, my sister, father, and I walked down the street to mingle with Presbyterian congregants who'd just witnessed my parents' performance. We generally arrived as Sunday school was ending but in plenty of time for the main sermon. As we stood around during the coffee-and-donut hour beforehand, I could feel countless eyes on us.

My mom's scorn for the Presbyterians was steeped in class consciousness, the dislike of the child of a divorced working mom for what she saw as a dull, snobbish, idle group of social climbers. Their faith had no passion, she said. Jesus wouldn't have approved of them. They, in turn, believed that, as a woman, my mom sentenced herself to hell by presenting herself as a preacher. My parents' religious schism underscored for me the arbitrariness of religious conviction, but even so, I loved my mother with a ferocious intensity and wanted her to be right. Why couldn't I see what she saw?

Because I doubted, she said. I failed to "walk by faith and not by sight."

How could I have faith, though, if I simply didn't? "Faith is the substance of things hoped for," said a Bible verse she liked, "the evidence of things not seen." No matter how strenuously I pretended otherwise, faith didn't materialize.

A FEW YEARS LATER, God told my mom in a dream that she was supposed to marry my stepfather. He was a postal worker who went to her church. I didn't really know him, but I was excited at the prospect of a different father. As I got to know him, my optimism grew: At last I would have a caring father, a respectful and interested father, a fun father, a down-to-earth father, a kind mail-carrier patriarch rather than a lecturing tax lawyer. Maybe God was nicer than I thought!

My mom, sister, and I had moved into the apartment complex where my future stepfather and stepsister (and, soon, quite a few more of my mom's church members) lived. Even though my stepfather and his daughter had another apartment exactly like ours two floors down, they soon moved in with us. Sometimes a church member would knock on our door, looking for my mom. They would draw back in shock when my stepdad answered the door in his bathrobe. Not long after my parents' divorce was final, my mom and stepfather were married.

If I sometimes thought my stepfather seemed a little overenthusiastic about my sundress or watched me strangely, it didn't seem like a big deal in comparison with his compassion, his attention, the way he talked to me like a confidant rather than a child. I was twelve when he molested me, a couple of months after they married. I was lying on my bed, upset about something that had happened at school. He seemed at first to be trying to console me. As I realized what was happening, I froze with dread, I'm not sure for how long—fifteen minutes, half an hour? Things slowly but steadily advanced and I didn't move. It could have been far worse, but it was bad enough. Luckily my mom and sister arrived home, unknowingly interrupting. Through the window, he saw them walking across the field. He put his clothes back on and left the room.

Dinner that night was agony. Afterward, I told my mom. We were alone in the kitchen, washing dishes. I don't remember the words I used.

"Well, I guess I have to divorce him," she said. My stomach roiled with feeling. My mom would do that, leave her husband, *for me*? I felt prioritized and cared for, but, in the next second, the warmth in my gut turned molten with despair. We'd been miserable with my father. We'd lived in fear. And my mom's embarrassment at shacking up with my stepfather before they married, at being judged by her congregation and uncertain of my stepfather's intentions, was something I couldn't imagine her having to go through again. There was also the question of money. Apart from the church, my mom hadn't worked since before I was born. Granny paid the biggest chunk of our bills. "No," I said, "don't do that."

"If he would do that with you," she said, "he would do it with someone else."

I stood, dish towel in hand, pondering the terrible koan of her

words. If he would do it *with* me, he would do it *with someone else.*
In this way of looking at things, my being a daughter deserving
protection seemed secondary to the possibility that her husband
might engage in sexual acts with someone else. I was twelve. Over
the years, I sometimes hoped to second-guess this interpretation,
but the fact that my mom occasionally referred to girls the same age
I'd been as tramps and home-wreckers didn't seem promising.
When I was in my early thirties, she mentioned the "slut niece" of a
man she'd long ago been involved with. She'd been convinced that
the man and his niece were sleeping together.

I'd had enough. "How old was his niece?" I asked my mom.

"Thirteen," she said.

My voice shook. "If a grown man has sex with a thirteen-year-
old girl," I said, "it is never the child's fault." She tried to return to
the subject of her former paramour's assholery, but I repeated myself, with stronger emphasis on "never."

"I understand what you're saying," she said, in a tone that suggested the opposite. After that conversation, I wrote the letter to
my mom and stepdad that led to years of silence between us. Mentioning what my mom had said that night years before as we stood
washing the dishes, I invited her to correct my interpretation of her
fear that he might "do this with someone else." "With," I wrote, "is
a word that inherently implies consent." My mom replied by urging
me to let go of these hurts and slights, as she called them.

WELL AFTER MIDNIGHT ON the night my stepfather molested
me, my mom and stepfather came into the room where my sister,
stepsister, and I were sleeping. My mom whispered that they wanted
to discuss what had happened. They wanted to explain. My stepfather had done what he did, she said, because of Angela.

Angela? When I was ten, when my parents were still married
and we lived in our old house, my mom had invited Angela, a sex
worker and cocaine addict who went to my mom's church, to stay in

my room and share my bed. My father didn't know. Every morning, for some number of weeks or months, I set my alarm so that I could wake Angela before he came in to wake me for school. She hid in my closet until he was gone. She also picked me up from school most days and took me to the arcade and, late at night, with booze and weed on her breath, she answered all my questions about sex. I adored Angela. But—my mom explained that night, as my stepfather stood silently by—the "devils had jumped off" Angela and into my mattress, where they'd lain dormant until jumping on my stepfather that afternoon.

In hindsight, this night must have been when I knew for certain I didn't believe in the Christian God, who always seemed to align with my mom and justify her desires. Demons had a way of showing up, as she told it, to underscore the wickedness or folly of whatever she didn't like. Like my Puritan forebears—and their Puritan enemies—she was certain that God took her side. Religion was a shield and a weapon. If someone had to suffer, it was not the believer.

OCCASIONALLY MY MOM WILL SAY, as though for the first time, that she suspects Zone, her grandfather, molested his daughters—Louise, at least, and maybe Granny, too. When I ask why she believes this, she points to the fact that Louise pulled a knife on Alma. "The mother is always the one the child blames," my mom says. I hear my experience as a heavy subtext, though she never explicitly connects this thesis to me.

Over the years, when asked about her relationship with Zone, my mom insisted she didn't have much of one. As a young girl, she followed him around with a hammer and tools, emulating him, pretending to be a carpenter. In later years, she listened to a radio show at Zone and Alma's house. That was about it. From time to time, I asked if Zone did anything *to my mom* that led her to believe he molested Louise and Granny. No, she always said. Finally, a few years ago, she acknowledged that Zone was "very sexual-minded." When she was about eight years old, he urged books on her that, my mom said, "I had no business reading." One was *Forever Amber*, a bestselling 1944 novel about a pregnant sixteen-year-old who sleeps her way from poverty into the arms of King Charles II. Her grandfather was grooming her. At the age of eight, she knew. I pressed her; I wanted her to say it: Why did she think Zone wanted her to read those books? "I don't know if he was trying to turn me to sexual things so he could molest me," she said. Zone's view of my mom warped her sense of herself as a girl and later her view of me.

Just a few months after my mom attributed my stepfather's behavior to demon possession, Granny warned me to watch myself for signs of mental illness. I wasn't brave enough to tell Granny I'd been molested, but I was in a rough place, not feeling particularly sane, when she told me about her sister. Did she see something of Louise in me?

"A mean-ass sonofabitch," Granny often called her father. I knew Zone abandoned his wife and daughters, ran off with other women, but no matter how I probed, Granny never described his malice in a way that brought it into relief for me. Maybe it wasn't that she couldn't evoke the depths of his cruelty but that she chose not to. After Louise was institutionalized, Granny moved in with her aunt and uncle. My mom suspects she was trying to get away from her dad.

I don't believe in demons that jump on someone because they slept in a bed that a sex worker slept in before them, but I do believe in patterns across generations that seem nearly supernatural in their virulence. I've seen them for myself, in my life and the world more broadly. Even scientists have found that improbable things tend to recur in families. Sexual abuse is one, which hardly seems fair. So is religious belief: Among identical twins raised separately, if one twin is a believer, the other is likely to be a believer, too.

LONG AFTER MY FEAR of conversion took root, I learned that my mom wasn't the only woman in Mary Parsons's line who became a preacher. For years, Granny's aunt and cousin "pastored the only church" in the Texas town of Stockard, until, as my mom put it, "they finally got a man to come in and take over." They were Baptists—and descendants of Mary Parsons.

My mom's grandmother through Robert, Rindia, was a "devoted Pentecostal 'holy roller,'" who donated all her and her son S.E.'s money to her church, a lavish Dallas forerunner of the megachurches of today. I'm also related, through Rindia, to a Baptist preacher who established a fringe North Carolina sect and advocated being "born again" and the laying on of hands. Robert's paternal great-great-grandfather was an unlicensed Methodist preacher. And there are plenty of us believers on my father's side, too. Of the ancestors I've found, Abraham Martin, Robert's great-grandfather through Charley, stands out for his comparative moderation. According to a history written in 1943, he was a Universalist. "He lived in the faith for fifty years and died in it," a faith with "a liberal view of God's mercy, much more so than that other faith that a large part of the human family was elected to be damned before the world was."

At the same time, there are unbelieving strains among my ancestors—precedents for my own doubt. Like her father, Granny was a lifelong atheist, or so she told me in her old age. When I mentioned this to my mom a few years ago, she was incredulous. "That's horseshit," she said.

I considered the evidence. I couldn't recall Granny doing a single thing that led me to believe she was a Christian. True, after her death I discovered that Granny invoked God in her 1943 letter to the husband of the woman Robert was cheating with. "I say a prayer every night," she wrote to Christine's husband, "for your Ray Lee and my little 3-year-old Sandy for I know that there is a God in heaven and just as sure as the day will dawn tomorrow their tragedy can be righted if we will all pray and try." Maybe the mention of God was strategic, or maybe she was in a period of trying to believe, which she later discounted. But when I was a kid and Granny attended services at my mother's church, she exuded an air of polite detachment, one that embarrassed me on my mom's account, because Granny so clearly didn't subscribe to what my mom was preaching, and embarrassed me on Granny's account, because I could tell the congregation judged her for not being full of the spirit.

At Granny's funeral, my stepfather related a dream she'd told him six or eight months before. She'd dreamed she died and went to heaven. She was shown to a mansion with ornate and gilded doors. Beyond them, she knew without looking, lay more rooms than she could count. This would be her eternal resting place.

"Were you excited?" he asked her. (Maybe this was it—maybe she would finally accept Jesus as her personal savior and Lord!) "Wasn't it great to see your reward?"

"Hell, no," Granny said. "Who's going to dust those goddamned doors?"

No sooner had these words left my stepdad's mouth and a laugh started to rise under the funeral tent than a strong wind came and blew the flowers off the coffin. The wreath slammed to the ground. And then it started to rain.

Chapter 26

VENERATION

———

OVER THE YEARS, AS I RESEARCHED MY ANCESTORS AND pondered their genetic and emotional legacy in me, I was increasingly drawn to them in a spiritual register. The impulse was steeped in fear at first, a reflexive echo of my mom's belief in generational curses brought on by our ancestors' sins and handed down as demons. To imagine a more positive connection to my family dead felt fraught, too, given all the pain I knew my ancestors had caused, outside and inside my family.

In 2013, as I usually do, I turned to books. Over the next few years, I read everything I could find on the history and practice of ancestor reverence, in all disciplines I encountered that remotely touched on the subject. I wanted to understand every form of ancestor worship that had ever existed, but, as I read, I kept losing track of the details of various faiths, practices, and mythologies. Soon I had to admit how grandiose and, at least for me, impossible my plan was. The stories of the Bible so dominated and shaped my understanding of theology that I'd never even properly learned the Greek and Roman myths. My mind had trouble with complex pantheons and intricate animist belief systems. I was never going to fully understand the significance of ancestors to the Yoruba people, the Melanesian people, or the Lenape people, or to people in ancient France, China, or Peru. It was hubris to pretend otherwise. I could only read around the edges and take in whatever stuck.

For a long while, my inquiry into the spiritual significance of ancestors didn't extend to attending any actual ceremonies. On the one hand, I longed for an understanding that transcended the theoretical. On the other, as a committed agnostic, I wanted to keep whatever I found at arm's length. But I also rejected the idea of participating in rituals as a dispassionate observer. I knew it would feel wrong to go into the heart of other people's ancestry work from a sociological place. I would participate only if I could enter in good faith, if the ceremony seemed like something I might end up embracing.

Complicating things further, I found that I had some unexpected subliminal allegiance to Christianity. Though I wasn't a believer, I carried forward the fear. I worried that it was dangerous to explore the kind of spiritual contact I'd been warned against, that I'd be opening my life to evil forces outside my control. What if my ancestors were like demons, unsafe to interact with?

My agnosticism had never hardened into atheism, despite a few months in college when, mostly to goad my mom, I pretended I was certain that there was no God. I'd always enjoyed the feeling of some mysterious divine energy connecting things, just not a world ruled by a punishing deity like the Christian God. I'd also had a number of uncanny experiences over the years and been amazed and terrified hearing of many others from old friends in Miami whose families practiced Santería or friends whose beliefs were explicitly witchy or pagan.

Occasionally, I had a sixth sense about some impending calamity that manifested as I was predicting it. One summer several years ago, I was pointing at some tall trees in the backyard during a thunderstorm, telling Max I had a bad feeling one of them would eventually fall. As he began to try to reassure me that the trees were healthy, one of them snapped. More than half of it fell directly toward us, grazing the gutter above the window we were looking through, before slamming down into the yard below. The night before, out of nowhere, I'd suddenly begun regaling some young friends of mine with the same fear as we sat out back in the wind while our dogs ran around. I'd never thought much about danger the trees might pose before that night. When my friends left, I felt embarrassed and old, and I resolved not to mention it to them again. After the tree fell, I wondered: Did I pick up on its distress?

Even leaving aside the possibility of malign spirits, I worried about a religious conversion. Would this ancestor obsession become my version of the church in the living room? Would I wind up hectoring friends, preaching to strangers, retreating from a world that did not share my beliefs? The prospect of considering any spiritual practice activated all kinds of neuroses rooted in my fundamentalist background, but the worst fear of all was that I'd end up feeling nothing, that this search for connection would end up like my failed efforts as a child to believe God heard me when I spoke to him. And so, for a very long time, I did not act. I wondered if I'd spend the rest of my life yearning for a relationship to my family dead that I was in practice unwilling to extend myself toward.

AND YET, DESPITE ALL my self-imposed strictures, over time I had a dawning sense of something good and true and numinous at the core of my ancestry compulsion, a desire to heal by accessing a kind of divinity that was uniquely mine. As I continued to read and search around over the years, it became increasingly clear that I was in good company. Ancestor-veneration courses for beginners were popping up in Brooklyn and Asheville and Portland and New Orleans. Tools for ancestor altars exploded on Etsy. Tumblr became a place where people shared their practices. General books for newbies like me began to appear. Rootwork practitioners of Southern Black conjure offered ancestral sessions online. LGBTQ+ ancestral-reverence workshops offered people a sense of belonging amid re-jection by living family.

The scholar of animism and paganism, Graham Harvey, ob-served with characteristic insight and humanity in his 2015 fore-word to the collection *This Ancient Heart: Landscape, Ancestor, Self* that, with our renewed interest in the relationship between the liv-ing and the dead, "Something curious is emerging from the heart of the modern world, something not only unexpected, but perhaps the opposite of what was expected." It wasn't so long ago in the Christian-dominated West that only Indigenous people (or those who preserved Indigenous traditions) held "the peculiar notion that dead people mattered." The idea that ancestors had relevance for the living was considered primitive and "supposed to have been abandoned." A foundation of modernity was the Protestant Chris-tian "rejection of the medieval idea of the 'communion of saints,'" as Harvey puts it, "that the living and dead could pray for each other as they formed one community worshipping their God." But while modernism foresaw a world in which religion went extinct, the op-posite has happened. People whose forebears turned away from the dead are seeking a connection again.

INTEREST IN ANCESTOR VENERATION first reentered the aware-ness of the dominant white culture in the West in the late 1800s, through Christian scholars who were researching funerary practices across the world. These scholars viewed ancestor-oriented tradi-tions as "'lower theologies,'" of interest because they were thought to reveal how "more enlightened religions, such as Christianity," developed. The historians Erica Hill and Jon B. Hageman explain in *The Archaeology of Ancestors: Death, Memory, and Veneration* that the "primitive" religion of ancestor veneration was believed to have naturally given way to a more sophisticated and evolved monothe-ism. (Let's pause here to consider that Christianity is a belief in a

faraway God who created the earth and all beings and later condemned humanity to death but then sought to save it by impreg-
nating a human woman with his son, who would have to die for the
salvation to take.)

In 1870, the first cultural anthropologist, Edward B. Tylor, described worship of human souls, including ancestors, as the first,
lowest, most "savage" attempt to develop "a philosophy of nature."
Disagreement soon erupted as to whether ancestor worship was the
first religion of humankind or a later development. Those in the
second camp contended that the concept of kinship emerged only
with agriculture. Sigmund Freud took this view, maintaining that
what he called totemism, a belief in a spirit or symbol that unites a
clan, preceded ancestor worship, and emphasizing fear of the dead
over reverence for them. Freud believed that ancestor worship
flowed from an earlier fear that the dead turned into demons. In
reality, "totemism" and ancestor veneration are not mutually exclusive but often linked, and fear of the dead usually persisted alongside veneration.

SCHOLARS DISAGREE ON THE extent to which Christianity intentionally disrupted pagan practices across Western Europe. Courtenay Raia, a historian of science whose brilliant and entertaining
2009 "Science, Magic, and Religion" UCLA class is available in full
online, observes that the church and universities affiliated with it
were the sole vehicle for intellectual life in the West until the medieval era. In the thirteenth century, as the early Middle Ages were
coming to a close, the writings of Aristotle reentered the West, creating a quandary for church leaders, who found much that they
wanted to draw on but also much that appeared to contradict the
Bible (and the Platonic lens through which the Bible had been in-
terpreted). Thomas Aquinas partly resolved the conflict by arguing
that the Bible did not and could not communicate everything about
God's creation and intentions and that theories like Aristotle's

could be accepted insofar as they did not directly conflict with the Bible. For centuries afterward, the church's policy of accommodation allowed contradictory philosophies to flourish, under the idea that only God knows all, that our reading of the Bible is imperfect and incomplete, and that earlier thinkers might offer valuable insight into the workings of the universe, to the extent that they did not directly oppose the words and will of God.

Consistent with this big-tent attitude, Raia argues, village priests in the provinces took a fairly hands-off approach throughout Christendom toward family and pagan traditions, until the crackdown that preceded the Inquisition. Common people went to church but did not have Bibles. They learned about Christianity from priests. Their personal practices coexisted with official church ritual but weren't endorsed or acknowledged by the church.

In *The Return of the Dead: Ghosts, Ancestors, and the Transparent Veil of the Pagan Mind,* Sorbonne professor emeritus Claude Lecouteux recounts the history of revenants—figures that were not ghosts but the dead returned, solid in body, to haunt and torment, and potentially harm, the living. He gathers records of Germanic and other traditions from Western Europe (excluding England, where pre-Christian records are elusive) that, collectively, involve commemorations of ancestors around the hearth and beliefs about what one should or should not do in relation to the dead. Belief in revenants and terror of them was commonplace in pagan Europe, Lecouteux finds, and closely tied to "worship of the dead and the family." In this world, the bonds between humans and the universe extended to the entire family, including ancestors. A goal was to reintegrate "the dead back into the family of the living," taming the dead through veneration and funeral practices.

Many Christians, especially charismatic Protestants like my mom, view the body and its kinship links with suspicion. Unlike Jews and Muslims, who claim a genetic tie to Abraham as well as a spiritual one, the relationship of most Christians to Abraham as a patriarch is limited to, as religious-studies scholar Jill Raitt puts it, the "bond of faith." Human "flesh is literally heir to sin" for Christians, and only "rebirth in Christ" brings release. In the early church, saints and martyrs took the place of ancestors, their relics and shrines replacing "the genetic relation of the family" with a new type of *patronus*. The "cult of the dead," as anthropologists call it, gave way to "the cult of the saints." The eminent historian of American religion Charles H. Long linked Christianity's insistence that we are "'born only from above'" with modernity and contrasted the absence of ancestral practices in the United States with the African diaspora in the Caribbean and South America, where traditional African religious rituals for ancestors often openly coexisted with Christianity.

Some Christians do honor their family dead. As my mother-in-law, Jane, has explained to me, in Orthodox Christianity "there's a veil between the living and dead, not a wall. The beloved dead are honored at a service nine days after death, forty days after, and yearly. A dish of cooked wheat and honey is served after the service. Orthodox people pray for their dead and put candles up in church at every service, for both the living and the dead. It's a mystical rather than intellectual way of understanding the world." In Catholicism and the liturgical Protestant churches, the dead elevated to sainthood are remembered on All Saints' Day, and prayers for the rest of the dead are held on All Souls' Day. But the idea of a direct ongoing personal relationship with the dead as entities that affect us directly and we them is not a component of religious life as I was taught it. Claude Lecouteux argues that with the disappearance of ritual burial, "The dead man is just that—a dead man—and his wishes are no longer of any importance."

ENGLAND OUTLAWED PRAYERS FOR the dead with the Elizabethan Settlement of 1559. The scholar Ronald Hutton, author of *Pagan Britain* and *The Stations of the Sun: A History of the Ritual Year in Britain,* as well as other writings, characterizes this abolition as the reformers' "longest and hardest struggle" against "traditional ecclesiastical rituals." The prayers persisted, partly because of "a profound fear for the fate of the family dead" and partly because families could conduct them at home. Violators kept the church courts busy through the 1560s. Prosecutions persisted into the 1580s. Ecclesiastical archives establish that on All Saints' Day in 1587, men in Nottinghamshire "'used violence against the parson'" to maintain their rituals. As late as the early nineteenth century in Lancashire, one family member would hold "a large bunch of burning straw on the end of a fork" while the rest of the family "knelt in a circle around and prayed for the souls of relatives and friends until the flames burned out."

Hutton casts doubt on the portrayal of All Hallows' Eve and Samhain—which have largely given way to Halloween in the States—as long-standing Celtic customs for venerating the dead across what are now England, Ireland, Scotland, and Wales. He speculates that "a prehistoric belief in the danger from supernatural forces at the turning of the pastoral seasons" was "reinforced by the arcane associations of the Christian feast of the dead" rather than being driven underground by the church. Still, connecting what little we know of the original traditions of All Hallows' Eve and Samhain with what we know of the traditions that survive as May Day, even Hutton concedes that "it seems hardly plausible that all the dread of the night came from the Christian festival."

Hutton expresses impatience with the contemporary ancestor-veneration movement in the West, pointing out that "more recent spiritual ancestors" are often neglected in favor of figures "who are ancient enough to lack faces, names and individual traits, unless we invent or dream those for ourselves." He suggests that post-hippie Westerners engage in exploitation by projecting fantasies onto the Iron Age Druids. "Why should we equate our ancestors, who paved the way for [contemporary] achievements and disasters, with traditional peoples elsewhere in the world who chose a different course?" he asks. "Why should we regard them as more wise and admirable than our forebears in the more recent past, or ourselves?" Fair questions, though it's not the case that everyone of European origin in the West who tries to feel their way back toward ancestor-honoring practices looks only to ancient forebears and not the recent dead. And I wonder if, in his efforts to be scrupulous given the lack of records, Hutton is overcorrecting on behalf of the church.

In other parts of Christendom, church leaders actively restricted practices related to the dead, including family dead. The late Oxford scholar Peter Brown contends in *The Cult of the Saints: Its Rise and Function in Latin Christianity* that the church in its earliest days probably didn't forbid traditions related to the family dead, which only later became branded as "'superstitious' contaminations" of official church doctrine. In the Mediterranean world of the late fourth and early fifth centuries, the Christian churches debated "superstition" around cemeteries. During that period, Ambrose in Milan and Augustine in Hippo tried to restrict funerary customs among their Christian congregations, "most notably the habit of feasting at the graves of the dead," including at family tombs. Augustine characterized these practices as pagan, although they'd "been accepted as authentically Christian in all previous generations." Soon the church became "an artificial kin group," onto which members were to transfer loyalties and obligations historically directed to the physical family. "Nowhere was this made more plain than in the care of the dead."

While I can't argue with certainty that the early church intentionally acted to eradicate family practices related to the dead and their veneration in what is now England, it demonstrably did so in places where more-extensive records survive. We can see, in more-recent history, ways the Christian church demonized ancestral practices as its missionaries landed in other parts of the world. An obvious example is how Western missionaries confiscated the relics of the Fang people, claiming they were worthless if not satanic, only to toss the sacred parts away and sell the carvings for a handsome sum. In the twentieth century, the U.S. government separated Native children from their parents, placing them into church-run boarding schools that forbade the children to speak their own languages, share ancestral wisdom, or observe their rituals. The right to practice Native religions on sacred sites in traditional ceremonies became law only in 1978 and is enforced inconsistently even now.

ONE OF THE MOST beautiful and persuasive books I know that speaks to the uninitiated of the spiritual importance of ancestors is Malidoma Patrice Somé's *The Healing Wisdom of Africa*. At age four, Somé was taken from his people, the Dagara, after his father made an agreement with Catholic missionaries. It was a deal, Somé writes, "in which I had no say, a deal he did not fully understand." Though his father pleaded for the boy's return, the priests kept Somé in the missionary school system until the age of twenty. He returned to his village then, as a man carrying "the marks of literacy on his body," literacy "literally beaten into him."

At first, he judged and pitied his own people. In the eyes of fellow villagers, Somé's Western literacy was a kind of poison, "a logic that was incompatible with the logic innate to the Dagara and other native peoples. It made me prone to doubt, incapable of trust, and subject to dangerous emotions such as anger and impatience." Soon, though, Somé found that the Indigenous values he began, belatedly, to acquire "gradually overshadowed the concepts learned in the course of my Western education, scaring away the notion that my own culture was primitive and doomed." Why, for example, if his people's practices were "devilish or satanic," could they bring healing to the sick that Western doctors could not?

Slowly, he became initiated in the ways of the Dagara, and his Western education was undone. "I was reconnected to the deep regions of my psyche and to all living things. I rediscovered my home in the natural world, which is the true home of all beings on earth." But the joy of his initiation had a painful outcome, too. To fulfill his name, Malidoma—"he who makes friends with the stranger," as he puts it—was sent back into the West. The elders, as he recalls, said something like, "'Having been exposed to this and that and successfully endured its pain, we now grant you the right to more trouble and tribulation for your own growth and for the fulfillment of the destiny associated with you. May the ancestors continue to stay by your side.'"

And so Somé continued his Western education and has devoted his life to bridging Indigenous cultures and modern ones, in part by teaching Westerners how to "find the deep healing they seek." This healing, he maintains, requires "addressing one's relationships with the visible worlds of nature and community and one's relationships with the invisible forces of the ancestors and Spirit allies." Somé's wisdom and lyrical insight made me yearn for the kind of communion he describes. At the same time, I didn't see a place for myself in the specifics of his spiritual cosmology and had trouble imagining how to achieve the reconnection he advocates without some existing community or structured approach. This continued to be the case as I read many histories, scholarship, and memoirs by and about the ancestral practices of other Black and Indigenous people.

In part, I struggled with questions around appropriation: My ancestors had already taken so much; would I now also take on spiritual traditions from the very people they persecuted? But even if I'd felt comfortable leaping into someone else's belief system and making it my own, my fundamentalist Christian background was both an impediment and the place I was unavoidably starting from. It was a reality I had to work through. Superimposing some complex religious structure on top of that background wasn't the solution—for me, at least. Was I interested in the Druids? Something more open-ended? What about the white-supremacist element in some pagan communities? I found a reason to reject everything I considered. Somehow, I had to escape my agnosticism and my intellectual searching. I needed to find an entry point through my heart.

Chapter 27

LINEAGE REPAIR

——

ALL HALLOWS' EVE EVENTUALLY BEGAN TO SEEM WEL-coming, in its historical sense as a time of the thinning veil between the worlds of the living and the dead. Living in the Northeast, especially after moving near woodlands in Queens, I reveled in the approach of fall. The temperature dropped. The leaves turned golden, then orange and red, and they sailed to the ground in the October wind. I hadn't been allowed to celebrate Halloween as a kid once my mom decreed it demonic, but mostly I'd felt deprived of candy and fun, not spirit. Outside of South Florida, I could see how the idea took hold that the dead might commune more easily with the living as the fall harvest gave way to bare trees and cold nights. I mulled my childhood affinity for graveyards and my mom's horror and disgust at my interest.

In 2018, after a couple of years' deliberation, I set up an ancestor altar as an All Hallows' supplement to my meditation practice. I laid out an embroidered cloth and some candles, rocks, gemstones, and shells. Alongside all this, I placed a glass of water, a photo of Granny, and one of Grandpa. They were the ancestors whose legacies I was most interested in connecting with and whose energy felt most manageable.

By then I'd spoken with some writers I admired who had established veneration practices. Two that stood out to me in their re-
laxed commitment to ancestor work were Honorée Fanonne Jeffers
and Sheree Greer, both of whom are Black and find inspiration in
African traditional religious practices while also doing things their
own way. "I don't identify with Yoruba/Ifá formally," Jeffers told me,
"but one of my good friends does, and so, on his advice, I began
keeping an altar. I'm a progressive, radical feminist Christian. There
are about five of us."

Rather than insisting on rules, I made it up as I went along. I sat
on my cushion in front of the altar. After my usual practice, I med-
itated on what might survive of Granny in myself and then, the
next day, on what I saw of Grandpa in me. The insights that came
were unexpected. Contemplating Granny, I had a sense of intense
and effortless witchy knowing that had been intentionally closed
off because of oppression and fear. Through Grandpa, I saw how I
could hold my jaw in a determined way that didn't involve clenching my teeth. I felt some surprising remnant in me of his humor
and firm, straight-backed way of asserting himself. I felt more confident after meditating on both of them, less frightened of what
contact with ancestors might bring.

I soon removed the photographs, but the altar became a fixture
in the room where I write, and I knew that I needed to figure out
how to go deeper. I returned to some writings from people doing
ancestor work whose lineages originated in England.

I REMEMBER REDISCOVERING AN essay from *This Ancient Heart*,
by Caitlin Matthews: "Healing the Ancestral Communion: Pilgrimage Beyond Time and Space." Matthews's mother was raised
by an aunt rather than her parents. The absence was "a continuous
sorrow" for her mother, one that had plagued her throughout her
eighty-five years of life. Growing up, Matthews also felt the absence

of a connection to her maternal lineage and was driven to "untangle my mother's sense of exile."

On family drives into the countryside during her childhood, Matthews felt a deep tenderness, a sense of participating in a broad embrace. The chalk of the downs filled her dreams, and she related to it as a spirit being. Later she discovered that some of her paternal ancestors had labored on that land at least as far back as the 1500s. To this day, she feels a deep kinship with "the bright bones of the exposed chalk downs," which she recognizes as her ancestral landscape.

With so many of us split from our homelands, whether in the move from country to city or between countries or continents, Matthews writes, our sense of exile from our ancestors is immense. So it's understandable that many children of what she calls the Celtic diaspora have tried to remedy this sense of disconnection by seeking refuge and wisdom in "the world's traditional cultures" or "the ancestral wisdom of their host country." But this approach can sometimes entail a needy, grabby, hungry-ghost energy toward those whose spiritual insight they seek. A New Zealand student of Matthews—a member of the Celtic diaspora—approached a group of Maori women and asked if she could learn their ways. "'When you understand your own traditions,'" the women said, "'come back to us, and we'll see.'"

SEARCHING AROUND ONLINE AT the end of 2018, I discovered a listing for an "ancestral lineage healing intensive" to be held in Black Mountain, North Carolina, a couple of months later, by an organization called Ancestral Medicine. "Everyone has loving and wise ancestors," the event announcement said, "and by reaching out for their support we access tremendous vitality for personal and family healing. In addition to supporting repairs with living family, our ancestors encourage healthy self-esteem and help us to clarify our

destiny, relationships, and work in the world." The description emphasized that the leaders would guide the rituals "in ways that are
psychologically grounded, ritually safe, and culturally mindful," and
that people "new to ancestor work, adoptees, and folks with a tough
experience of family are all warmly welcome."

I'd never traveled as an adult for a spiritual event, but the description resonated with what I was seeking. And I'd been to Black
Mountain. My mom lived nearby, outside Asheville, and Granny
was buried nearby. My stepdaughter, away in school in Chapel Hill,
had moved to the area with her mom, stepdad, and brothers several
years before. I'd already begun to feel that Western North Carolina
was determined to have a role in my life, whether I wanted the connection or not, and after coming to this conclusion I'd discovered
that ancestors of mine on multiple lines once lived in the region. So
I signed up, bought a plane ticket, reserved a place to stay, and ordered *Ancestral Medicine,* a book by Daniel Foor, the founder and
director of the organization that put together the retreat.

Foor is of German and English ancestry and descended from
early settlers and colonizers in the Americas. He's a therapist, and
he advocates what he calls a nondogmatic approach to ancestor and
earth reverence. Reading his book in preparation for the intensive,
I learned that Foor developed his practices by seeking "the Earth-
honoring ways of my older European ancestors"; studying with a
Buryat Mongolian shaman; regularly participating in Native ceremony, of the Lakota style, and with the Native American Church;
and studying and becoming an initiate of the Ifá/Òrìṣà religious
tradition of the Yoruba people. Earlier, he lived in North Africa and
studied Islam in Sufi orders. In the book, he says that his approach
does not borrow from or purport to represent any of the traditions
he's studied. Instead, the teachings and practices are intended to
"emphasize cross-cultural similarity" and "aim to be widely accessible and free from the constraints of any specific tradition." No
particular religious identity is required, he writes; "nor do you need
to see yourself as a particularly religious person in order to love and

honor your ancestors." I've found Foor's writings and teachings indispensable as a starting point, though I haven't worked with him directly. (And I was concerned when, in late 2020, a group of students formally training with Foor to be certified in his methodology cut ties with him and the Ancestral Medicine organization, citing criticisms of the culture and his approach.)

Foor lists the following four assertions as ones that most Indigenous peoples and animists share and that are foundational to his approach: Consciousness continues after death; not all of the dead are equally well; the living and the dead can communicate; and the living and the dead can strongly affect one another. Reading this, I was not at all certain that I could accept these, but I felt I could go to the intensive in good faith, open to possibility, while also recognizing that I might get there and find myself unbelieving and alienated.

Foor's emphasis is on connecting with "well" ancestors rather than our most immediate ancestral dead. The idea is that, as in ancient Greece and Rome (and many ancient and currently practiced religions around the world), untended ancestors can cause harm, intentionally or unintentionally, whereas ancestors who have been properly honored and tended in death have joined earlier ancestors as something akin to family deities and are powerful spirit allies. Those of us from colonial backgrounds, who come from Europeans whose ancestors abandoned healthy ways of dealing with family dead, Foor says, may need to reach back a thousand years or more to find an ancestor who's integrated with those who are deeply well in spirit. Anyone descended from Indigenous people, whose spiritual practices remained intact until the last few centuries, likely won't have to go back so far, Foor writes, because most Indigenous cultures emphasize tending to family dead as an important facet of the wellness of the family and the larger community. Ceremonies ensure that the dead are well after death, that they are integrated with those who died before.

Doubt and fear fought for my attention as I read. So I was relieved that Foor offers (as he puts it) ritual safety tips, such as guidance for focusing on one lineage at a time. At the same time, as is my way, I felt constrained by the rules. I didn't love the insistence on focusing initially on one of four lines based solely on assigned biological sex: mom's mothers, dad's fathers, mom's fathers, or dad's mothers. What about my mother's father's mother, or my father's father's mother? Or my ancestor Mary Parsons? But the idea is to start with the four core lineages, analyzing the wellness of each and then choosing one—ideally the most well one—to work with first.

WANTING TO GAUGE WHETHER I could spend a weekend doing this, I set up a session with an Ancestral Medicine practitioner listed on the organization's website. I chose someone local, with a background in Christianity: Lindsay Sudeikis, a former nun who lives in Brooklyn. As our Skype session approached, I felt trepidation about attempting to seek solace in spirits that I'd been taught were demonic. I also worried that I wouldn't connect to anything for the full hour.

We began (as I expected from Foor's book) by assessing each of my lineages. For each, I closed my eyes and pictured the line and evaluated its wellness among the recent dead. Then I looked to the dead of a few hundred years ago, and then, purely using intuition or imagination, to the ancient dead. I didn't seem to access anything concrete, but I had a sort of gut sense of the wellness of each line at these stages, and I decided not to worry whether this sense was more intellectual, based on my knowledge and experience of people in the lines, or based on some other kind of insight or knowing. It all seemed a little abstract, although I did connect colors to some lines—green to the ancient section of my father's father's line, and a deep purple-blue to my mother's mother's.

Once I concluded that my mother's mother's people were in the best shape, Lindsay led me in an effort to connect with a "deeply well" ancestor on the line. Again I was afraid that I would see nothing, feel nothing, and for what felt like several minutes I didn't. But as I tried to look backward into the lineage, a sort of fairy insect appeared. She had a fat blue-green body like a caterpillar, large blue wings, and a blue human face. I was too fascinated to be shocked. Fairies had not been part of my fantasy life since I was four or five years old, and in any case, this figure looked nothing like Tinker Bell or Thumbelina. She was thick and sturdy, handsome rather than wispy (a bit like a figure in the Book of Kells or another illuminated manuscript from the monasteries of Ireland, Scotland, and England, but more earthy). I was relieved that something had come forward, whether from my imagination or the world of the spirits, and amazed that it was this being. I didn't think of myself as a visually inventive person. Lindsay said that the fairy may have been a deity who helped my ancestors. She instructed me to ask the fairy to take me to a well ancestor on the line.

Next I saw a woman with blond hair in a simple hut with a straw roof. She was baking bread on the hearth in the middle of the room and radiated kindness and nurturing. Everything about her surprised me, her motherliness most of all. Lindsay instructed me to ask her if she was an ancestor on the line. I had the feeling she was. I asked if she was well with all those on the line who'd come before. Again I had the "yes" feeling. Then I was to ask if she could and was willing to help me. She was, she said. But I wasn't sure that I could feel a connection with her. I had trouble believing that this gentle maternal figure would be my best guide to this line.

So I asked her to take me back further, to another well ancestor. What came next was an intense and radiant image, an enormous face in the sky like a god: a woman with dark hair, in a tunic for battle. I later realized she looked a bit like my great-aunt Louise, who'd died in the mental hospital. With Lindsay's help, I asked the questions. Yes, the warrior was an ancestor on the line and well with all those who'd come before. Yes, she could help me. Lindsay asked where I would place her in space and time. My best guess was somewhere on what's now the border of England and Scotland, in the first century A.D. I was drawn to the warrior but afraid.

That night, a cold I'd been fighting burgeoned into terrible chills. Lying awake under the covers, shivering, my teeth knocking together so that the noise scared the cats and worried the dog, I was terrified that, in going against my Christian upbringing, I'd opened some demonic portal I'd never be able to close. Over the coming days, I looked for excuses to skip the intensive. But no one I consulted about it backed up my desire to stay home. "I think you should go," Max said, knowing that I'd been skirting ancestral ceremonies, while longing to go to one, for years. "I think you'll be able to handle whatever comes up," said my stepdaughter, then twenty-five, always preternaturally wise.

AT THE INTENSIVE, our leader, Shannon Willis, explained that we could ask spirits to dial back energy if it was too much. And so, as we dropped into the ritual, I did that. Instead of appearing to me as a warrior, the well spirit appeared as a benevolent light in the shape of an eye—a deep-purplish-blue iris glowing in the sky. Below, I sensed, a cauldron was boiling in a ceremony in a clearing in the woods beneath mountains like the ones on the horizon in Black Mountain.

I had a feeling of belonging and peace, the sense of a personal connection to divinity. It came to me that Mary Parsons (who is not, past Granny's mother, a matrilineal ancestor) was only one of many women in Granny's background persecuted as witches because of their forthrightness, their communication with spirits, and their connection with animals. I saw that some of my own anxiety and depression could be traced to the shutting off of some of these impulses in myself. At the same time, I felt that the more recent dead were terrified that I was connecting to our witchy history, and that the fear and sickness I felt after seeing the warrior ancestor was theirs, not mine. I remembered that Maud, the name I'd given my-self, means "powerful battler." So did Louise, the middle name I'd been given in honor of my father's grandmother but also a name I shared with Granny's sister, who in portraits looked so much like the warrior.

Later I encountered an essay by the environmental scientist, educator, musician, and community organizer Lyla June Johnston, who is of Native (Diné and Tsétsêhéstâhese) and European lin-eages. Growing up in Taos, New Mexico, she was considered a "half-breed" and taught to forget the "pale-skinned mothers and fathers" of her father's family, who carried "violence in their blood and avarice in their smile." One day, though, sitting "in the ceremo-nial house of my mother's people," a revelation came from her Eu-ropean grandmothers and grandfathers, a song "of their life before the witch trials and before the crusades," before serfdoms, the plague, and the guillotine, "the vast and beautiful world of Indige-nous Europe. This precious world can scarcely be found in any lit-erature, but lives quietly within us like a dream we can't quite remember." The European women slaughtered as witches were the medicine people of old Europe, Johnson saw; after being "raped and tortured for so many thousands of years," Indigenous Europeans forgot who they were and only knew to conquer or be conquered. She resolved to stop being ashamed of her European ancestors and instead to honor them by reclaiming all that was lost—their con-nection to the earth most of all.

AT THE INTENSIVE, WHENEVER someone asked Shannon how we knew we weren't making everything up, she encouraged us to let our imagination go, to be playful and curious. A teacher from an intensive I would attend in Brooklyn at the end of 2019, the profes-sor and Hebrew priestess Taya Mâ Shere, had another answer, too. Why should we assume, she asked, that whatever we might imagine about our ancestors would be separate from their legacy in us?

At Shannon's instruction, we began what Foor calls "the prayer for the lineage between." The process is to ask the guide to contain, or cocoon, all the unwell dead, from the oldest unwell ancestor to the last person who died. Shannon called it "the most loving and compassionate time-out ever," and emphasized that while we would invite and make space for our guides to do the work, the healing itself was a project that the guide, not we, took on. The cocoon I saw for this line was shimmering gold.

The teachers I've worked with in this tradition have emphasized that the well ancestors themselves handle the healing. The living hold space for the well ancestors to do their work by maintaining contact, showing reverence, and tending the altar, but do not directly engage with the unwell dead, who can be dangerous. The more our own unresolved trauma and patterns are connected to a line, though, the more difficult it can be to maintain that distance.

Foor writes of the immense cultural impact of the unhealed energy in all our ancestral lines. Holding ghosts in a state of unforgiveness makes things worse. So there's a "forgiveness practice" that's been one of the most emotional, transformational, and often difficult parts of the intensives for me. Sometimes the forgiveness is more aspirational than actual, as when I emailed the practice from my second intensive (in Decatur, Georgia, in June 2019) to my mom, saying:

> I have been working through some things recently and I wanted to share a forgiveness practice with you that has brought me a lot of peace. I'm sure you have your own ways of achieving the kind of healing this has brought me—I'm pretty intimately familiar with your relationship with Jesus, having heard approximately 1 million of your sermons over time!—and I hope that you can accept and respect mine, even if it doesn't entirely fit with your approach. I have practiced the following forgiveness practice toward Granny and her

maternal line, and since you're part of that line I wanted to extend the practice to you, too.

Then I wrote (using Foor's template as filtered through Shannon) that I forgave her, Granny, Alma, "'and all my grandmothers on this line, for all the harms, both real and imagined, intentional and unintentional, known and unknown, from this moment in time to all moments in time, and I release you from all of these.'" At the intensives, participants say this to other participants about their own line three times and then turn it around and imagine the line offering forgiveness. I included that in my email to my mom, too. "'I accept your forgiveness of me for all the harms, both real and imagined, intentional and unintentional, known and unknown, from this moment in time to all moments in time, and I accept your release of me from all of these.'"

Synchronicities came up. On my way to Decatur, I discovered that the Airbnb I had booked was on Martha Avenue. Martha was Granny's name. My hope was to emerge from that weekend with this lineage "healed" all the way down through Granny, but when I got there, I felt that the well ancestors on the line were telling me that I needed to work on my father's mother's line, and I was annoyed and resistant. I'd always identified Grandma and her line with my pallor and lack of vigor and love of beautiful spaces and objects, and I'd always judged and condemned these things in myself. It was precisely for this reason, the well ancestors on my mom's mother's line seemed to say, that I needed to work with the well ones through Grandma.

My feelings toward Grandma had already been softening. I'd always associated her with cardinals—because of some decorative china plates and figurines and the bird feeder hung from a tree that you could see from the kitchen and the family room windows—and as I'd worked on this book the preceding winter, before and after the first intensive, I'd seen them everywhere, flashes of red in the

snow, at my feeders, in the trees in the woods when I was out walking the dog. And then, in the spring, I'd thought of Grandma as the
cabbage white butterflies flitted over wildflowers and clover and the
herbs in my backyard. They were small, simple, unobtrusive, and, in
their ease of movement, beautiful. As I began to work with the line,
I traced to these women a habit of clenching on my lower right side,
something I'd always connected to being yelled at by my father.
Sometimes it unclenched during the intensive and pain rushed in.

The ancestors on these lines had some other rules for me. They
forbade me to use this book to crusade against Christianity. They
would not be well, they said, and thus neither would I, if I used my
talents to hector people in that way and to work against the beliefs
that had brought them comfort in hard times.

After the intensive, I began working with the teacher Larisa
Noonan, who comes from a Christian fundamentalist background.
With her help, I met the guide on the line, a blindingly pale, tall,
thin, red-haired woman in a pale-bluish-violet dress, with a crown
that I came to understand represented spiritual riches. She radiated
peace and empathy. What happened? I asked her. Where did compassion go in these women, these Baileys and their foremothers
who enslaved people? I felt the reply rather than heard it. The lack
of empathy in the recent line was the precise inverse of what is possible, she told me. The lightness and nonattachment and love of
beauty that I perceived in the line and sometimes in myself, and
dismissed as frivolous, was medicine for me. I could continue to be
compassionate in the world and also move through it with lightness, like a butterfly or cardinal. I could take joy in beauty. Like
Grandma, when my time comes, I could choose to let go of life with
grace.

At the intensive in Brooklyn in December 2019, I was glad to
land in the small group of the healer and writer Langston Kahn. I'd
listened to several of his talks and interviews online, and I admired
his willingness to reckon with all the facets of his ancestors and
their backgrounds, including his ancestors who were enslaved and

his Swiss grandmother, who, he discovered long after her death, had written a letter for him when he was a child to be read when he (as she knew he would) "writes his book."

In one drop-in, I asked my mother's mother's line what to do about my mom, about the anger I felt toward her because of her political opinions and the fear I felt over her health issues and her unwillingness to deal with them. I heard Granny's voice for the first time since her death. "You know your mama is just gonna do what she's gonna do," Granny said, "and there ain't a damn thing you can do about it." I smiled as hard as I cried. Granny had said this so many times during her life. Maybe now I could take it in.

Part Eight

CREATIVITY

Chapter 28

THE NAMESAKE

—

I'VE ALWAYS BEEN DRAWN TO STORIES OF ARTISTS UNKNOW-ingly devoting their creative work to the problems of their ancestors, their extended family back through time, and discovering the synchronicity when the work is done. This repetition feels so *true* to me, so *inevitable,* it's like magic through the centuries, a coincidence so uncanny, it must be something else.

Maaza Mengiste's novel *The Shadow King* centers on a group of Ethiopian women fighting Italian soldiers during Mussolini's brutal occupation. As she started to write, Mengiste was filled with conviction that women really had taken up arms against the invaders. When the book was nearly done, she mentioned to her mother how excited she'd been while writing to find a photograph of a woman in uniform. "It confirmed what I had always thought: that these women really existed," Mengiste told her. And then her mother revealed that Mengiste's great-grandmother had demanded her father's gun and gone to war. Mengiste had never heard the story in all her years of work on the book.

The novelist Naomi Alderman's critical retelling of the story of Jesus, *The Liars' Gospel,* was inspired by a passage from Josephus that she later learned had also preoccupied her grandfather. "He had the same question mark in the margin," she wrote, "the same part bracketed where we both, I imagine, made the same frown at the same moment. So it seems as though my family has been after this hare for a while."

Frank Ching's *Ancestors: 900 Years in the Life of a Chinese Family* is a tribute that might have been received as the opposite by his forebears during their lives, even though it traces his lineage back thirty-four generations to the poet Qin Guan, a common ancestor of his mother and father. Ching had left China as a young boy and wasn't able to return until after his father's death. On that trip, he was given a fragile, thread-bound volume of the family genealogy that had belonged to his father. Awed by the book, Ching soon learned it was far from comprehensive. One relative had been executed in the Shanghai purge of 1927 and stricken from the records in an act of family preservation. Whole clans could be slaughtered because of one person's actions, a punishment that could extend to nine generations of a family. People thought to have disgraced the clan through the most minor of infractions were also removed. Ching's clan records abound with stories of "filial sons," but those who selflessly attended and brought honor upon their parents, any "unfilial sons" have been forgotten.

Like many children of his era, Ching was inculcated in the Confucian duty to parents, filial piety, "'the root of all virtue.'" Our bodies, "in every hair and bit of skin, are received by us from our parents" and so, according to *The Book of Filial Piety*, we owe our parents everything. We live to serve and honor them. By these metrics, Ching and his book are filially un-pious. In *Ancestors*, he reveals his unhappy relationship with his father, his feeling of alienation from his family's past. He lays bare all kinds of disputes that reverberate through the centuries. In an earlier era, he could very well have been stricken from his official family records for his writing.

Yet it was Ching, this son of dubious filial virtue, who wrote stories animating his lineages. It was Ching who found the grave of the family's patriarch, the scholar and poet Qin Guan, who'd "died in disgrace" and been forgotten. And, by extension, it was also Ching who enabled all of Qin Guan's descendants to resume the tradition of gathering at the grave each April to honor their ancestor on Tomb-Sweeping Day—to make "the report to the ancestors," as another descendant put it, "to tell them how we are doing and how they still live on in us." These rituals were outlawed after the Cultural Revolution, but seekers like Ching helped restore them. He may earn low marks for filial piety by traditional Confucian acting-as-human-mosquito-netting standards, but philosophically and spiritually it's hard to imagine someone embodying the virtue of honoring ancestors more fully.

So often, our recurring preoccupations, our seemingly random decisions and obsessions, point us where our attention needs to be.

"MAUD" IS A NICKNAME NOW, one most of my friends call me. It started as a pen name, a sort of homage to Maude Newton, my mysterious great-great-aunt. When Grandpa died in the fall of 2008, I lost my only known source of information about Maude, and my research into her and the rest of the Newtons intensified. Wallace Newton, Grandpa's first cousin, was able to tell me that Maude had been a schoolteacher, but not much more.

I somehow had never thought to search newspaper archives for her married name, Maude Simmons. When I did, I found treasure: a photo of Maude in 1977, at age ninety-two, sitting in a "King Midget" car. This vehicle, billed as "the World's Most Affordable Car," was assembled from a kit, although hers reached the Mississippi Delta in completed form. The picture accompanies a profile of Maude by James Dickerson for the *Delta Democrat-Times*.

According to this article, Maude was about seventy-nine years old when, nine years or so after she retired from the public school system, she saw a *National Geographic* ad seeking Midget Motor

Corporation dealers. She responded, volunteering herself as the dealer for Sunflower County, Mississippi. The company was enthusiastic and sold her a car at the discounted rate of five hundred dollars.

Maude was eighty or so, according to Dickinson's account, when the car was shipped down on a train from Ohio. Main Street was "filled with curiosity seekers" when it arrived. Despite her excitement, Maude had no idea how to use it. "It was my first car," she said. "And I couldn't drive an inch," but she learned. She recounted her hesitancy over becoming a King Midget dealer. "My family didn't want me to do it. I listened to them for about a year. Then I wrote the company anyway and told them to send me a car." Everything about this story delighted me, apart from Maude's disapproving Mississippi Delta family, though I related most to that.

Dickerson describes Maude's house as filled with "stacks of books and magazines," another commonality. She told him that she met her husband in Indiana, where she had a job in an architectural office. "'I learned how to do house plans there,'" she explained. "'In fact, I did the plans for this very house I'm living in right now.'"

She also remembered teaching in Southern Mississippi "'when we had Halley's Comet.'" She said, "'That was 1910, the year Mark Twain died. When the comet came over we all went outside to have a look.'" I'd gone through a phase of devouring Mark Twain's nonfiction in the years before I read this, so I knew he was born shortly before the comet passed and that he'd died the day after its return. "It will be the greatest disappointment of my life if I don't go out with Halley's Comet," he'd said. "The Almighty has said, no doubt: 'Now here are these two unaccountable freaks; they came in together, they must go out together.'" Like most people, Maude, who was born in 1884, got to see the comet only once. She died in 1981, at the age of ninety-seven.

Finding this article, I allowed myself to hope that she really was a kindred spirit.

WITH THIS NEW INFORMATION, I dug deeper. I knew Maude's family was poor, at least during her childhood. Her father died when she was twenty years old. Four years later, in 1908, Maude somehow graduated from Grenada College, a Methodist girls' college in Grenada, Mississippi, with a bachelor of letters degree. I don't know how she was able to attend, unless on scholarship.

In the *Delta Democrat-Times* profile, Maude implied that she met her husband at an architectural office prior to 1910 and returned to Mississippi before that year, but the records I've found show that she married Simmons in Elkhart, Indiana, in 1912. In 1915, the couple ran a solicitation in *The American Contractor* as the architectural firm Simmons & Simmons. The ad revealed that Maude Newton (whose middle name was Corona) had, at one time, dropped the Maude!

> Simmons & Simmons, architects, have opened an office. . . .
> The members are Royal Leonard Simmons and his wife, Corona Newton Simmons. Mr. Simmons has had twelve years' experience in the profession. Mrs. Simmons is a graduate of the Grenada, Miss., college, and has taken a course in advanced designing and engineering. A number of Elkhart bungalows were designed by her. The new firm will be pleased to receive samples and trade literature.

Reading this, I felt sad. Maude was so close to escaping Mississippi and doing her own thing, I thought, but the Delta sucked her back in.

My research led to another Newton descendant, Mike Newton, my third cousin twice over—his Newton great-great-grandfather was the brother of my great-great-grandfather, and his Ricketts great-great-grandmother was the sister of my great-great-grandmother. In reply to an email from me, Mike consulted with his father, John, who described Maude as "an intellectual, and a teacher, and very precise in her speech." He considered her the smartest of all the Newtons. He knew the story of Maude's split from her husband, but not as one in which, as my grandfather put it, she "threw pepper in her husband's eyes until he stopped coming around." John knew it as a tragedy for Maude.

> Early in her life she left home with an architect and went to Missouri. They had an argument and she left and came home by herself to Drew. That probably caused quite a stir in that small town. The worst was yet to come. . . . The architect visited Drew to make amends with Maude. Grand Newt [my third great-grandmother] and Ethel [Maude's sister] would not let him enter the house. They lied to him and told him Maude never wanted to see him again. He left and was never ever heard from. Grand Newt and Ethel never shared this story with Maude but did do so with my father's family.

It's impossible to know the real story of the end of Maude's marriage. The 1920 census falsely identifies her as widowed—maybe that was the story in the community for a time—but the 1930 and 1940 censuses indicate that she was divorced. By 1930, her ex-husband, Royal, had remarried.

I tend to believe the pepper story, because it strikes me as one my family in the mid-century Mississippi Delta would have wanted to paper over with something less odd and more ladylike. Maybe I also lend more credence to that version because it's the one Grandpa remembered. The fact that such different but equally dramatic versions were handed down on different lines interests me in itself. Maybe both things happened—Maude tossed pepper in her husband's eyes and then he came back and her mother and sister turned him away, and then different Newton nephews reflexively preserved the details that jibed with their preexisting impressions of my great-great-aunt.

One thing the Newtons of earlier generations always seemed to agree on was that the lineage produced an unusual number of, as John put it, "old maids," a course I could easily imagine having decided on for myself—or, courtesy of my undocile personality, being chosen. The preponderance of unmarried daughters traces at least as far back as the children of Jesse Newton, my fourth great-grandfather, likely son of the unmarried Sally Newton.

MAUDE TURNS OUT TO have been *a writer* of sorts. In 2010, I discovered that the Mississippi Department of Archives and History maintained a "Maude C. (Newton) Simmons collection," devoted to newspaper articles, local interest items, and letters, some of them published in the Drew, Mississippi, newspaper from 1960 to 1970. Her "Drew Doings" column "concerned a variety of subjects, including births, deaths, church and school news, politics, sports, topics of community interest, visitors, and poetry composed by Simmons or published authors."

Were the archives mostly church-supper bulletins? Or opinion? Whatever else they might be, one thing was certain: They were civil-rights-era dispatches from the very town where, in 1955, Emmett Till was lynched, and from the state and era where the 1963 murder of civil-rights activist Medgar Evers led a sickened Eudora Welty to, for once, discard her reticence, sit down at her desk, and write, in a single impassioned rush, her short story "Where Is the Voice Coming From?"

I was nervous to read Maude's writing but also eager. The library said the microfilm was too badly eroded to be copied under the normal procedures, so I hired a Delta researcher and veteran civil rights activist, Jan Hilegas, to take a look at the archives. She returned paper copies of the writings she thought would interest me. The first article, published January 4, 1968, in Indianola's *Enterprise-Tocsin,* offered a survey of New Year's celebrations, customs, and superstitions from around the world. The second, published November 14, 1968, opens with "My walking marathon," a section on car trouble. "Such a wonderful age with efficiency (?) the order of the day!" it begins, before launching into her motor travails. Her King Midget was out of commission for four months. The company kept shipping the wrong parts. And then, she wrote, "At the voting precinct, Nov. 5th, if I didn't have enough trouble deciding how to vote, a member of the shop said, 'I have good news for you. The mechanic broke the parts.'"

I laughed. Then I realized the timing. Maude had trouble deciding how to vote the year independent segregationist presidential candidate George Wallace carried the state.

Soon came a dispatch about the Newton family's history in Mississippi, about fishing and playing with "little Negro boys on the plantation," until "a crop failure from cutworms" forced the family to move. After their father died, her teenage brothers "carried on the farming and later added Newton Brothers General Store."

In the end, everything I feared was in the packet. In notes for one article, Maude excoriates Lyndon Johnson's "fuzzy-thinking" and "wishy-washy policies." Later she contrasts him unfavorably with Barry Goldwater, who "had the integrity and stability to vote against the civil-rights bill and the nuclear test ban treaty—the latter the first step in giving up our sovereignty to become a member of a One World Government." In another article draft, she advocates defying the Civil Rights Act. Otherwise, she warns readers, "Your little girl will be integrated with little Negro boys and grow up on intimate social terms." Maude would still have been teaching in Drew, and her column would have been running, in 1965 when a Black family that enrolled their children in the town's white school district woke to gunshots fired through all their windows after they refused to return their children to the Black school. She retired around 1968.

Elsewhere, Maude claims that "Congress is planning to pass a voting bill that will discriminate against the white people in six

Southern States. Mississippi is one of them." She says that she has it "on good authority" that "an average of 70 Negroes go every day to Indianola to register. It is a well-known fact in the South that scores of Negroes do not know their ages. This will make it possible for many under voting-age to register and vote." In another *Enterprise-Tocsin* column, in a Deep South "but I have Black friends" hat trick, she writes:

> Many, many years ago my mother ran a hotel in Drew and later moved into a private home and kept boarders. Naturally, she had to have a colored houseboy [*sic*], which was the custom in those days.
>
> This particular colored houseboy of hers moved to Chicago. He still lives there. Through the years, being a porter on the Santa Fe passenger train, he has had the opportunity to attend the Pasadena Tournament of Roses. And I am happy to say he always sends me a copy of the Pasadena Tournament of Roses Pictorial. I received my 1970 copy the other day.
>
> This "relationship" does not stem from decisions handed down by the U.S. Supreme Court.

In Maude's position, I'd view the annual gift from Chicago as an indication that her mother's former employee didn't exactly pine for his old life waiting on my great-great-grandmother and her boarders in the Delta, but that doesn't seem to have occurred to Maude.

THUS DID IT TRANSPIRE that, in naming myself Maud Newton, I'd accidentally honored the parts of my family history that trouble me most. The disappointment I felt reminded me of a biography I reviewed that revealed the Southern writer Flannery O'Connor relished racist jokes.

The critic Sadie Stein, whom I later met and liked (and who has

Arkansas roots on her mother's side), responded to my review, observing that my and others' surprise over O'Connor's racism seemed "disingenuous." I saw where she was coming from and appreciated the critique; on reflection, though, the most accurate description would have been "willfully naïve." I'd known the likelihood that O'Connor, having grown up in Georgia during the Jim Crow era, was racist, but I'd chosen to hope she'd applied her stringent values and astringent perspective to white supremacy. In the case of both Flannery O'Connor and Maude Newton, I'd hoped so hard, I'd nearly convinced myself my fantasy was true. But both Maude and O'Connor actively fed the systemic racism from which they benefitted.

In retrospect, I realized that when I was in elementary school, the Drew newspaper that had originally published Maude was revived. My father bought a subscription that turned up each week at our house in Miami. He often pointed out things of interest to him while my sister and I were eating breakfast. I wonder now if my father mentioned back then that Maude Newton had written a column for the paper and if that's how she became lodged in my mind as someone whose story was worth digging up.

Whatever the cause of my original interest, Grandma's horror at my curiosity fueled my persistence. My research was an act of defiance, an attempt to unearth what she wanted to hide. It was also a desire to find a precedent in my father's family for myself. Maude was a reject; so was I.

Ironically, I believe now that Grandma's resistance to my interest in Maude was partly a result of the things Maude wrote that I myself find unconscionable. Before she died, Grandma believed having the Confederate flag on the Mississippi state flag was an embarrassment. She threw away fifty years of her mother's plantation journals. Whatever nostalgia she may have had for her childhood, she realized that defending the segregated South was offensive. I suspect she'd also come to think it was wrong. I know she would approve of the new state flag with the magnolia—"look at those magnolias!" she'd said once, when I persisted in asking about Maude. But trying to change the subject only intensified my curiosity.

I'm sorry that Maude's writing turned out to be what it is, but I'm not sorry I found it. As the world shows more clearly every day, pretending racism doesn't exist doesn't make it go away. Giving myself her name deepened and sharpened a reckoning I knew from my youngest years was inevitable.

Chapter 29

BENEFICIAL AND
MALIGNANT CREATIVITY

—

IN MY YOUNGER YEARS, I VIEWED STORYTELLING AS AN inherently positive part of myself, something to be proud of that came from my mom. But Maude also told stories, dangerous stories, and so did my father. One in particular he told again and again. It was his own "Negro boy on the plantation" fable, intended to bolster his maxim that Black and white children should never mix.

As my father told the story, when they were boys he often played with Mann, the son of his grandmother's (Mama T.'s) onetime housekeeper. One day, my father was counting his quarters in front of Mann, a "game" almost comically on brand. When Mann left, my father discovered he was missing a quarter. He counted several times to make certain but still came up short. Soon Mann came whistling up the street with a six-pack of Coke.

At that time, a six-pack cost—here my father paused for dramatic emphasis, to give his young listeners a hint that this was a time for deductive reasoning—exactly a quarter. My father asked Mann where he'd gotten the six-pack, and Mann said he'd bought it. My father asked where he got the money. Mann said he'd saved it up. Because of the missing quarter, my father knew Mann was lying. The adults agreed. Mann was punished, and my father never played with him again. Thus, my father said, no Black child could be trusted, ever. This was the lesson my sister and I were to take from his experience.

Even as a child, I realized Mann was a strawman (though I didn't know the word). The fact that this one child had supposedly stolen a quarter from my father didn't mean that every Black kid stole quarters. Also, having played Monopoly with my father, I could easily imagine him counting his change and lording it over his grandmother's servant's son. My sympathies lay with Mann, who in my father's story had the temerity to take action against him. The only time I'd been brave enough as a kid to do the same, at age three or four, I was taking cough medicine that made me hyperactive. I bit my father on the nose. Then I mouthed "I hate you" at him in the mirror, not realizing he could see. The spanking he gave me didn't dent my sense of triumph.

MY FATHER EASILY FILLED the role of "racist parent" when I was a child. But my mom sat by as my father told my sister and me that story. In his presence, she neither endorsed nor rebutted it. When he wasn't around, she despaired over and mocked his racism.

But a few years ago, I mentioned the story of Mann and the quarter, and my mom told me it wasn't true. My father made it up. He told her when they were dating that he'd gotten Mann in trouble for stealing a quarter that had never even gone missing. He thought it was funny. He also thought it was courtship material, apparently. Judging by the fact that my mom married him, it seems he was right. By email, I reminded my mom that my father used the Mann story to persuade my sister and me that Black children were inherently untrustworthy, to persuade us of the necessity of segregation. I asked her: "Since he'd already told you it wasn't true, what did you think when he told it to us? Did you ever ask him to stop lying about it? Or did you consider telling us? What did you think when he told us that we couldn't watch *Sesame Street*? Or when he cut Black children out of our storybooks? What did Granny think?"

My mom didn't reply to the question about the Mann story but said this:

> I thought he was stupid about *Sesame Street*. That's why I let you watch it anyway. I didn't want you to be "culturally deprived," which is what you would have been.
>
> I was absolutely disgusted at his cutting pictures out of your books. He didn't care what I thought. I guess I figured in your little hearts that you would know his actions amounted to nothing in your life attitudes. I think I thought (as usual) that he was an "ass of a man," like Abigail's husband in First or Second Kings (exact words the KJV version uses regarding Abigail's husband). I don't know if Gran was ever aware of it. If so, she would just have thought like I did: he was an ass totally. And all the arguing in the world wouldn't change that. Besides, I tried my best to avoid arguments with him so you and [my sister] wouldn't have to live in any more strife than you already did. I always felt as if you both "knew" about him and dismissed his rants.
>
> Maybe I was wrong, but I never felt as if either of you really respected him or wanted to be like him or his prejudices.

I followed up with more questions, but she didn't answer them.

The adults in the 1950s Delta believed my father's story about Mann. Or at least they pretended to believe him. But the truth was the opposite of the moral my father sought to impart. The white boy was the perpetrator, the unsafe and dishonest figure. The Black boy was punished for buying himself a six-pack of Coke and walking happily down the street with it.

AS I PONDERED MY MOTHER'S complicity in my father's deceit, I also mulled my own. When I was in high school, my father introduced my sister and me to two different girlfriends. "My friend," he called each of them, in their absence. He instructed us not to mention them to each other.

Over the years, we saw them regularly and did as he said. My grandparents visited, met the girlfriends, and followed suit. Friends of mine saw him out with different women, at the movies, at dinner. When I was thirty, he introduced me to another girlfriend, who I later learned was a little younger than I was. It became clear that, from my father's perspective, one of my primary roles on visiting was to help him juggle all the relationships by perpetuating his lies.

One of his girlfriends shared my sister's name, and another shared my (given) name. I suppose this made lying about seeing "us" easier. His longest-term girlfriend, Jenny, did not share either of our names but was under the impression that our father spoke with and visited my sister and me constantly. "When she asks you about my visit to New York," he coached me once, as we were heading to her place, "just go along with it." Another time, he instructed me to pretend Max and I were staying with him even though we were at Max's grandmother's apartment. He later explained that the girlfriends believed my sister still lived in Miami and was getting a graduate degree in accounting at Florida International University. (In reality, my sister had moved to Massachusetts in her early twenties, didn't speak to him, and would never have studied that.)

Max and I last visited my father in 2001, for Christmas. In a phone call beforehand, my father ran down the particular untruths we were to tell each woman. When I called Max to fill him in, he surprised me by saying he wouldn't lie to enable my father's womanizing. I was thirty years old, a feminist and women's-studies minor, and the idea of refusing to help my father string women along had never occurred to me. After a shocked silence, I agreed and rang my father to tell him.

At first, my father shouted and lectured. "I take umbrage at your use of the term 'womanize,'" he said. I encouraged him to look up the definition. He insisted that Jenny was "too fragile" to handle the truth. I laughed and hung up. In the end, he grew conciliatory, assuring me that no questions would arise, no lies would be necessary.

Weeks later, Max, my father, Jenny, and I set out on a ninety-minute drive to Christmas Eve dinner at Jenny's sister's house. Five minutes in, Jenny began to cry. She said it would be our last Christmas together, because my father wouldn't marry her. Then she asked why my sister couldn't be with us.

I'd told my father I wouldn't lie for him, but apparently I was not immediately going to come forward with the truth. I heard myself telling Jenny that I wouldn't answer questions about my sister. "You'll have to ask my father," I said, bowing to his dictates even as I claimed to reject them. In the moment it felt like the greatest defiance imaginable.

Jenny asked if I'd been on the phone with my father one night when an operator interrupted a call at her request. She knew my father and I spoke all the time, she said. (In reality, we spoke once a week, on average, for about twenty minutes, when we were both at work.) But what about then? "Sorry," I said. "I don't know what you're talking about. I don't know about that."

Jenny turned to my father, her face blotchy with anguish. "You lied!"

"If you don't shut up, Jenny," he said, slamming his hands on the wheel, "I'm going to turn this car around."

It was a flashback to my childhood. "Sorry," I whispered to Max in the backseat, and he took my hand. We careened along the interstate. Jenny wept and asked my father where my sister lived. He told her to be quiet. Finally, as we turned in to Jenny's sister's driveway, my father offered an answer that technically didn't contain a lie. "Well, if you go to FIU, you must live in Miami," he said (implying my sister lived in Miami without explicitly saying she did).

His manipulation enraged me. "That's it," I said. "We're not staying."

Jenny's family rushed out to greet us. I'd never met her mother or sisters before. "Merry Christmas!" they shouted. Jenny sobbed into her sister's sweater. "They just got here," she said, "and now they're leaving!"

The family supported her to the door in her crying and went inside. Max tried to arrange alternate transportation, but taxis were scarce, ride-hailing apps did not exist, and Max's brother, who lived an hour's drive away, was, very reasonably, enjoying Christmas Eve dinner of his own. So we knocked on the door, after all, as the others assembled at the table. We were led to the sofa, given plates, and encouraged to help ourselves from the platters in the kitchen.

On the drive home afterward, Jenny asked about my sister again. "She's not here because she's in Massachusetts," I said. "Where she lives."

Jenny turned around to look at me. "She doesn't live with your mother anymore?"

No point in holding back at that stage. "My mom moved to North Carolina six years ago."

A long silence passed. I squeezed Max's hand. My father's watch ticked. "Why would you lie to me about that?" Jenny asked him.

"I don't know, Jenny," my father said. "I just don't know."

A few minutes later, Jenny changed the subject. Wasn't the baby at dinner cute? Didn't my father love him?

Several months later, I had a work voicemail from Jenny. She was weeping. She wanted to apologize, she said, if she'd done something wrong at Christmas.

Back in New York, I didn't see a way to have a relationship with my father without getting entangled in his toxicity. I sent a letter cutting off contact. I said I would be willing to communicate about the past, present, and future of our relationship but only by letter. He left a voicemail for me at work. We were "both professionals," my father said, and "as professionals, we should settle this like professionals." When I didn't succumb, he told his parents I'd made up the Christmas Eve story. I was "troubled," he said, because I "came from a broken home." ("He's the one who broke it," my mom said, her voice vibrating with colossal sass and annoyance, when I told her this.)

My grandparents believed him. Grandma discouraged the broader family from seeing me. Grandpa, in the early stages of Alzheimer's, soon forgot to be mad, but my relationship with Grandma was still strained when she got sick. In our last conversation, neither of us mentioned my father. At the end of her life, when she was unable to speak, I focused on wishing her ease and peace.

SO MANY NIGHTS I sat in my father's study, flooded with dread. When I was nine years old, his disapproval focused on my math grades, but I knew one day he'd discover that sharing his genes didn't make me a genius. Eventually, I'd be unmasked as an ordinary person of reasonable intelligence. He would see that I was, by his metrics, fundamentally defective.

And he did. I was careless and lazy, he said. I needed to put my nose to the grindstone. In high school, there was no excuse for my trouble with physics. When I was kicked by a horse and limped for a time, my father was embarrassed to be seen with me. Later, when I was in college, I needed to lose weight. I styled myself poorly. I should wear high heels on campus, grow my hair out, and wear more dresses. After my overactive thyroid made my hands shake and eyes bulge, he berated my mom for her "defective genes."

But my dad married my mom in part to compensate for deficits of his own. People found her charming. He must have hoped they would view him more favorably by extension and that his children would inherit her charisma. I hoped so, too. "You're just like your goddamned daddy" was one of the most hurtful things my mother could say to me as a child; later I learned it was something Granny said to her.

My father seemed to strive to be unpleasant. In restaurants, if he thought the meal was taking too long, he'd clomp to the kitchen, bang on the door, demand an update. My sister and I would stare at the table when the server brought our plates. His tips were abysmal. Sometimes he left a quarter. If my mom put extra money on the table, he pocketed it. He shouted at grocery-store cashiers, parking-lot attendants, school guidance counselors—anyone who disappointed or inconvenienced him, which nearly everyone did. When meeting people he believed to be his social inferiors, he reveled in giving them his "dead fish" handshake. But on occasion during my childhood, I saw him alienate people by accident. I wondered if he could tell they didn't like him and if it hurt his feelings. I felt embarrassed for him, watching him "uhhhh" through conversations, gesticulate as stiffly as I did, speak with the same strange deliberation, but with no apparent intuition as to other people's reactions. Looking back, I can see he was nervous that I might take after him socially. I was a strange, anxious child, but I always had friends, and he was relieved by this.

His lack of common sense, especially in anger, was remarkable. My mom likes to tell the story of the time when a toilet wouldn't stop running, so he hit the tank with a hammer and shattered it. (Ever thrifty, he apparently put it back together with aquarium glue.) He made coffee by boiling the grounds in a saucepot and pouring liquid from the resulting sludge. After the divorce, when my sister and I were at his house, he'd put us to bed and then sneak out. We didn't mind being left alone. We snooped through his things, found lingerie and a letter from a girlfriend. We ate ice cream. But after a break-in one night when we weren't there, he put key-operated dead bolts on our bedroom doors. Then he locked us in from the hallway, leaving no escape but the windows, which opened toward Bahama shutters that wouldn't have left much room for wriggling out. "Good night, y'all!" he'd say, as he extracted the key. "Daddy loves you!" Soon his car would be pulling out of the garage, into the night.

His house during those years was perpetually infested with huge flying water bugs. They lived in the bathrooms, the pantry, the toaster oven. Many mornings, he'd start making cheese toast for my sister and me and, as the heat clicked on, we'd hear the roaches scrabbling. He'd remove the bread and cheese, douse the toaster oven with Raid, wait a minute or so, and put the toast back in to cook. Sometimes bugs staggered out. Other times they crackled and twitched as cheese dripped down. The toast tasted like burnt cheddar, dirty pennies, and cheap drugstore sunscreen that gets in your mouth when you sweat. Even as a teenager, I was too afraid of his anger to protest.

UNTIL I CUT OFF contact with my father, I downplayed my writing in a way that still bleeds into how I live my life now, a bifurcated existence, one foot in the work I love and the other in a job I'm good at, which affords me a paycheck and benefits. Much of my impulse to write comes from my mom. She endlessly read me books as a child and was always highlighting books of her own. Later, she brought me stacks of library books, sometimes seven one day and seven more the next, and helped with my papers. For many years, she wrote, too—sermons that got longer and funnier and more passionate when she was in the pulpit. But her love was for the performance of storytelling, not the writing. My obsessive commitment to putting words on the page, the way I construct pieces of writing, is much more influenced by my father. Throughout my childhood, he jotted notes in legal pads, read heavy law books, wrote and published articles. When I was seven or maybe eight, he decided to write a legal treatise, the first in its subject area. He was the parent I saw, night and day, sitting at his desk, writing paragraphs, crossing them out, and writing new ones. It was his job. After it was published, he updated his book every year, page proofs littering the floor around the desk in his study.

In many ways, my father's writing is the opposite of what I like to read and try to write. I lean toward straightforward language and active verbs, whereas he uses passive voice and legalese even in personal correspondence and casual conversation. In 2004, after he and I had been estranged for three years, he sent my sister and me photocopies of a letter addressed to us, making the case that our mother was to blame for their divorce, as if that would persuade us to get in touch.

> Most regrettably we have had little contact during the past year and I must acknowledge my bewilderment in this regard.
>
> In this connection my thoughts reverted back to the [attached] 1/20/84 letter from Mommy to me setting out the reasons from her perspective for the divorce. As this was indeed only 9 months after the divorce it is perceived same would offer the most accurate and true state of mind concerning the divorce and the events leading up to it.

I suspect he sent my grandparents the original letter and that he wrote it to convince them that he was reaching out and we were the ones to blame for the rupture. If he felt anguish at our absence from his life, he didn't specifically express it. He did sign off with love.

I remember telling my parents at four or five years old that I planned to be a writer. My father seemed to take me seriously, which made me feel that being a writer was possible. Recently, I discovered that he sent Granny a copy of a short story I'd written in high school. "I wanted you to see Rebecca's story," he wrote, in a note I found amid papers that my mom sent me. Later he viewed my creative pursuits as a boondoggle, possibly unsavory. And I imagine if he had it to do over again, he would have tried to eradicate those ambitions at the first sign of them, just as he hammered the head off my sister's brown-skinned toy, just as he forbade me to play guitar and my sister to play with a football. But it was too late. He encouraged my writing before he discouraged it. His certainty that I could achieve whatever I set out to do was a powerful force. I'm grateful to him for that.

Nowadays I trace fundamental aspects of the way I write to my Newtons—the way I return to subjects again and again, from different angles, explaining my thoughts and feelings to myself as I go and then building them into an argument to satisfy myself and anyone else who might, along the way, be persuaded. I suppose it's a less intrusive counterpart to my father's urge to appear at the foot of someone's bed in the middle of the night with a lit flashlight under his face to say, ". . . and furthermore." My insistence on understanding my family's enslaving history is also a legacy of my Newtons. If my father's racism hadn't been as clear-cut as his grandfather's, maybe I would have been able to overlook it, explain it away, conveniently forget. I'm not glad he raised me in such an explicitly white supremacist way, but I'm grateful that he made it impossible for me to move through life without the level of ignorance I might have had otherwise. He highlighted a trauma our people wrought, in a way I couldn't forget or ignore.

Sometimes people ask if I think there's a chance I'll reconcile with my father. After all, I once was estranged from my mom, so why not reconnect with him, too?

I care about my father and wish him happiness. I've largely made peace with our history. But I don't regret that we're estranged. I don't see a way to have a healthy relationship with someone whose life was so steeped in manipulation and falsehoods that he saw it as my duty to perpetuate them. I'm realistic about what's possible for my father in this life and what's safe for me. I feel sad sometimes that we've never known a pure, healthy father–daughter love, but contact with him at this point would be a form of self-harm.

The day I told my father, back in 2002, that I couldn't have a relationship with him anymore, Grandpa emailed me. "It must be serious to cut your roots," he said. "Better think about it long and hard."

That, at least, is a patriarchal directive I think it's safe to say I've fulfilled.

Chapter 30

ROOTS

———

TOWARD THE END OF GRANDPA'S LIFE, I LEARNED THAT he, like me, had struggled with depression. After he died, I ended up with copies of a few booklets he'd made, little pieces of paper stapled together, smaller than three-by-five index cards. One of them is titled "February Must Be Met." I believe it was a devotional he mentioned delivering late in life, when he must have known his mind was slipping, to his Sunday School class.

> February is not the best month of the year. It is an in-between month, a short bridge between winter and early spring. Every year when I reach it, I feel that winter will not be boss much longer, and for that I am glad. I also feel within my life the stirrings of spring. February will carry me to March, and March will bring longer days, brighter days, and will lead me safely to April mornings. February is my path to spring's return.
>
> In this I find a lesson. There is in every life a February time. It stands between our times of barrenness and our times of increased hope. It is not very exciting. It lacks autumn's glory and spring's festooned splendor. It is just there, a pause,

a connection, a bridge between loss and gain, a road that leads from emptiness to fullness.

I can't remember Grandpa invoking the Bible even once in my presence, but here he finds solace in the knowledge of Jesus's difficult times. Jesus, too, felt sadness, frustration, and a sense of failure, Grandpa writes. Some of his days, like some of ours, were "round-shouldered and slow of foot." He cried out to his father, feeling forsaken. But no matter how impatient we are to see the end of February malaise, we have to wait it out. "Nor would it be good if all days were soft like April mornings or radiant like October afternoons. Nature has February times, and so does man."

Reading this for the first time a decade ago, I felt, as I often did growing up, that I didn't know my grandfather nearly well enough. Over time, his words have taken on a new comfortable resonance—the feeling of a conversation we've left off but are still in the midst of having.

HUMANS ACROSS THE WEST long for connection but have never been more polarized or fearful. We face many dangers, including the possibility of extinction because some of us have insisted, over generations, on seeing ourselves as separate from the earth and the rest of our nonhuman kin.

Malidoma Patrice Somé—who was removed from his community as a boy, to be taught in church schools, and had to learn the ways of his people as a grown man—describes the idea in an Indigenous society of "dire consequences" when "problems that are intended for a collective solution are held personally and privately." He argues that "the way Western societies approach accountability takes a painful toll on the individual," isolating them, condemning them forever, leading them to self-destructive behavior or hostility.

Conversely, in an Indigenous society, accountability means "something like a deepening of the connection with the thing or the person you wronged. If you cause harm to someone, accountability means doing something that brings you close to the person on a regular basis for as long as you live." Indigenous societies dispense with the idea of individual perfection, he says, and embrace the idea of human fallibility.

And when someone dies, mourning and ritual are imperative and collective. The spirit of the deceased attains wellness through the grief that carries them "from one realm to another." They will continue to serve the community as an ancestor, so the community "does all it can to ensure that their spirit makes it safely to their new home."

From this perspective, all our dead who have not been properly grieved and elevated are unwell ghosts cluttering up the spirit realm, preventing us from accessing the wisdom of our ancestors and the best way forward for ourselves. Whether or not we believe in the existence of spirits, on a metaphorical level we can see the consequences of our individualism and disconnectedness all around us. Giving deep consideration to our family dead is a way of reconnecting with the larger circle of humanity, even if we don't believe that the dead can hear us, even if we consider this kind of connection to be purely psychological. For myself, the distinction between imagination and spirituality has come to seem less like a bright line than a continuum.

At times I've found myself projecting concepts from Christianity onto the ancestor work. For a while I found myself in a fundamentalist finger trap, sourly contemplating the potential for "salvation." If helping our family dead to be well, and helping ourselves to be well in the process, would really solve everything, then how did all the ills in the world take root in the first place?

My teacher Larisa Noonan, also raised fundamentalist, understands questions like this. The goal, she says, is not salvation but the removal of confusion, the return of connection and clarity. We can see more clearly where we need to go, how we may best live, if we know precisely, in our bones, who and where we came from.

Through this work, I've reached a place where I feel that the line of my mother's mother's people is well, where their blessings can flow directly to me and sometimes through me. Over time, after many years of anxiety, I developed a sense of both of my grandmothers with me, one over each shoulder, blessing me and this book as I worked. And now as I write these last pages, I have the sense of all my grandparents, and some more-distant ancestors, gathered in a kind of benediction.

Spending time with my ancestors is exciting and scary, joyful and sad, expansive to the edges of the universe and confining as the pain in my jaw. Grappling with their legacies is something I know I will never do perfectly. Making this reckoning as explicit as possible releases me from the idea that I will ever be free of this history. My understanding of the power of all our ancestors for each of us and all of us will continue to take shape in me as long as there is breath in my body.

At least that long.

ACKNOWLEDGMENTS

———

THANK YOU: TO MY AGENT AND IDEAL READER, JULIE BARER, without whom I would never have been brave enough to let my work be everything I didn't know I wanted it to be. To my editor, Andrea Walker, whose edits pushed me ever closer to the true flame of this book, who encouraged my unconventional and sprawling approach to research, who told me to start the book with my father, who never flinched as my approach got more out-there, and whose edits made this book what it is. To Rachel Ake for a gorgeous cover that exceeded all my hopes. To the whole Random House team: Andy Ward, Robin Desser, Emma Caruso, Melanie DeNardo, Benjamin Dreyer, Dennis Ambrose, my unnamed but brilliant copy editor, and everyone else who worked so hard on this book. To my independent publicist, Michael Taeckens, an old friend with a deep understanding of language and readers, for his help moving this book into the world. To Nicole Cunningham and everyone at The Book Group for support and encouragement. To William Boggess, for friendship and help with the proposal. To Elizabeth Bachner, for the texts and phone calls, for sharing her own family stories and spectacular writing with me and for reading at least five drafts of this book and always responding excitedly, no matter what a mess they were. To Carrie Frye, a wonderful friend whose novels-in-progress are marvels, for being the supportive writing partner to whom I reported "done" or "not done," at times daily, over many of the years I worked. To Maaza Mengiste, for detailed draft notes on language and silence and so much more that I will continue to ponder after the book is published; for entrusting me with her own novel draft, which required no notes at all; for flowers when I needed them most; and for our always cherished Queens outings. To Laila Lalami, for her gently tenacious and entirely indispensable suggestions, for her own excellent and inspiring work, and for her many years of friendship. To Sarah Smarsh, straight-shooting sister of my heart, for single-handedly fixing some of the boggiest paragraphs in an early unfinished draft with a few deft maneuvers that I kept in mind as I worked on the rest. To Casey N. Cep, for smart, intricate suggestions throughout, and informed, patient pushback on many of my assertions about Christianity; the book is vastly stronger for her critique, and any shortcomings that remain on this front are entirely my own and not for lack of her trying. To my dearest fellow Miami expat Rahawa Haile, for sharing a little of her brilliant new work with me as we wrote, and for making time for phone calls and cafecitos. To Lizzie Skurnick, for telling me years ago, as I kept berating myself for spending time on genealogy when I was trying to finish a novel, that "your family is your work," even though I wasn't ready to hear her. To my eternal sugar sister, Lauren Cerand, for savory galettes and backyard cocktails, for her stories about her own grandparents, for gold forged with fire, and for the magic of her presence. To Emma Garman, for always picking up the phone across the pond even though getting me to stop talking is never easy, and for her friendship and encouragement. To Alexander Chee, one of my most cherished muses, for everything always. To Kellie Wicker-Downes, D. E. Rasso, Gina Briggs, and Stephany Aulenback, for all the heart-to-hearts over the years about family history. To the Yaddo Foundation, for the gift of two weeks to do nothing but write. To the incredibly talented friends I made at Yaddo. I don't think I'm allowed to list you here, if I understand the rules correctly, but I will carry your work and our time together in my heart always. To the magnificent writers Honorée Fanonne Jeffers and Sheree Greer, each of whom generously shared glimpses into her own ancestral practices. To Garrard Conley, for his friendship and his courageous and generous writing about the intersection of family and religious intolerance. To Emily Raboteau, for insights on the essay that formed the seed of this book; I've held them close over the years. To Saaed Jones and Celeste Ng, for sharing family stories with me as I began work on this book. To Terry Teachout, who encouraged me more than a decade ago to read William Maxwell's *Ancestors* as I mulled whether and how to write about my own family. To Kate Christensen, Phillip Connors, Jason Kerr, and Patrick and Teresa Nielsen Hayden, for early encouragement. To ancestry buff and U.S. diplomat Carl Budd for the tool that helped me find my great-grandfather Charley's death certificate. To the much-missed Awl, and especially to Alex Balk, Choire Sicha, and Carrie Frye for providing a safe space to cultivate the kind of writing that turned into this book, and to Alex for his brilliance and our twenty years of friendship. To Adam Sternbergh, for allowing me to write about my religious childhood for *The New York Times Magazine,* and for knowing enough about charismatic Christianity to shape my work for the better while letting the weird, true stuff stay. To Claire Gutierrez, for accepting and editing a Lives piece that, despite its brevity, is one of my favorite pieces of my own writing. To Hugo Lindgren, for inviting me aboard during his tenure at *The New York Times Magazine,* and to Jon Kelly and Willy Staley for editing my weekly mini-columns there. To Christopher Beha, for inviting me to write at length about genealogy for *Harper's* and editing me so precisely, and for his own thoughts about family. To Tom Jenks and Carol Edgarian of *Narrative Magazine* for publishing my work so beautifully and prominently. To Bill Tipper for his thoughtful editing at *B&N Review* and his friendship. To Nicole Chung, for republishing and interviewing me at Catapult about a newsletter I wrote on white supremacy in my family, and for the inspiration of her own writing. To John Freeman, for featuring a micro-essay about my father at the *Granta* website back in 2008. To Chris Lehmann, for inviting me to write my very first piece of published writing (not counting my high school literary magazine) and for setting the example himself. To my old friend Antonio Ginatta, editor of the high school literary magazine, for calling me at age seventeen to tell me that two of my (not very good) poems had been accepted though only one could be published. To my high school English and creative writing teachers, John Kendall and the late Marianne Kjos; my late English professor David Leverenz; my friend and former law school professor Lyrissa Lidsky; and my City College writing teachers, Aram Veeser, Salar Abdoh, and Linsey Abrams, all of whom encouraged my writing and intellectual foraging in various ways. To my late therapist, Dan Cohen—without whom this book would not exist—for painstakingly helping me see, forty-five minutes at a time, how I might live open-heartedly in the world without feeling like a crustacean lacking a shell. To my current therapist, Jacky Frost. To Dan Cayer, Larisa Noonan, and Ethan Nichtern, for their wisdom and teaching. To Sarah-Lu and Lydia, my sisters in ancestral seeking and deeper earth connection. To Dominick Guerriero, Langston Kahn, Shannon Willis, Daizy October, and Jeanna Kadlec, who served as guides or teachers for me of one kind and another. To Melissa Oaks and Matthew Pickelle, for arranging the two-month leave of absence from my other job at a crucial point and generally being awesome, and to my current manager and all my colleagues there for understanding my occasional need for time away for creative work. To Rebecca Federman and Melanie Locay of the Allen Room at the New York Public Library, for invaluable research tips, a quiet place to work on weekends and weeknights for several months, and a dedicated cubby for my research during that time. To the researchers at the Local History and Genealogy section of the New York Public Library's Irma and Paul Milstein Division of United States History, for answering endless obscure questions. To the genealogical researchers at the Dallas Public Library, who expanded my knowledge of so many things, including how my great-grandfather came to kill a man with a hay hook. To Jason Bordeaux, Jan Hillegas, and Judy Russell for their genealogical research. To Ira Beare for Northampton research assistance, and Julie Bartlett Nelson of Northampton's Forbes Library for background on records relating to Mary Parsons. To Shaker Samman for his excellent fact-checking work on the book as a whole and Brendan O'Connor for some crackerjack targeted facts fine-tuning. Any errors that remain are mine alone. To CeCe Moore for expanding my early understanding of genetic genealogy. To the cousins I've found through genetics, especially Matthew Ware, James Pylant, Deborah Hampton-Miller, and Kristin and Reed, and the cousins I've found through genealogy, especially David Newton, Barbara Grider, and the late Wallace Newton. To Jane, Margaret, Karen, and Ariel, and the rest of the dog-run crew, for the pup fun and welcome distractions from writing. To Marco Navarro for the wisdom about Queens and trees. To chosen family who met up for dinners or long-distance visits and believed the book would get done: Vicky and Christian Zabriskie; Kellie and Greg Wicker and my godson, Graham; Elizabeth and my goddaughter, Aurelie; Darice and Walter Moore; and Mark Sarvas, Jennifer Carson, and Clara. To my late friend Nelson Almeyda. To Max, my partner in life, love, and making art while working a day job, for his kindness, intelligence, and sense of humor over decades, for knowing my work and brain well enough to serve in a pinch as my default thesaurus, for jokingly suggesting the perfect title of this book, and for understanding why I almost never went out to dinner or a movie with him for seven years. To my stepdaughter, Autumn, for her wisdom and love, and the gift of her time. To my brilliant, hilarious, and incisive sister, without whom I don't know how I would have gotten through childhood, who remains a delight and a balm in my life at middle age. To my mother-in-law, Jane, for her love and notes and insight and enthusiasm. To my stepsister, Christina, a fellow seeker. To my beloved sister-in-law, my brothers-in-law and their partners, and my niblings, aunt, uncle, and cousins, for their acceptance, love, and in many cases forbearance. I will refrain from dragging in all their names. To my stepfather. To my late grandparents, especially my granny. And to my mom—our paths and beliefs have taken different directions, but if I wrote the book as I intended, my love for her shines on every page.

NOTES

————

xiv **growing up in 1970s Miami**   I now know and gratefully acknowledge that I grew up on the land of Native nations, including the Tequesta people, the Calusa people, and the Taino people, and today the Seminole people and Miccosukee people. I acknowledge that these peoples and their elders were the original stewards of this land.

xiv **dismal family parcel in the Mississippi Delta**   To the best of my knowledge, this land was Choctaw land. Under the care of the Choctaw people, it undoubtedly had a very different feeling than it did when largely abandoned but planted with fields of cotton for picking by machine.

PART ONE   GENEALOGY

CHAPTER 1. A DOORWAY

4 **bottoming out**   Kristen V. Brown, "Ancestry Pulling Health DNA Test Just over a Year After Launch," *Bloomberg,* Jan. 14, 2021 ("cut jobs as sales of DNA tests slowed"); Nicole Wetsman, "Layoffs at Genetic Testing Companies Reflect the Changing Market," *The Verge,* Feb. 6, 2020; Kate Gibson, "Americans Are Losing Interest in At-Home DNA Ancestry Testing," CBS News website, Feb. 7, 2020.

5 **don't know our own history**   See Chapter 22, "Disconnection," and Chapter 26, "Veneration."

CHAPTER 2. NOT FORGOTTEN

10 **a hay hook in downtown Dallas**   I acknowledge that the area now known as Dallas, like Grand Prairie and North Texas as a whole, was originally land tended and sporadically occupied or used by many Native peoples, including the Kilkaapoi, Wichita, Tawakoni, and Jumanos.

10, 13 **the "difficulty"** "Killed with Hay Hook—Murder Charge Filed," *Daily Times Herald,* June 13, 1916; "Charles Bruce Trial Set," *The Dallas Morning News,* June 15, 1916; "Order Release of Charles Bruce," *The Dallas Morning News,* June 17, 1916.

10 **"the trouble between the two men"** "Killed with Hay Hook—Murder Charge Filed," *Daily Times Herald,* June 13, 1916.

10 **Charley's name, for instance** I'm unsure whether Charley Bruce's given name was William Charles Bruce or Charles William Bruce. He went by Charles or Charley/Charlie and was generally identified that way, including on his draft card and death certificate and in newspaper reporting of his marriage and the hay-hook incident. In the 1880 census he is listed as Charles William Bruce. But in one census and on two of his children's birth certificates he's identified as William Charles Bruce, and one of his grandchildren is named William Charles Bruce. His eldest son, my grandfather Robert, wrote a request to the state of Texas for his birth certificate in 1966 and gave his father's name as William Charles Bruce, though Robert's own death certificate identifies his father as Charlie Bruce.

12 **born in Georgia, in 1879** He was probably born in or near Dawsonville, on Tsalaguwetiyi (Cherokee) or Yuchi (S'atsoyaha) land, but I'm not certain.

12 **Doctors said** "Skull Is Crushed as Truck Is Hit," *The Dallas Morning News,* Nov. 3, 1935. According to this article, doctors initially thought S.E. would not survive. My mom recalls being told that, when he did live, they predicted he would be paralyzed.

12 **received an insurance settlement** *Bruce v. Miller,* Dkt. No. 18969-E/A, Dist. Ct., Dallas County, 14th Judicial Dist., May 5, 1936 (order approving a $4,400 settlement to be held by the court); *Bruce v. Miller,* Dkt. No. 18696-A, Dist. Ct., Dallas County, 101st Judicial Dist., May 13, 1936 (order approving payment of $1,466 in attorneys' fees from the $4,400 settlement and disbursement of $934 to Rindia Bruce, with an unknown portion of that earmarked for "all of the doctor and hospital bills including nursing and medicine" rendered to S.E. as of that date); *Bruce v. Miller,* Dkt. No. 18696-A, Dist. Ct., Dallas County, 14th Judicial Dist., July 17, 1936 (order approving payment to Rindia of $2,000 from the trust fund held by the court for S.E., who was still a minor).

12 **a forerunner to today's megachurches** W. K. McNeil, "Rex Humbard Family Singers," *Encyclopedia of American Gospel Music* (New York: Routledge, 2005), p. 338, noting that in 1939, Pastor Albert Ott's Bethel Temple Church was "the largest Assembly of God church in America"; David W. Spence, Landmark Nomination of the Bishop Arts Building, 408 West Eighth Street, submitted to the Dallas Landmark Commission, Mar. 29, 1999, noting that the Bishop Arts Building was owned by Ott until the early 1960s, when the area became less "homogeneous, tightly-knit, and safe" and hypothesizing that Ott "of Bethel Temple, a prominent Oak Cliff church, may have decided that renting to the lower class did not befit a minister." There is no record of Rindia's gift to the church, only my mom's memory of what her parents told her.

13 **"a preliminary hearing"** "Charles Bruce Trial Set," *The Dallas Morning News,* June 15, 1916.

13 **articles in other papers** "Farmers' 6-Year Feud Ends in Murder Charge," *The Dallas Dispatch,* June 13, 1916; "Killed with Hay Hook—Murder Charge Filed," *Daily Times Herald,* June 13, 1916.

13 **which newspaper you believe** "Farmers' 6-Year Feud Ends in Murder Charge," *The Dallas Dispatch,* June 13, 1916; "Killed with Hay Hook—Murder Charge Filed,"

Daily Times Herald, June 13, 1916; "Order Release of Charles Bruce," *The Dallas Morning News,* June 17, 1916.

14 **"the sharp point"**   "Killed with Hay Hook—Murder Charge Filed," *Daily Times Herald,* June 13, 1916.

14 **"testimony in [Grimes's] trial"**   "Farmers' 6-Year Feud Ends in Murder Charge," *The Dallas Dispatch,* June 13, 1916.

14 **"mistreatment of a 'female relative'"**   Ibid.

14 **acting in self-defense**   "Order Release of Charles Bruce," *The Dallas Morning News,* June 17, 1916.

15 **on Grimes's case—twice**   *Grimes v. State,* 141 S.W. 261, Nov. 29, 1911; *Grimes v. State,* 160 S.W. 689 (1913).

17 **"they figured there would never be"**   Skip Hollandsworth, "Patient Observation," *Texas Monthly,* June 2010.

17 **"exhaustion from manic depressive insanity"**   Charles Bruce, Death Certificate, July 13, 1927, File No. 25469, Wichita County, Texas State Department of Health, copy on file with author.

17 **confirmed to me that he's buried**   Elizabeth J. Boyt, certified paralegal, Office of General Counsel, Texas Dept. of State Health Service, Open Records Request No. 18809, Apr. 18, 2011, confirming that "'the burial log at North Texas State Hospital, Wichita Falls Campus, shows that a Charles Bruce, date of death July 13, 1927, is buried in plot #65. The log actually shows "Chas," but as that is the preferred abbreviation for Charles, I believe this is the correct information for your relative.'" I acknowledge that Charley is buried on Kiikaapoi and possibly Wichita and Numunuu (Comanche) land.

CHAPTER 3. LIKE A LENTICULAR PRINT

20 **oldest form of logic**   Staffan Müller-Wille and Hans-Jörg Rheinberger, *A Cultural History of Heredity* (University of Chicago Press, 2012), p. 1.

20 **"ancient logic such as genus"**   Ibid.

20 **"of noble birth"**   Plato, *Plato in Twelve Volumes,* vol. 12, trans. Harold N. Fowler (Cambridge, Mass.: Harvard University Press; London: William Heinemann, 1921; Perseus Digital Library), 12.174(e)–12.175(a).

20 **"has had countless thousands of ancestors"**   Ibid.

20 **questioning the value of pedigrees**   Juvenal, *Juvenal and Persius: With an English Translation,* trans. George Gilbert Ramsey (New York: William Heinemann, 1918; Perseus Digital Library), p. 159.

20 **"Boast a Fabius"**   Ibid.

21 **"so worn by age"**   François Rabelais, *The Complete Works of Rabelais: The Five Books of Gargantua and Pantagruel,* trans. Jacques Le Clercq (New York: The Modern Library, 1936), pp. 39–40.

21 **"Genealogy? That's like those people"**   Christine Kenneally, *The Invisible History of the Human Race: How DNA and History Shape Our Identities and Our Futures* (New York: Viking, 2014), p. 19.

21 **who once described fictional characters**   E. M. Forster, *Aspects of the Novel* (London: Edward Arnold, 1927), p. 75.

22 **the province of royalty**   François Weil, *Family Trees: A History of Genealogy in America* (Cambridge, Mass.: Harvard University Press, 2013), p. 10.

22 **their own siblings or close cousins**   Ker Than, "King Tut Mysteries Solved: Was

Disabled, Malarial, and Inbred," *National Geographic,* Feb. 17, 2010; Marwa Awad, "Egypt's King Tut Born of Incestuous Marriage: Tests," *Reuters,* Feb. 17, 2010; Niraj Rana, "Tutankhamun Parents Were Cousins, Not Siblings," *The Times of India,* Feb. 20, 2013.

22 **To represent the relationships**   Nadieh Bremer, "Royal Constellations," Visual Cinnamon website, October 2016.

23 **crucial to their prestige and position**   Rosalind Thomas, *Oral Tradition and Written Record in Classical Athens* (Cambridge Studies in Oral and Literate Culture, 1989), pp. 107, 155–157, 173.

23 **some French and German royal lines claimed**   Jill Raitt, "Spiritual Relations, Bodily Realities: Ancestors in the European Catholic Tradition," *Ancestors in Post-Contact Religion: Roots, Ruptures, and Modernity's Memory,* ed. Steven J. Friesen (Cambridge, Mass.: Harvard University Press, 2001), p. 221.

23 **nine bound volumes**   Alexander Chee, conversation with Maud Newton, notes on file with author, Oct. 4, 2014.

23 **The books are filled with**   Maud Newton, Tumblr blog post, "The Begats," Oct. 6, 2014, including a selection of images posted with Chee's permission.

23 **"blue-eyed, blond-haired American girl"**   Alexander Chee, "Portrait of My Father," *Granta* website, Mar. 11, 2009.

23 **A generation after the Revolution**   Weil, *Family Trees,* pp. 57–58. As Weil writes elsewhere in *Family Trees,* in the sixteenth century, bourgeois European merchants started emulating aristocrats and creating their own genealogical records, but even then the practice was not by and large imported to the American colonies until the 1800s. Some early colonists used Bibles to record their marriages and progeny, but "ascending," or backward-looking, genealogies were rare.

23 **"despise pedigree"**   Ibid., pp. 46, 54.

24 **"made himself so conspicuous"**   Nathaniel Hawthorne, *The Scarlet Letter* (Boston: James R. Osgood and Co., 1878), pp. 8–9.

24 **"Anglo-Saxon purity"**   Weil, *Family Trees,* p. 120.

24 **"extremely remote connection"**   Charlotte Perkins Gilman, The Living of Charlotte Perkins Gilman, (University of Wisconsin Press, 1991), p. 1.

24 **passing down Bibles, heirlooms, or memorabilia**   Alison Light, *Common People* (University of Chicago Press, 2015), Preface.

25 **"My father was a white man"**   Frederick Douglass, *Narrative of the Life of Frederick Douglass, an American Slave: Written by Himself* (Boston: The Anti-Slavery Office, 1845), p. 2.

26 **white people married Osage**   David Grann, *Killers of the Flower Moon: The Osage Murders and the Birth of the FBI* (New York: Doubleday, 2017).

26 **The novelist Celeste Ng's great-grandfather**   Maud Newton, "The Family Tree: Celeste Ng," *Tin House* website, Nov. 6, 2014.

27 **Genealogy is so embedded**   Oftentimes, members of the church run out of known relations but still need people to baptize, and so people who aren't family members end up getting swept in. In this way, cultural icons such as Anne Frank have notoriously and very controversially been baptized; the church has publicly repudiated this practice, but conversations I've had with LDS members suggest baptism of non-relatives continues all the same in many LDS communities.

30 **"directed almost exclusively toward establishing"**   H. L. Mencken, *Prejudices: First Series* (New York: Knopf, 1919), p. 332.

30 **evidently considered himself to qualify**   Terry Teachout, *The Skeptic: A Life of H. L. Mencken* (New York: Harper Perennial, 2002); Fred Hobson, *Mencken: A Life*

(New York: Random House, 1994); D. G. Hart, *Damning Words: The Life and Religious Times of H. L. Mencken* (Grand Rapids, Mich.: Eerdmans, 2016).

PART TWO   GENETIC GENEALOGY

CHAPTER 4. SKELETONS AND MAGNOLIAS

33 **Gulf Coast town**   The town was Long Beach, Mississippi, which I acknowledge as Chahta Yakni land.

38 **a website devoted to**   The site was called Miami Stories, and it no longer exists.

CHAPTER 5. FAMILY SECRETS

37 **Gulf Coast town**   The town was Long Beach, Mississippi, which I acknowledge as Chahta Yakni land.

41 DREW'S LAST COTTON BUYER   Ruth Jensen, "Drew's Last Cotton Buyer Goes Out of Business," publication and date unknown, but likely *Sunflower County News,* 1976.

43 **"granted a license to retail spirituous"**   Biographical and Historical Memoirs of Drew County, Arkansas (Goodspeed Publishing Company, 1890), p. 929. I acknowledge that Drew County is on Ogaxpa land. And if Jesse was born in Duplin County, North Carolina, he most likely came into the the world and was raised on Skaruhreh/Tuscarora and/or Lumbee land.

43 **and a boy who was orphaned**   Ibid., p. 948.

43 **"an honored citizen of that bailiwick"**   Josiah Hazen Shinn, Pioneers and Makers of Arkansas (Washington, D.C.: Genealogical Publishing Company, 1908, p. 195.

43 **Jesse also enslaved six people**   1860 U.S. Census, Drew County, Ark., slave schedule, Spring Hill Township, p. 262 (handwritten number scratched out; 262 stamped), Jesse Newton, slave owner, NARA microfilm publication M653, roll 29.

44 **"We had the same problem"**   Wallace Dolphin Newton, letter to Maud Newton, Sept. 5, 2009.

44 **according to *Texas Hill Country Magazine***   Max McNabb, "The Newton Boys: Charming Texas Outlaws Who Robbed 85 Banks & Half a Dozen Trains," *Texas Hill Country,* June 25, 2018.

44 **some similar names and close proximity**   According to various citizen genealogist sources online, the Newton brothers were descended from: their great-grandfather James Sutton Newton, who was born in South Carolina in 1800 and died in Calhoun County, Arkansas, in 1868; their grandfather Jesse James Newton, who was born in 1831 and died in 1896 in Calhoun County, Arkansas; and their father, James Willis Newton, who was born in 1854 in Calhoun County, Arkansas, and died in 1933 in Uvalde County, Texas. See, for example: James Sutton Newton, Find a Grave, Memorial 20626294, added July 21, 2007; Jesse James Newton, Find a Grave, Memorial ID 92409122, added June 23, 2012; James Willis Newton, Find a Grave, Memorial ID 42010119, added Sept. 15, 2009; Gregory Newton, "Re: The Newton Gang, Late 1800's," Genealogy.com, July 26, 1999. My Newtons descend from my fourth great-grandfather Jesse W. Newton, and his son, my third great-grandfather James S. Newton, who died of disease during the Civil War at age 28, six days before his second son, my second great-grandfather, James Alexander Newton, was born; the names represented by the "W" and "S" initials are unknown.

My Jesse Newton migrated from North Carolina to Drew County, Arkansas, which is now just over an hour's drive from Calhoun County, Arkansas, where the other Jesse Newton lived.

CHAPTER 6. DNA SLEUTHING

45 **asking about my family's connection**   Name withheld for privacy, Ancestry.com messages to Maud Newton, Mar. 7, 2019, Mar. 19, 2019, Aug. 15, 2020.

46 **background in pattern recognition**   Kevin Kinchen, Ancestry.com message to Maud Newton, Aug. 4, 2013.

47 **"the myth of the 1870 Brick Wall"**   Shannon Christmas, "Pre-1870 African American Genealogy Is Real," Through the Trees Tumblr, July 28, 2020; Shannon Christmas, "Ancestry.com IS for Black People: The True Story of How to Research African American Family History—Part I," Through the Trees Tumblr, Feb. 25, 2021; Shannon Christmas, "Ancestry.com IS for Black People: The True Story of How to Research African American Family History—Part II," Through the Trees Tumblr, Feb. 26, 2021; Shannon Christmas, "Ancestry.com IS for Black People: The True Story of How to Research African American Family History—Part III," Through the Trees Tumblr, Feb. 27, 2021.

47 **"an unmarked door"**   Shannon Christmas, "Pre-1870 African American Genealogy Is Real," Through the Trees Tumblr, July 28, 2020.

47 **as of January 2021, the site**   Matthew Ware, ancestry composition results, 23andMe, Jan. 2021.

47 **Ware has learned**   Matthew F. Ware, email to Maud Newton, June 27, 2013.

47 **"I believe that gift"**   Deborah Hampton-Miller, 23andMe message, Feb. 28, 2014.

47 **As of January 2021, 23andMe**   Deborah Hampton-Miller, ancestry composition results, 23andMe, Jan. 2021.

48 **According to 23andMe originally**   Maud Newton, ancestry composition results, 23andMe, 2010.

48 **My mother was 100 percent**   Sandy Bruce, ancestry composition results, 23andMe, 2013.

48 **The second account**   Maud Newton, ancestry composition results, 23andMe, 2015.

48 **percentage settled for a time**   Maud Newton, ancestry composition results, 23andMe, 2017; Maud Newton, ancestry composition results (second account), 23andMe, 2017.

48 **Then, in 2019**   Maud Newton, ancestry composition results, 23andMe, 2019; Maud Newton, ancestry composition results (second account), 23andMe, 2019.

48 **As of January 2021, I have been assigned**   Maud Newton, ancestry composition results, 23andMe, Jan. 2021; Maud Newton, ancestry composition results (second account), 23andMe, Jan. 2019.

48 **The closest ancestor might be**   Debbie Parker Wayne, Percentage of Shared Autosomal DNA, presentation PDF, DebbieWayne.com, accessed May 15, 2021; CeCe Moore, Forensic Genealogy Course, Dallas, Tex., March 2015.

48 **denounced in the site's forums**   Various discussions, 23andMe forums, now removed, last accessed 2015; HHRoyalThrowaway, comment on "Ancestry Composition Algorithm Update (v5.9) Has Now Rolled Out to All V5 Chip Tested Users (Official Release)," 23andMe, Reddit, posted by U/Spacemutant14, 2020 ("This one seems way off"); Noah678, comment on Ibid. ("this is very inaccurate for me");

JohnBoddy, comment on Ibid. ("Maybe I'm shit at math, but something about this update seems very off"); Hippielilthang, comment on Ibid. ("It seems like something went horribly wrong"); Kirlie, comment on Ibid. ("The previous version seemed more accurate").

49 **AncestryDNA breaks down regions differently** Maud Newton, ethnicity estimates, AncestryDNA, 2012–21.

49 **While about 15 percent of adults** Nikki Graf, "Mail-in DNA Test Results Bring Surprises About Family History for Many Users," Pew Research Center, Aug. 6, 2019.

49 **"ancestry-informative markers"** Alex Wagner, *Futureface: A Family Mystery, an Epic Quest, and the Secret to Belonging* (New York: One World, 2018), pp. 284–285, 298.

50 **"wants a *yes* or *no*"** Ibid., pp. 294, 304.

50 **"flossy statistics"** Ibid., p. 305.

50 **"Possibly inaccurate to the point"** Ibid., pp. 286, 309.

50 **"classified using political borders"** Ibid., p. 286.

50 **True, Burma** Ibid., p. 284.

50 **"At what point was Burmese blood"** Ibid., p. 286.

50 **The major testing companies' reference samples** Amadou Diallo and Brishette Mendoza, "The Best DNA Testing Kit," Wirecutter, *The New York Times*, last updated Oct. 26, 2020.

50 **"newfound ancestral lands"** "DNA Travel, It's a Trip," 23andMe blog, Jul 5, 2017. See also "Travel As Unique As Your DNA," Airbnb website, last accessed May 15, 2021; "Explore Your Ancestral Homeland," Heritage Tourism, Ancestry-ProGenealogists, last accessed May 15, 2021.

50 **"handpicked hotels, authentic cuisine"** Our Heritage Tours, Go Ahead Tours website, last accessed May 15, 2021.

50 **only 1,980 "reference individuals"** Reference data sets, ancestry composition scientific details, 23andMe website, last accessed May 15, 2021.

50-51 **"Only white people can steal you"** Mina II Society, Twitter post, Jan. 12, 2018.

51 **more than 30,000 Indigenous African DNA samples** Diallo and Mendoza, "The Best DNA Testing Kit."

52 **"gift deed"** Sally Newton, Deed of Gift, Duplin County, North Carolina Deed Book 8A, dated Aug. 14, 1810, filed July 1823, p. 137.

52 **"a very close fit"** Jason Bordeaux, email to Maud Newton, Sept. 23, 2014.

52 **"Sally Newton having been delivered"** Duplin County Court Minutes, Duplin County, North Carolina, Jan. 19, 1808. Bordeaux observed that the entry in the minutes "is brief compared to others. Usually there is at least one or two men who post the bond. Sometimes the man who caused the pregnancy and his relative or sometimes the woman's family. There are a LOT of entries during this period in Duplin that say things like this: 'James Smith guilty of begetting a bastard child upon the body of Jane Doe.' That's just an example. Unfortunately, we don't get details like this for Sally Newton." Jason Bordeaux, email to Maud Newton, Sept. 27, 2014.

52 **"with public knowledge or a complaint"** Dave Tabler, "Bastardy Bonds," Appalachian History blog, Nov. 13, 2018.

52 **"asked to declare the name"** Betty and Edwin Camin, North Carolina Bastardy Bonds (Mount Airy, N.C.: B. J. and E. A. Camin, 1990).

53 **"Illegitimacy was very common"** Jason Bordeaux, email to Maud Newton, Sept. 27, 2014.

53 **"made her mark"**   Sally Newton, Deed of Gift, filed July 1823, p. 137.

53 **an announcement in the newspaper**   Petition for Partition, *The North Carolinian,* Fayetteville, N.C., July 5, 1845.

53 **an additional 0.2 percent**   Relative Finder, 23andMe, last accessed May 15, 2021.

CHAPTER 7. A UNIVERSAL FAMILY TREE

55 **"everyone in the world outside"**   Christine Kenneally, *The Invisible History of the Human Race: How DNA and History Shape Our Identities and Our Futures* (New York: Viking, 2014), p. 247.

55 **Kenneally imagines them**   Ibid., p. 252.

56 **"a library of ancient genomes"**   Ibid., p. 253.

56 **"a unified humanity"**   Eva Botkin-Kowacki, "How a 400,000-Year-Old Skull Fragment Hints at Ancient 'Unified Humanity,'" *The Christian Science Monitor,* Mar. 14, 2017.

56 **"Our family tree was rooted"**   Carl Sagan and Ann Druyan, *Shadows of Forgotten Ancestors* (New York: Ballantine Books, 1993), p. 412.

57 **"from the hardscrabble Adirondack frontier"**   Joan Didion, *Where I Was From* (New York: Vintage Books, 2004), p. 94.

57 **"a blinding and pointless compaction"**   Ibid., p. 4.

57 **"pragmatic and in their deepest instincts"**   Ibid., p. 5.

57 **"What hurts is not just"**   David Treuer, *The Heartbeat of Wounded Knee: Native America from 1890 to the Present* (New York: Riverhead, 2019), p. 451.

58 **"Twenty little centuries flutter away"**   Mark Twain, *The Innocents Abroad, or the New Pilgrims' Progress* (Hartford: American Publishing Co., 1869; University of Virginia Library, Electronic Text Center), p. 336.

58 **A fantastic counterpoint**   *They Are We,* directed by Emma Christopher (2014; Brooklyn, N.Y.: Icarus Films, 2015).

59 **In our first conversation**   CeCe Moore, telephone interview with Maud Newton, notes on file with author, June 26, 2013.

60 **John had always admired Jefferson**   CeCe Moore, "DNA Test Spurs Surprising Discovery of Great Grandfather Thomas Jefferson," Your Genetic Genealogist, Sept. 30, 2011.

61 *The Genetic Detective*   First season directed by Remy Weber, performed by CeCe Moore, ABC, 2020.

62 **Moore wasn't involved in the case**   Heather Murphy, "Technique Used to Find Golden State Killer Leads to a Suspect in 1987 Murders," *The New York Times,* May 18, 2018; Heather Murphy, "Genealogists Turn to Cousins' DNA and Family Trees to Crack Five More Cold Cases," *The New York Times,* June 27, 2018; Jacey Fortin, "In Serial Rape Case That Stumped Police, Genealogy Database Leads to Arrest," *The New York Times,* Aug. 23, 2018.

62 **I was aware of Parabon's "Snapshot"**   Jordan Pearson, "Police Released a Suspect Photo Based on DNA from a Decades-Old Murder," Motherboard, *Vice,* Jan. 26, 2017; Carrie Arnold, "The Controversial Company Using DNA to Sketch the Faces of Criminals," *Nature,* Sept. 9, 2020.

62 **a "green light"**   Antonio Regalado and Brian Alexander, "The Citizen Scientist Who Finds Killers from Her Couch," *MIT Technology Review,* June 22, 2018.

62 **In 2019, GEDmatch changed its policy**   Judy G. Russell, "GEDmatch Reverses Course," The Legal Genealogist blog, May 19, 2019. But see Judy G. Russell, "The Choice That Really Isn't," The Legal Genealogist blog, May 22, 2019.

63 **Back in 2013, Moore was as ardent** CeCe Moore, telephone interview with
    Maud Newton, notes on file with author, June 26, 2013.

CHAPTER 8. TAKING A BITE

64 **"turn to forensic evidence"** Alondra Nelson, *The Social Life of DNA* (Boston:
    Beacon Press, 2016), p. 166.
64 **"There has just got to be"** Community Thread, 23andMe website, date un-
    known. While the 23andMe Community forums have been removed, this ex-
    change existed at least as far back as 2013, when I included it in an article for
    Harper's magazine. Maud Newton, "America's Ancestry Craze," *Harper's*, June
    2014.
64 **"really smarter than others"** RyanMD, Community Thread, 23andMe website,
    date unknown.
66 **But the U.S. Food and Drug** Peter Loftus, "Genetic Test Service 23andMe Or-
    dered to Halt Marketing by FDA," *The Wall Street Journal*, Nov. 25, 2013.
66 **By agreement with the FDA** Julia Belluz, "The FDA Ordered 23andMe to
    Stop Offering Users Unapproved Health Tests. Now It's Back," *Vox*, Oct. 21, 2015;
    Aditi Pai, "Two Years After FDA Letter, 23andMe Finally Relaunches Consumer
    Genetic Testing in US," MobiHealthNews, Oct. 22, 2015.
66 **23andMe has added tests** "FDA Allows Marketing of First Direct-to-
    Consumer Tests that Provide Genetic Risk Information For Certain Conditions,"
    U.S. Food & Drug Administration website, Apr. 6, 2017.
66 **A controversial breast-cancer-risk test** Editorial Board, "Why You Should Be
    Careful About 23andMe's Health Test, *The New York Times*, Feb. 1, 2019.
66 **One 23andMe user was devastated** Dorothy Pomerantz, "23ndMe Had Devas-
    tating News About My Health. I Wish a Person Had Delivered It," *Stat*, Aug. 8,
    2019.
66 **Another user credited the site** Shaheen Pasha, "23andMe Revealed a Condi-
    tion It Took My Doctors Six Years to Diagnose," *Quartz*, Nov. 27, 2013.
67 **She's studied the disproportionately large** Maud Newton, conversation with
    Margaret Pericak-Vance, Director, John P. Hussman Institute for Human Genom-
    ics, May 22, 2013.
67 **In 2021, the company announced** Ancestry Team, "Ancestry Deepens Focus on
    Family History; Will Discontinue AncestryHealth," Ancestry.com website, Jan. 14,
    2021; Discontinuation of AncestryHealth, Ancestry.com, last accessed May 15,
    2021; Staff Reporter, "Ancestry to Discontinue NGS-Based AncestryHealth Ser-
    vice," GenomeWeb, Jan. 15, 2021. The company will discontinue access to Ancestry-
    Health for existing customers after July 2021. Presumably this data will remain
    available to AncestryHealth and its partners, including Quest Diagnostics, Illu-
    mina, and PWNHealth.
68 **the "empathy gene"** Maud Newton, "America's Ancestry Craze," *Harper's*, June
    2014. See also "The Genetics of Empathy," 23andMeBlog, June 6, 2017, and accom-
    panying user comments; "New Research on the Genetics of Empathy, and How It
    Relates to Autism," 23andMeBlog, Mar. 12, 2018, and accompanying user com-
    ments. Most discussion and debate about results now occurs off the site. See, e.g.,
    "What Is Your Rs53576 (Empathy Gene)?" 23andMe, Reddit, 2020 (exact date un-
    known), and accompanying comments.
68 **Some scientists compare** Maud Newton, "A Conversation with Misha Angrist,
    Publisher of His Genome," *The Awl*, Jan. 10, 2011.

PART THREE   NATURE AND NURTURE
CHAPTER 9. IT SKIPS A GENERATION

73 **A friend thought**   Comments on a post at the Language Hat blog inspired by a post on my own blog including this and more of Granny's expressions spurred a number of other suggestions and speculations from language lovers, including that the expression could have been taken from or inspired by the Appalachian musical *Li'l Abner* or that it could be a reference to sharpshooting. "Talking Texan," Language Hat, Sept. 25, 2009, and accompanying comments. See also "Like We Say Back Home," MaudNewton.com, Sept. 20, 2009. For more of Granny's expressions, see Maud Newton, "Grannyisms: Like We Say Back Home," Medium, May 8, 2021.

74 **"diagnosis of hopelessness"**   Richard Noll, *American Madness: The Rise and Fall of Dementia Praecox* (Cambridge, Mass.: Harvard University Press, 2011), pp. 3–4.

75 **"the most frequently diagnosed"**   Interview with Richard Noll, "The Rise and Fall of American Madness," Harvard University Press blog, Jan. 30, 2021.

75 **According to Louise's death certificate**   Louise Johnston, Death Certificate, Feb. 1, 1943, File No. 8499, Kaufman County, Texas State Department of Health, copy on file with author.

75 **"We are sorry this girl"**   Wm. Thomas, M.D., Superintendent, Terrell State Hospital. Letter to Mrs. Z. H. (Alma) Johnston, undated carbon copy to Mrs. Robert Bruce, postmarked Feb. 3, 1943, on file with author.

75 **Alma's draft response**   Alma Johnston, draft letter to Dr. Wm. Thomas and staff, n.d., on file with author. A reply from the hospital arrived later that month. R. C. Sloan, M.D., Acting Superintendent, Terrell State Hospital. Letter to Mrs. [Z]. H. (Alma) Johnston, Feb. 22, 1943, on file with author.

75 **The obituary was brief**   "Louise Johnston Dies," Newspaper Publication Unknown, n.d., clipping on file with author.

76 **When she got pregnant again**   Sandy Bruce, emails to Maud Newton, Apr. 12, 2007 (noting that "Granny told me this long after I was grown. As far as I know Mammy didn't get in any trouble—don't know if anyone missed the infant. The way they dressed back then, a woman could probably hide pregnancy pretty easily under all the clothes. She hit the baby's head on the back door stoop"), Apr. 14, 2007, and Apr. 18, 2007 (noting that "Gran never talked about her much at all after she died . . . except to drop the bomb about the infant on the doorstep").

76 **"Mammy was rather a fearsome lady"**   Ibid., Apr. 14, 2007.

76 **"Each Johnston carried a can"**   Ibid., Apr. 12, 2007.

76 **"It is not too hard to believe"**   Ibid., Apr. 14, 2007.

77 **Among Granny's papers after her death**   Robert Bruce and Martha Johnston, "Marriage Licenses," *Dallas Morning News*, Oct. 29, 1939. The address given for the two is the same.

78 **On the phone years later**   Sandy Bruce, telephone conversation with Maud Newton, around 2011, author's memory.

78 **"was their most outstanding designer"**   Sandy Bruce, email to Maud Newton, Feb. 16, 2007.

79 **Researching further,**   Robert Bruce and Martha Johns[t]on, Marriage Record, Dallas County, No. 20401, filed Nov. 14, 1939, and reflecting that the marriage occurred Nov. 13, 1939, and the marriage license was granted Oct. 27, 1939.

79 **I also learned that Robert**   Robert Charles Bruce and Nettie Ma[e] Mason, Marriage Record, Dallas County, No. 106626, married Aug. 24, 1925, filed Aug. 26, 1925; Robert Charles Bruce and Clara Mae Brantley, Marriage Record, Bryan

County (Oklahoma County Marriage Records 1890–1995, Ancestry.com, Film No. 002194754), Apr. 19, 1930; Robert Charles Bruce and Rose Marie Emily Camiani, Marriage Record, Rockwall County (Texas, Select County Marriage Records 1837–1965, Ancestry.com, Film No. 17971), license granted and marriage performed July 3, 1937.

79 **"in or about or upon"**   *Rose Marie Bruce v. Robert Bruce*, Dkt. No. 41818-C, 68th Judicial Dist. Ct., Dallas County, Mar. 31, 1939. Quite a few of the cases involving Robert and his family, including this one, were decided by Judge Sarah T. Hughes, who later came to nationwide fame for swearing in Lyndon B. Johnson on Air Force One after John F. Kennedy's assassination. She also handled the first two cases involving Robert Bruce's brother S.E.'s insurance settlement, which their mother, Rindia, reportedly gave to her and S.E.'s church. (See Chapter 2, Notes 6–8.) My mom remembers Robert taking her to meet Hughes at some point in the 1960s. Hughes also presided over the three-judge federal panel that overturned Texas's abortion law in *Roe v. Wade*. "Sarah T. Hughes (1896–1985)," State Bar of Texas website, last accessed May 15, 2021.

79 **At some point Robert wept**   Sandy Bruce, emails and conversations with Maud Newton, 2007–2020.

80 **"to cook him a steak"**   Sandy Bruce, conversation with Maud Newton, Apr. 2018.

81 **And Alma's great-grandmother was abandoned**   Court Record, appointment of a tutor (guardian) for John Milton Kinchen, St. Helena Succession Bin M-4, p. 20 (uploaded by Ancestry.com user JPB419, June 14, 2012), May 12, 1823, noting that "the reputed father of the heir, having abandoned the wife and infant child before her death . . . had continued to do so ever since."

81 **The first, from Robert to Christine**   Christine Weber (née Barta), letter to Robert Bruce, 1939, on file with author.

81 **Next came Robert's letter**   Robert Bruce, letter on file with author, Sept. 11, 1943.

81 **For the third letter**   Martha Bruce, draft letter on file with author, n.d.

82 **Granny divorced Robert**   *Martha J. Bruce v. Robert Bruce*, Dkt. No. 76039-F, 116th Dist. Ct., Dallas County, Feb. 10, 1944.

84 **Granny married an older, well-off man**   R. Smith Alexander and Martha Johnston Bruce, Marriage Record, Dallas County, No. 91952, license granted Apr. 19, 1929, married Apr. 30, 1949, filed May 2, 1949.

85 **One of the things that surprised me**   Martha Alexander (née Johnston), scrapbook, on file with author, December 1940.

86 **"really a good guy"**   Ray Lee Bruce, telephone conversation with Maud Newton, July 31, 2015.

86 **"hereditary structures"**   Anne Ancelin Schützenberger, *The Ancestor Syndrome: Transgenerational Psychotherapy and the Hidden Links in the Family Tree* (New York: Routledge, 1998, digital print in 2010), p. 121.

86 **"genetic variants do not *cause*"**   Gregory L. Stuart, et al., "Genetic Associations with Intimate Partner Violence in a Sample of Hazardous Drinking Men in Batterer Intervention Programs," *Violence Against Women*, 20, no. 4 (2014), pp. 385–400.

87 **"similar to heritability for divorce"**   Tim Spector, *Identically Different: Why We Can Change Our Genes* (New York: Overlook Press, 2012), p. 213.

CHAPTER 10. AN IMPULSE TO LEAP

91 **"gave me back my bras"**   Sandy Bruce, conversation with Maud Newton, author's memory, 2015.

91 **She also had a serious beau** Sandy Bruce, various conversations with Maud Newton, author's memory, 2012–1019.

94 **"the archaic heritage of human beings"** Sigmund Freud, *Moses and Monotheism* (1939), in *The Complete Psychological Works of Sigmund Freud*, vol. 23 (London: The Hogarth Press, 1952), p. 99.

94 **In her 1998 book** Anne Ancelin Schützenberger, *The Ancestor Syndrome: Transgenerational Psychotherapy and the Hidden Links in the Family Tree* (New York: Routledge, 1998, digital print in 2010), p. 45.

94 **"psychological heredity"** Ibid., pp. 105–106.

94 **The most popular book** Mark Wolynn, *It Didn't Start With You* (New York: Penguin Publishing, 2017).

CHAPTER II. THE IDEA OF HEREDITY

99 **"a happy state of health"** Michel de Montaigne, "Of the Resemblance of Children to Fathers," *The Complete Works*, trans. Donald M. Frame (New York: Alfred A. Knopf, 2003), p. 701.

99 **"in greatest horror"** Ibid., p. 697.

99 **"the propensity to this infirmity"** Ibid., p. 702.

100 **"seed from which we are produced"** Ibid., p. 701.

100 **"had an aversion to medicine"** Ibid., p. 703.

100 **A Christian reinterpretation of the scheme** Tim LaHaye, *Spirit-Controlled Temperament* (Wheaton, Ill.: Tyndale House, 1993).

101 **"hereditary factors"** Ibid., p. 2.

101 **"You're Born with It!"** Ibid., pp. 1–4.

101 **"Temperament Can Be Modified!"** Ibid., pp. 7–9.

102 **"We can be fairly sure"** John Waller, *Heredity: A Very Short Introduction* (Oxford University Press, 2017), p. 1.

102 **"the seed of gods"** Ibid., p. 3.

102 **The God of the Old Testament** Genesis 2:22–24.

102 **"Verily, We created"** Qur'an 76:2, trans. Yusuf Ali.

102 **It's hard to generalize too broadly** Noga Arikha, *Passions and Tempers: A History of the Humours* (New York: Harper Perennial, 2007), p. 6; G.E.R. Lloyd, "Introduction," *Hippocratic Writings*, trans. J. Chadwick and W. N. Mann, et al. (New York: Penguin Books, 1983), p. 10.

102 **"from the whole body"** "The Seed," *Hippocratic Writings*, trans. I. M. Louis, pp. 320–322.

103 **"pangenesis"** Justin E. H. Smith, *The Problem of Animal Generation in Early Modern Philosophy* (Cambridge University Press, 2008), p. 3.

103 **The author of "On Airs, Waters, and Places"** "On Airs, Waters, Places," *Hippocratic Writings*, trans. J. Chadwick and W. N. Mann; see, for example, pp. 159–169.

103 **The Hippocratics also emphasized** Ibid.

103 **known for his triangle theorem** Many scholars hold that scientific views attributed to Pythagoras often reflect opinions of his followers. And like the Hippocratics, Pythagoras's disciples espoused conflicting ideas that come to us mostly secondhand.

103 **"mystical vapors"** Siddhartha Mukherjee, *The Gene: An Intimate History* (New York: Scribner, 2016), p. 21.

103 **Essentially, Mukherjee characterizes Pythagoras** He's not alone in this, but

some scholars contend that the record is unclear. See, for example, Smith, *The Problem of Animal Generation,* p. 5.

103 **"vital heat"** Aristotle, *Generation of Animals,* trans A. L. Peck (Cambridge, Mass.: Harvard University Press, 1942), p. 191.

104 **"only in the sense"** Ibid., p. 113.

104 **"soul" and "knowledge"** Ibid., p. 121.

104 **It's unclear whether parents passed along** The historian Jenny Davidson concludes that Aristotle was "agnostic on the question" of acquired characteristics being passed down to children, which seems true. Jenny Davidson, *Breeding* (New York: Columbia University Press, 2009), p. 21. John Waller argues that Aristotle "accepted the heritability of acquired characteristics. Waller, *Heredity,* p. 6. My hunch is that Aristotle thought it could happen but didn't find it easy to account for in his scheme.

104 **"outline of a scar"** Davidson, *Breeding,* p. 53.

104 **"mutilated parents"** Ibid., p. 71.

104 **Aristotle did allow** Waller, *Heredity,* p. 6; Mukherjee, *The Gene,* p. 27.

104 **He also held** Waller, *Heredity,* pp. 8–9.

104 **In *On the Nature of Man*** "On the Nature of Man," *Hippocratic Writings,* trans. J. Chadwick and W. N. Mann, pp. 264–265.

104 **"in the correct proportion"** Ibid., p. 262.

104 **calling epilepsy "hereditary"** "The Sacred Disease," *Hippocratic Writings,* trans. J. Chadwick and W. N. Mann, pp. 240–241.

105 **Humoral theory of disease** Arikha, *Passions and Tempers,* p. 66.

105 **Ascribing these bodily fluids** Kushner, Irving, M.D., "The 4 Humors and Erythrocyte Sedimentation: The Most Influential Observation in Medical History," *The American Journal of the Medical Sciences,* 346, no. 2 (Aug. 2013), pp. 154–157; Ingvar Johansson, Niels Lynøe, and Walter de Gruyter, *Medicine & Philosophy: A Twenty-First Century Introduction* (Berlin: De Gruyter, 2008), p. 24.

105 **even their proportions** We can't know for sure that humoral theory originated from watching blood separate, but we do know that the Hippocratics were devoted to observation.

105 **"the humoral characteristics present"** Arikha, *Passions and Tempers,* pp. 9–14.

105 **"groundless despondency"** Aristotle, *Problemata,* trans. E. S. Forster, *Works of Aristotle,* Vol. VII, edited by W. D. Ross (Oxford: Clarendon Press, 1927), p. 954–955.

105 **six "non-natural things"** Staffan Müller-Wille and Hans-Jörg Rheinberger, *A Cultural History of Heredity* (University of Chicago Press, 2012), p. 2.

106 **"rare disorders as purely natural phenomena"** Axel Lange and Gerd B. Muller, "Polydactyly in Development, Inheritance, and Evolution," *The Quarterly Review of Biology,* 82, no. 1 (Mar. 2017), p. 9.

106 **"the child will resemble the father"** Muhammad al-Bukhari, *The Hadith* (London: Global Grey, 2019), p. 1210.

107 **"anonymous late thirteenth-century text"** Waller, *Heredity,* p. 17.

107 **"impressive evidence of creative force"** Kate Millett, *Sexual Politics* (1970; New York: Columbia University Press, 2016), p. 28.

107 **"a desire for strawberries"** Davidson, *Breeding,* pp. 21–23.

107 **Courts generally rejected** Silvia De Renzi, "'The Hereditary,' Resemblance, and Family Ties," *Heredity Produced: At the Crossroads of Biology, Politics, and Culture, 1500–1870,* eds. Staffan Müller-Wille and Hans-Jörg Rheinberger (Cambridge, Mass.: MIT Press, 2007).

107 **In a story from Genesis** Genesis 30.

107 **"ardent and obstinate imagination"**   Ambroise Pare, *On Monsters and Marvels*, trans. Janis L. Pallister (University of Chicago Press, 1982), p. 38.

108 **"while drunk a man is clumsy"**   Plato, *Plato in Twelve Volumes*, Vols. 10 & 11, trans. R. G. Bury (Cambridge, Mass.: Harvard University Press; London: William Heinemann Ltd., 1967 and 1968), 6.775d.

108 **"her ideas, beliefs, intelligence, intellect"**   Davidson, *Breeding*, p. 21.

108 **While people had long known**   The notion of biological inheritance was imported from the law, but the questions that arose in the flesh-and-blood context were new.

108 **"nothing was so fixed"**   De Renzi, *Heredity Produced*, p. 63.

108 **"white Paper or Wax"**   John Locke, *Some Thoughts Concerning Education* (1693), eds. John W. Yolton and Jean S. Yolton (Oxford: Clarendon Press, 1989), p. 265. As Jenny Davidson observes, Locke also held "that individual children possess 'various Tempers, different Inclinations, and particular Defaults.'" Davidson, *Breeding*, p. 40.

108 **"shaped the makeup of offspring"**   De Renzi, *Heredity Produced*, p. 63.

109 **"the history of "hereditary"**   Carlos López Beltrán, "The Medical Origins of Heredity," *Heredity Produced*, p. 106.

109 **"part of the organic constitution"**   Ibid., pp. 100–111.

109 **"inheritance capacity"**   Roger J. Wood, "The Sheep Breeders' View of Heredity Before and After 1800," *Heredity Produced*, p. 241.

109 **"as the central problem of biology"**   Müller-Wille and Rheinberger, *A Cultural History of Heredity*, p. 74.

109 **"very rare deviation"**   Charles Darwin, *On the Origin of Species: A Facsimile of the First Edition* (1859; Cambridge, Mass.: Harvard University Press, 1966), pp. 12–13.

110 **"the true carriers of hereditary properties"**   Rasmus G. Winther, "Darwin on Variation and Heredity," *Journal of the History of Heredity*, 33, no. 3 (Winter 2000), pp. 425–455.

110 **to construct a model"**   Mukherjee, *The Gene*, pp. 51–53.

111 **"knowledge regime of heredity"**   Müller-Wille and Rheinberger, *A Cultural History of Heredity*, pp. 136, 138.

111 **"economic and social preconditions"**   Ibid., p. 136.

CHAPTER 12. GENES EXPRESSING THEMSELVES

112 **"the socialisation of the selective breeding"**   Victoria Brignell, "The Eugenics Movement Britain Wants to Forget," *New Statesman*, Dec. 9, 2010.

113 **"good genes"**   Ryan Teague Beckwith, "Donald Trump Loves to Talk about His 'Good Genes,'" *Time*, Sept. 12, 2017; Katie Rogers, "In the Pale of Winter, Trump's Tan Remains a State Secret," *The New York Times*, Feb. 2, 2019.

113 **when you "connect two racehorses"**   Sammy Nickalls, "Trump Believes in Eugenics, According to Trump's Biographer," *Esquire*, Sept. 29, 2016.

113 **"the racehorse theory"**   Jonathan Chait, "Trump's Lifelong Obsession with His Superior DNA Is Being Put to the Test," *New York Intelligencer*, Oct. 11, 2020.

113 **"there are superior people"**   Nickalls, "Trump Believes in Eugenics," *Esquire*.

113 **"If you can breed cattle"**   Richard Dawkins, letter to the Scottish *Herald*, Nov. 20, 2006. In 2020, Dawkins doubled down in a tweet. "It's one thing to deplore eugenics on ideological, political, moral grounds. It's quite another to conclude that it wouldn't work in practice. Of course it would. It works for cows, horses, pigs,

dogs & roses. Why on earth wouldn't it work for humans? Facts ignore ideology." Richard Dawkins, Twitter post, Feb. 16, 2020.

114 **"trying to convince a skeptical"**   Tim Spector, *Identically Different: Why We Can Change Our Genes* (New York: Overlook Press, 2012), p. 10.

114 **"met a few rare identical twins"**   Ibid., p. 19.

114 **"each gene is of tiny"**   Ibid., p. 17.

114 **"not by one gene"**   Ibid., p. 18.

114 **compares our genes to sheet music**   Sharon Moalem, *Inheritance: How Our Genes Change Our Lives and Our Lives Change Our Genes* (New York: Grand Central Publishing, 2014), p. 35.

114 **The hardest thing to explain**   Ibid., pp. 28–33.

115 **"collection of molecules"**   Carl Zimmer, *She Has Her Mother's Laugh: The Powers, Perversions, and Potential of Heredity* (New York: Penguin Publishing, 2019), p. 430.

116 **taken place in the pancreas**   Steven Pinker, *The Blank Slate: The Modern Denial of Human Nature* (New York: Penguin Putnam, 2002; reprint, New York: Penguin, 2016), p. 434.

116 **an ongoing study of Holocaust survivors**   See, for example, Rachel Yehuda, et al., "Influences of Maternal and Paternal PTSD on Epigenetic Regulation of the Glucocorticoid Receptor Gene in Holocaust Survivor Offspring," *American Journal of Psychiatry*, 171, no. 8 (Aug. 2014), pp. 872–880.

116 GHOSTS OF FAMILY TRAUMA   John DeMont, "Ghosts of Family Trauma Haunt Descendants," *The Chronicle Herald*, Sept. 19, 2018.

116 CAN WE INHERIT MEMORIES   Elizabeth Rosner, "Can We Inherit Memories of the Holocaust and Other Horrors?" *The Daily Beast*, Sept. 23, 2017.

117 **commonly called the "Dutch Hunger Winter"**   Carl Zimmer, "The Famine Ended 70 Years Ago, but Dutch Genes Still Bear Scars," *The New York Times*, Jan. 31, 2018.

117 **"sensationalistic claims to global dismissals"**   Rachel Yehuda and Amy Lehrner, "Intergenerational Transmission of Trauma Effects: Putative Role of Epigenetic Mechanisms," *World Psychiatry*, 17, no. 3 (Oct. 2018), pp. 243–257.

117 **Joy DeGruy describes in her 2005 book**   Joy DeGruy, *Post Traumatic Slave Syndrome* (Portland, Ore.: Joy DeGruy Publications, 2017).

117 **"use the strengths we have gained"**   Joy DeGruy, "Post Traumatic Slave Syndrome," Joy DeGruy website, last accessed May 15, 2021. Some Black scholars, including Ibram X. Kendi, have argued that the notion of Post Traumatic Slave Syndrome is a racist idea, saying that "Black people as a group do not need to be healed from racist trauma. All Black people need is to be freed from racist trauma." Ibram X. Kendi, "Post-Traumatic Slave Syndrome Is a Racist Idea," *Black Perspectives*, June 21, 2016. But see Ta-Nehisi Coates, *Between the World and Me* (New York: Random House, 2015), and Guy Emerson Mount, "Is Post Traumatic Slave Syndrome Stamped from the Beginning?" *Black Perspectives*, June 28, 2016.

118 **"regardless of our background or skin"**   Resmaa Menakem, *My Grandmother's Hands: Racialized Trauma and the Pathway to Mending Our Hearts and Bodies* (Las Vegas: Central Recovery Press, 2017), pp. 7–13, 14.

118 **He points out that poor white**   Ibid., pp. 57–65.

118 **"whose paternal grandfathers lived through"**   Zimmer, *She Has Her Mother's Laugh*, pp. 427–428.

119 **taught male lab mice to fear**   Ewen Callaway, "Fearful Memories Passed Down to Mouse Descendants, *Scientific American*, Dec. 1, 2013.

119 **"Smelling it made them more likely"** Zimmer, *She Has Her Mother's Laugh*, pp. 429–430.

119 **In one study, rat babies** Molly Webster, "The Great Rat Mother Switcheroo," *Radiolab*, WNYC website, Jan. 10, 2013.

119 **"separated from their mothers for hours"** Zimmer, *She Has Her Mother's Laugh*, pp. 429–430.

120 **Morgan Jerkins's conjecture** Morgan Jerkins, *Wandering in Strange Lands: A Daughter of the Great Migration Reclaims Her Roots* (New York: Harper, 2020), pp. 24–29.

120 **"there must be something inside sperm"** Zimmer, *She Has Her Mother's Laugh*, pp. 429–430.

120 **"'best people'"** Ibid., p. 83.

120 **"'the feebleminded'"** Ibid., p. 84.

120 **"'carefully worded sterilization law'"** Ibid., p. 86.

120 **His bestselling 1912 book** Henry Goddard, *The Kallikak Family: A Study in the Heredity of Feeble-Mindedness* (London: Macmillan, 1912).

120 **"a primal myth"** Stephen Jay Gould, *The Mismeasure of Man* (1981; New York: W. W. Norton, 1996), p. 198.

120 **"the same troubles"** Zimmer, *She Has Her Mother's Laugh*, pp. 478–480.

120 **"every feeble-minded person"** Ibid.

PART FOUR PHYSICALITY

CHAPTER 13. GRANDMA'S EYES

126 **she recorded in letters** Sandy Bruce, various letters, on file with author, 1973–76.

130 **In an undated eight-page** Pearl Beasley, "Daddy Joe," joint letter with John Beasley to family, n.d., on file with author, p. 3.

132 **"that part of the body"** Dan Cayer, Alexander Technique lessons, date unknown.

135 **she corrected me** Sandy Bruce, email to Maud Newton, Oct. 1, 2019.

CHAPTER 14. THE FAMILY FACE

139 **"I knew this photo of Earl"** Sven Birkerts, *The Other Walk: Essays* (Minneapolis: Graywolf, 2011), p. 87.

139 **"I'm the self-portrait"** Saeed Jones, *Prelude to Bruise* (Minneapolis: Coffee House Press, 2014), p. 77.

139 **"For a brief moment"** Maud Newton, "The Family Tree: Saeed Jones," *Tin House* website, Dec. 11, 2014.

140 **In her memoir, *The Mistress's Daughter*** A. M. Homes, *The Mistress's Daughter* (New York: Penguin Books, 2007).

140 **"When I look in the mirror"** Jennifer Teege, *My Grandfather Would Have Shot Me* (New York: The Experiment, 2015), p. 41.

140 **"I saw my jaw, my nose"** Dani Shapiro, *Inheritance: A Memoir of Genealogy, Paternity, and Love* (New York: Knopf, 2019), p. 61.

140 **"uncanny resemblance"** Aaron, "Look-Alike Competition: Win a Family Photo Shoot!" MyHeritage blog, June 3, 2015.

141 **"looked as if they were"** Neal Ungerleider, "Ancestors, Inc.: Inside the Remarkable Rise of the Genealogy Industry," *Fast Company*, July 15, 2015.

141 **"I am the family face"** Thomas Hardy, "Heredity," *Moments of Vision and Miscellaneous Verses* (London: Macmillan, 1917).

141 **It's even possible** Stefano Vaglio, "Chemical Communication and Mother–Infant Recognition," *Communicative & Integrative Biology,* 2, no. 3 (Feb. 2009), pp. 279–281; "Newborn-Senses," Children's Hospital of Philadelphia, last accessed May 15, 2021.

141 **"a son in his own likeness"** Genesis 5:3 (Revised Standard Version).

141 **"Rabbi, who sinned"** John 9:2 (RSV).

141 **"wives give birth to children"** Hesiod, *Works and Days,* in *Theogony; Works and Days, Testimonia,* trans. Glenn W. Most (Cambridge, Mass.: Harvard University Press, 2006), p. 225.

141 **"a large forehead are sluggish"** Aristotle, *History of Animals,* vol. I, trans. A. L. Peck (Cambridge, Mass.: Harvard University Press, 1965), p. 39.

141 **By the eighteenth century, the mother's** See, e.g., Jenny Davidson, *Breeding* (New York: Columbia University Press, 2009).

142 **"child forecast"** Amram Scheinfeld, *You and Heredity* (New York: Frederick A. Stokes, 1939), pp. 91–96; see also pp. 62–90.

142 **Scheinfeld surveyed musical ability** Ibid., pp. 234–279.

142 **"mental defectives"** Ibid., p. 360.

142 **"reared unwittingly by"** Ibid., p. 354.

142 **"can undoubtedly eliminate"** Ibid., p. 381.

143 **"the most important, most wondrous map"** Robin McKie, "'The Wondrous Map': How Unlocking Human DNA Changed the Course of Science," *The Guardian,* June 21, 2020.

143 **"a history book"** Francis S. Collins, "Remarks at the Press Conference Announcing Sequencing and Analysis of the Human Genome," National Human Genome Research Institute, Feb. 12, 2001.

143 **"the human genetic blueprint"** Craig Venter, White House event, June 26, 2000.

143 **"Genes are not the whole story"** Venter, *A Life Decoded* (New York: Viking, 2007), p. 258.

143 **"talk alike"** Tim Spector, *Identically Different: Why We Can Change Our Genes* (New York: Overlook Press, 2012), p. 41.

143 **"major genetic influences"** Ibid., p. 38.

143 **appear to be strongly genetic"** Ibid., p. 11.

144 **"enormous sacks of sagging skin"** Sharon Moalem, *Inheritance: How Our Genes Change Our Lives and Our Lives Change Our Genes* (New York: Grand Central Publishing, 2014), p. 45.

144 **"bloated and disfigured"** Ibid., p. 29.

144 **"the genetic workmanship"** Ibid., p. 11.

145 **"a condition in which"** Ibid., p. 12.

145 **"feel the texture of your skin"** Ibid., p. 7.

145 **"our most important biological trademark"** Ibid., p. 11.

146 **"monozygotic (identical) twins"** Sharon Moalem, Tumblr post, Jan. 25, 2015.

146 **I do, as 23andMe suggests** Maud Newton, Health and Traits, 23andMe, last accessed May 15, 2021.

146 **My husband Max's test correctly suggests** Max Clarke, Health and Traits, 23andMe, last accessed May 15, 2021.

147 **my ring finger is longer** Maud Newton, AncestryDNA, last accessed May 15, 2021.

147 **My mother's eyes**   Sandy Bruce, Health and Traits, 23andMe, last accessed May 15, 2021.

CHAPTER 15. MUGSHOTS FROM DNA

148 **In 2014, I learned of efforts**   Sara Reardon, "Mugshots Built from DNA Data," *Nature*, Mar. 20, 2014.

148 **I found the prospect chilling**   Andrew Pollack, "Building a Face, and a Case, on DNA," *The New York Times*, Feb. 23, 2015.

148 **"occasionally consults for law-enforcement"**   Mark Shriver, Bio, Penn State Department of Anthropology website, last accessed May 15, 2021.

148 **"superficial traits belie our interconnectedness"**   Mark Shriver, "It's All Relatives: The Science of Your Family Tree" panel, 2014 World Science Festival, May 29, 2014.

149 **Back then, when Shriver's research**   Peter Claes, et al., "Modeling 3D Facial Shape from DNA," *PLOS Genetics*, 10, no. 3 (Mar. 2014), e1004224; Reardon, "Mugshots Built from DNA Data."

149 **"take reasonable efforts"**   Permission form for DNA face-mapping study, Penn State University Anthropological Genomics Lab, on file with author, June 2014.

150 **"the crime of WBB"**   Randall Pinkston, "It's All Relatives: The Science of Your Family Tree" panel, 2014 World Science Festival, May 29, 2014.

150 **"a couple people"**   Mark Shriver, interview at Penn State, notes on file with author, Aug. 1, 2014.

151 **He lauded a federal law**   Genetic Information Nondiscrimination Act, P.L. 110-233 (2008).

151 **"the first civil-rights bill"**   Peter Aldhous, "US Outlaws Genetic Discrimination," *New Scientist*, Apr. 28, 2008.

151 **parents in Palo Alto**   *Chadam v. Palo Alto Unified Sch. Dist.*, 666 F. App'x 615, 616 (9th Cir. 2016), reversing in part and remanding *Chadam v. Palo Alto Unified Sch. Dist.*, No. C 13-4129 CW (N.D., Cal. Jan. 29, 2014). The federal District Court had dismissed the family's claims, but the Ninth Circuit revived the case in part and returned it to the lower court for further consideration. The family ultimately settled with the school district for $150,000. Elena Kadvany, "Update: School Board Approves DNA Privacy Settlement," *Palo Alto Weekly*, Aug. 20, 2018.

151 **In recent years, life-insurance companies**   Christina Farr, "If You Want Life Insurance, Think Twice Before Getting a Genetic Test," *Fast Company*, Feb. 17, 2016.

151 **A bill proposed by congressional Republicans**   Sharon Begley, "Employers Demand Workers' Genetic Test Results," STAT, *Scientific American*, Mar. 10, 2017.

151 **"face morphology analysis"**   The French Homicides, Parabon NanoLabs website, last accessed May 15, 2015; "Parabon Snapshot Helps Investigators Solve Double-Homicide Cold Case," *Cision PR Newswire*, Jan. 4, 2017.

152 **"highly associative with blue eyes"**   Ellen Graytak, "Generating a Suspect's Mugshot from Solely DNA," June 6, 2016.

152 **MyHeritage invited people to upload**   Esther, "New: Introducing Deep Nostalgia—Animate the Faces in Your Family Photos," MyHeritage website, Feb. 25, 2021.

152 **"moving too quickly to market"**   Jordan Pearson, "Police Released a Suspect Photo Based on DNA from a Decades-Old Murder," *Vice*, Jan. 26, 2017.

152 **"quite focused on selling tests"**   David Murrell, "Some Philly-Area Police De-

partments Have Used DNA to Create CGI Sketches of Suspects," *Philadelphia Magazine*, Dec. 9, 2019.

152 **"obsessively collect[ing]"** Heather Dewey-Hagborg, "Sci-Fi Crime Drama with a Strong Black Lead," *The New Inquiry*, n.d.

153 **The police identified a young New Orleans filmmaker,** Jim Mustian, "New Orleans Filmmaker Cleared in Cold-Case Murder; False Positive Highlights Limitations of Familial DNA Searching," *The New Orleans Advocate*, Mar. 12, 2015.

153 **CeCe Moore identified** CeCe Moore, "Unraveling the Twisted Case of Angie Dodge," ISHI News, Feb. 11, 2020.

PART FIVE TEMPERAMENT

CHAPTER 16. GRUDGING KINSHIP

157 ***The Dallas Morning News* featured her** March Wilson, "Cat Club Expanding," *The Dallas Morning News*, Dec. 1, 1968.

157 **denounced it as "horseshit"** Sandy Bruce, conversation with Maud Newton, author's memory, June 2017.

159 **Daddy was married thirteen times, I think** Sandy Bruce, email to Maud Newton, Feb. 16, 2007.

161 **"I was the only child"** Sandy Bruce, email to Maud Newton, June 20, 2003.

163 **the "ever-present mud"** "Grand Prairie Historical Recap," City of Grand Prairie website, last accessed May 15, 2021.

164 **a court opinion** *Grimes v. State*, 141 S.W. 261, Nov. 29, 1911.

164 **appeared in newspapers around the state** "Killed with Hay Hook; Murder Is Charged," *The Paris Morning News*, June 14, 1916; "Killed with Hay Hook; Murder Is Charged," *Waxahachie Daily Light*, June 13, 1916; "Peritonitis Caused Death," *Corsicana Daily Sun*, June 13, 1916; "Defendant Exonerated," *The Austin American*, June 18, 1916 (misidentifying Charley as James Bruce and George as Henry Grimes but briefly describing the story and Charley's exoneration).

164 **But the neighbors came forward** See above, Chapter 2, and accompanying endnotes.

165 **Robert married Nettie Mae Mason** Robert Charles Bruce and Nettie Ma[e] Mason, Marriage Record, Dallas County, No. 106626, Aug. 24, 1925.

165 **on the same page in the census** 1920 U.S. Census, Justice Precinct 8, District 0110, Dallas, Texas, Roll T625_1794, Page 5B, Robert Bruce, son of Charley Bruce, House No. 104, and Nettie Mae Mason, daughter of Sam P. Mason, House No. 105.

165 **the 1922 Dallas City Directory** A significant amount of the information I've learned about Robert and the women he married comes from the Dallas City Directory. As a concession to space, I haven't cited the directories in notes.

165 **Dallas clothing manufacturers** Patricia Evridge Hill, *Dallas: The Making of a Modern City* (Austin: University of Texas Press, 1996), pp. 130–161.

166 **When they wed, Nettie's mom** Bonnie Mason, Death Certificate, Aug. 12, 1929, File No. 39268, Dallas County, Texas State Department of Health, noting duration of her illness, in Texas Death Certificates, 1903–1982, at Ancestry.com.

166 **Charley was struggling with bipolar disorder** Charles Bruce, Death Certificate, July 13, 1927, File No. 25469, Wichita County, Texas State Department of Health, copy on file with author, noting duration of his illness.

166 **Nettie gave birth to a daughter** Bonnie Katharine Bruce, Birth Certificate,

May 27, 1926, File No. 29206, Dallas County, Texas State Board of Health, Texas Birth Certificates, 1903–1932, at Ancestry.com

166 **"my daddy loved children"**   Sandy Bruce, email to Maud Newton, Apr. 14, 2007.

167 **"Tell Sandy Daddy loves her"**   Robert Bruce, letter on file with author, Sept. 11, 1943.

167 **He divorced Nettie**   *Robert Charles Bruce v. Nettie Mae Bruce*, Dkt. No. 80676-A, 14th Dist. Ct., Dallas County, July 25, 1929.

167 **By the 1930 census**   1930 U.S. Census, Precinct 7, District 0135, Dallas, Texas, Bonnie K. Bruce, Roll 2322, Page 3B, Image 811.0.

168 **A marriage certificate attests**   Robert Charles Bruce and Clara Mae Brantley, Marriage Record, Bryan County (Oklahoma County Marriage Records 1890-1995, Ancestry.com, Film No. 002194754), Apr. 19, 1930.

168 **According to her death certificate**   Bonnie K. Bruce, Death Certificate, Feb. 2, 1932, File No. 6159, Denton County, Texas State Department of Health, in Texas Death Certificates, 1903–1982, at Ancestry.com.

168 **"the deadly scourge of childhood"**   Evelynn Maxine Hammonds, *Childhood's Deadly Scourge: The Campaign to Control Diphtheria in New York City, 1880–1930* (Baltimore: Johns Hopkins University Press, 2002).

CHAPTER 17. CHASING THE DREAM

169 **"Bonnie Katherine Bruce"**   The newspaper misspelled her middle name as "Catherine."

170 **Skilled dress cutters like Robert**   Patricia Evridge Hill, *Dallas: The Making of a Modern City* (Austin: University of Texas Press, 1996), pp. 130–161.

170 **"condoned brutal tactics"**   Ibid., p. 131.

171 **They divorced that June**   *Robert Bruce v. Clara Mae Bruce*, Dkt. No. 21853-F, 116th Dist. Ct., Dallas County, June 24, 1936.

171 **Robert married a younger woman**   Robert Charles Bruce and Rose Marie Emily Camiani, Marriage Record, Rockwall County (Texas, Select County Marriage Records 1837-1965, Ancestry.com, Film No. 17971), July 3, 1937.

171 **Rose Marie obtained an injunction**   *Rose Marie Bruce v. Robert Bruce*, Dkt. No. 41818-C, 68th Judicial Dist. Ct., Dallas County, Mar. 31, 1939.

171 **They officially divorced in May**   Ibid., May 3, 1939.

173 **He was a card-carrying socialist**   "Socialists Launch Recall Petitions," *The Dallas Morning News*, Sept. 1, 1913.

173 GARMENT CUTTERS WILL CELEBRATE   *The Dallas Morning News*, June 11, 1941.

173 **Organized labor, to the extent**   Hill, *Dallas*, pp. 130–161.

174 **Granny divorced Robert over his affair**   *Martha J. Bruce v. Robert Bruce*, Dkt. No. 76039-F, 116th Dist. Ct., Dallas County, Feb. 10, 1944.

174 **he and Christine applied**   Robert Charles Bruce and Christine Weber, Marriage License, Rockwall County (Texas, Select County Marriage Records 1837–1965, Ancestry.com, Film No. 30236), Feb. 21, 1944.

174 **Christine filed the first of many**   *Christine Bruce v. Robert C. Bruce*, Dkt. No. 84480, 101st Dist. Ct., Dallas County, Sept. 6, 1944.

174 **they secured another marriage license**   Robert Charles Bruce and Christine Bruce, Marriage Record, Rockwall County (Texas, Select County Marriage Records 1837–1965, Ancestry.com, Film No. 28789), Jan. 9, 1945.

174 **Robert who filed for divorce** *Robert C. Bruce v. Christine Bruce,* Dkt. No. 92239, 101st Dist. Ct., Dallas County, June 29, 1945.

174 **Petitioned for divorce three more times** *Christine Bruce v. Robert C. Bruce,* Dkt. No. 3629, 95th Dist. Ct., Dallas County, Aug. 30, 1946; *Christine Bruce v. Robert C. Bruce,* Dkt. No. 33022, 68th Dist. Ct., May 24, 1949; *Christine Bruce v. Robert C. Bruce,* Dkt. No. 37522, 68th Dist. Ct., Oct. 14, 1949.

174 **newsy Oak Cliff shopping circular** "Fishing Party Brings Back Proof," *Shopping News of Oak Cliff* (Dallas, Tex.), May 16, 1947.

174 **Christine divorced Robert for good** *Christine Bruce v. Robert C. Bruce,* Dkt. No. 37522-C, 68th Dist. Ct., Dallas County, May 24, 1950.

175 **Robert married Olgie Evelyn York** Robert Charles Bruce and Olgie Evelyn York, Marriage Record, Dallas County, June 1, 1950.

175–176 **"apparently followed an argument"** "Man in Fair Condition After Shot in Stomach," *Daily Times Herald,* July 24, 1950. According to *The Dallas Morning News,* Evelyn was taken to the county jail and later released on a $2,500 writ bond. "Shooting Victim Reported in Fair Condition Monday," *The Dallas Morning News,* July 24, 1950.

176 **Robert was well enough** *Robert C. Bruce v. Olgie Evelyn Bruce,* Dkt. No. 46847, 116th Dist. Ct., Dallas County, Oct. 26, 1950.

176 **married Vera Fern Sebastian** Robert Charles Bruce and V. Fern Sebastian, Marriage Record, Dallas County, Jan. 29, 1951.

177 **"harmony duo"** "Future Stars' Contest," program announcement, *Dallas Morning News,* Aug. 6, 1937.

177 **"Daddy did more dress designing"** Sandy Bruce, email to Maud Newton, Apr. 12, 2007.

177 **His obituary claims** "Robert C. Bruce, 62, Leading City Realtor," *The Arizona Republic,* Apr. 24, 1970.

177 **a man with his name married** Robert Charles Bruce and Delores Lillian Preston, Marriage Certificate, Maricopa County (Arizona, County Marriage Records 1865–1972, Ancestry.com, Film No. 78361), Jan. 3, 1952.

177 **"Robert Bruce of Grace and Grace"** See, for example, "Keith Taylor Takes Lease on Warehouse," *The Arizona Republic,* Feb. 28, 1954; "Furniture Firm Leases Building," *The Arizona Republic,* Mar. 14, 1954; "Grace and Grace Report Two New Business Leases," *The Arizona Republic,* June 13, 1954; "Company Leases McDowell Site," *The Arizona Republic,* Dec. 5, 1954.

177 **evidently married for the tenth and final time** So far I haven't found any official record of the marriage itself or of a divorce from Delores. But see Julia E. Harlacher, Death Notice, *The Arizona Republic,* Oct. 5, 1955. Julia was Eleanore's mother, and the notice refers to her as mother of "Mrs. Robert C. Bruce." Later, Eleanore is also referred to as Robert's wife in his will and his reported obituary, among other places.

178 **"Robert C. Bruce, widely known"** "New Real Estate Office Opened," *The Arizona Republic,* June 19, 1955.

178 **"My dad was the FIRST"** Sandy Bruce, email to Maud Newton, Apr. 12, 2007.

178 **"be installed as a member"** "Bruce to Become Industrial Realtor," *The Arizona Republic,* Apr. 25, 1965.

178 **One year, he was named** "Realtor of the Year," *The Arizona Republic,* Nov. 14, 1965.

178 **By 1968** "Officers Elected by Realty Board," *The Arizona Republic,* Oct. 16, 1968; "Robert Bruce on IDC Board," *The Arizona Republic,* Jan. 22, 1967.

178 *The Arizona Republic* **relied on him**   Robert C. Bruce, "Home Sales Boom," *The Arizona Republic,* Dec. 29, 1968; "Realtor Week Starts," *The Arizona Republic,* May 18, 1969, extensively quoting Robert; "Buyer Urged to Inspect Land," *The Arizona Republic,* Apr. 27, 1969, extensively quoting Robert.

179 **ROBERT C. BRUCE, 62**   *Arizona Republic,* Apr. 24, 1970.

179 **attributed his death**   Ibid.

179 **his death certificate**   Robert Charles Bruce, Death Certificate, Apr. 23, 1970 (document misplaced and not on Ancestry.com—requested another copy).

180 **"professed to attain perfect love"**   "The Closing Scenes at Lumpkin Camp Ground," *The Atlanta Constitution,* Sept. 3, 1886.

182 **"A dictatorship, not a democracy"**   Maud Newton, MaudNewton.com, Dec. 1, 2003.

CHAPTER 18. EMOTIONAL RECURRENCES

184 **In a 1972 letter to friends**   Kurt Vonnegut, *Letters* (New York: Dial Press, 2014), Kindle, Nov. 2, 1972.

184 **"terrific depressions"**   Ibid.

185 **"a Great Writer's child"**   Nanette Vonnegut, "Writing," Nannette Vonnegut website, last accessed May 15, 2021.

185 **"allowed for sexual sterilization"**   Ibid.

185 **"At the root"**   Ibid.

185 **"all about family"**   Jennifer Bowen, "The Rumpus Interview with Nanette Vonnegut," *The Rumpus,* Nov. 12, 2012.

185 **"manic depression"**   Mark Vonnegut, *Just Like Someone Without Mental Illness Only More So* (New York: Delacorte, 2010), p. 5.

185 **"creativity and craziness"**   Ibid., p. 6.

186 **In my early thirties, I discovered**   Kay Redfield Jamison, *Touched with Fire: Manic-Depressive Illness and the Artistic Temperament* (New York: Free Press, 1996).

186 **"illness—driving me to the verge"**   Ibid., p. 231.

186 **"Wollstonecraft, like many Enlightenment"**   Charlotte Gordon, *Romantic Outlaws: The Extraordinary Lives of Mary Wollstonecraft & Mary Shelley* (New York: Random House, 2015), pp. 215–216.

186 **"My mind slumbers"**   Jamison, *Touched with Fire,* p. 231.

187 **"For no reason"**   Ibid., p. 28.

187 **"could be attributed to"**   Staffan Müller-Wille and Hans-Jörg Rheinberger, *A Cultural History of Heredity* (University of Chicago Press, 2012), p. 121.

188 **"evidence of Mendelian inheritance patterns"**   Ibid., p. 122.

188 **In his memoir, *Boy Erased***   Garrard Conley, *Boy Erased* (New York: Riverhead, 2016).

189 **Esmé Weijun Wang's *The Collected Schizophrenias***   Esmé Weijun Wang, *The Collected Schizophrenias* (Minneapolis: Graywolf, 2019), p. 24.

189 **"evolutionary-genetic paradox"**   Bernard Crespi, Kyle Summers, and Steve Dorus, "Adaptive Evolution of Genes Underlying Schizophrenia," *Proceedings of the Royal Society B: Biological,* 274, no. 1627, pp. 2,801–2,810.

189 **"the evolutionary development"**   Wang, *The Collected Schizophrenias,* p. 24.

190 **"the channel by which we receive"**   Plato, *Phaedrus and the Seventh and Eighth Letters,* trans. W. Hamilton (Middlesex, England: Penguin, 1974), pp. 46–47.

190 **One study purported to find**   "Psychologists Discover Oxytocin Receptor Gene's Link to Optimism, Self Esteem," *Science News,* Sept. 14, 2011.

190–191 **Exercise can lead to a decrease**   Elisa Grazioli, et al., "Physical Activity in the Prevention of Human Diseases: Role of Epigenetic Modifications," BMC Genomics, 18, no. 8 (Nov. 2017), n.p.

191 **Physical activity may also improve cognition**   Jansen Fernandes, Ricardo Mario Arida, and Fernando Gomez-Pinilla, *Neuroscience & Behavioral Reviews*, 80 (Sept. 2017), pp. 443–456.

191 **Despite a rush of enthusiasm**   Jill Sakai, "Study Reveals Gene Expression Changes with Meditation," University of Wisconsin-Madison website, Dec. 4, 2013.

191 **so far efforts to pinpoint**   Ivana Buric, et al., "What Is the Molecular Signature of Mind-Body Interventions? A Systemic Review of Gene Expression Changes Induced by Meditation and Related Practices," *Frontiers in Immunology*, 8, no. 670 (June 2017), n.p.

192 **"is asked to explain"**   Robert Wright, *Why Buddhism Is True* (New York: Simon & Schuster, 2017), pp. 78–79.

192 **"showed full awareness"**   Yaïr Pinto, "When You Split the Brain, Do You Split the Person?" *Aeon*, Sept. 26, 2017.

192 **"provided strong evidence for materialism"**   Ibid.

193 **Two prominent evolutionary psychologists**   Douglas T. Kenrick and Vladas Griskevicius, *The Rational Animal: How Evolution Made Us Smarter Than We Think* (New York: Basic Books, 2013).

193 **"Visited by over a Million People"**   Wright, *Why Buddhism Is True*, p. 94.

194 **"associated with motivation and emotion"**   Ibid., p. 80.

194 **"Your habitual tendencies get knotted up"**   Ethan Nichtern, *The Dharma of the Princess Bride* (New York: FSG Books, North Point, 2017).

195 **"do not just select for"**   Karola Stotz, "Extended Evolutionary Psychology: The Importance of Transgenerational Developmental Plasticity," *Frontiers in Psychology*, 5, no. 908 (Aug. 2014), n.p.

195 **"Our souls as well as"**   Carl Jung, *Memories, Dreams, Reflections* (New York: Vintage Books Edition, 1989, VIII, "The Tower.")

195 **"I feel very strongly"**   Ibid.

196 **but in *The Red Book***   Carl Jung, *The Red Book: Liber Novus A Reader's Edition*, trans. Sonu Shamdasani (New York: W. W. Norton, 2009).

196 **"those initial fantasies and dreams"**   Jung, *Memories, Dreams, Reflections*, VI, "Confrontation with the Unconscious."

196 **"Doing a schizophrenia"**   Jung, *Combat* interview (1952), *Jung Speaking: Interviews and Encounters*, ed. William McGuire and R.F.C. Hull (Bollingen Series, Princeton, N.J.: Princeton University Press, 1977). pp. 233–234.

196 **"Turn to the dead"**   Jung, *The Red Book*, p. 344.

196 **"general principles from his fantasies"**   James Hillman and Sonu Shamdasani, *Lament of the Dead: Psychology after Jung's Red Book* (New York: W. W. Norton, 2013), p. 17.

PART SIX   INHERITANCE

CHAPTER 19. HEIRLOOMS AND DISINHERITANCE

207 **"MOMMY"**   Maud Newton, handmade card, on file with author, 1981.

207 **"You will remember"**   Sandy Bruce, letter to Richard Newton, III, Jan. 20, 1984.

208 **"all of your many suspicions"**   James R. Chandler, III, Bender, Bender, Chandler & Adair, P.A., letter to Richard Newton, III, June 23, 1986.

208 **"All propertys that I may own"** Robert Bruce, holographic will, Oct. 13, 1944.

208 **When Robert died** Robert Bruce, last will and testament, Jul. 20, 1961.

209 **"He told me he was"** Sandy Bruce, email to Maud Newton, Feb. 16, 2007.

210 **"Also enclosed"** Richard Newton, III, letter to Maud Newton , 2013.

210 **"Children living when the will"** "Arizona Law Digest," *The Martindale Hubbell Law Directory,* Vol 5. 101st Edition (Summit, N.J.: Martindale, 1969), p. 115.

CHAPTER 20. MONSTROUS BEQUESTS

215 **"my beloved wife Nelly McGee"** Davis McGee will, Jones County (Ga.), Jones County Probate Records Estate Book, A.P. 244, probated Feb. 3, 1817. I acknowledged that this is Mvskoke land.

215 **"land, stock, and property"** Joseph McGee will, Holmes County (Miss.), 213 record of wills, Vol. 1, 1833–1888, probated Nov. 18, 1850. I acknowledge that this, like most of the land my ancestors settled in Mississippi, is Chahta Yakni land. I have much to learn about my Southern ancestors' involvement in taking Native land and killing and displacing Native people, on this land and beyond.

216 **whatever "lot"** Ibid.

216 **enslaved a total of ten people** 1860 U.S. Census, Holmes County (Miss.), slave schedule, Tchula Beat, John W. Bailey, slave owner, p. 115.

216 **nineteen people listed alongside his name** 1860 U.S. Census, Holmes County (Miss.), slave schedule, Tchula Beat, Jordan Bailey, slave owner, p. 115.

217 **The Baileys, said to be** Bessie M. Mottley, "The Descendants of Benjamin Bailey Born in Augusta County, Virginia, 1755: First Lieutenant in Virginia Militia in Revolutionary War 1778, Died in Chesterfield County, Virginia, 1818," prepared 1958–1961, on file with author, p. 1. I acknowledge that he probably settled on Monacan land, Powhatan land, Arrohatec land, and/or Appamattuck land.

217 **"one of the most zealous"** Ibid.

217 **"inherited a religious fervor"** Ibid.

217 **"Never was there a clearer case"** Frederick Douglass, *Narrative of the Life of Frederick Douglass, an American Slave: Written by Himself* (Boston: The Anti-Slavery Office, 1845), pp. 118–119.

218 **both of Grandma's Bailey great-grandfathers** Richard Thomas Bailey, Sr., Bailey Cemetery, Find a Grave Memorial 24028393, died May 21, 1899; John William Bailey, Sergeant, Mississippi 38th Infantry, Company A, Index to Compiled Confederate Military Service Records; Mississippi Confederate Grave Registry, died May 21, 1909.

219 **"The size of those mules!"** John Beasley, "Daddy Joe," joint letter with Pearl Beasley to family, n.d., on file with author, p. 6. I acknowledge that this is Chahta Yakni land.

219 **"an example for me and others"** John Beasley, letter, p. 5.

220 **someone whose grandparents had been sharecroppers** Name withheld for privacy, email to Maud Newton, Feb. 17, 2016.

220 **"Fewer than one out of five"** Isabel Wilkerson, *The Warmth of Other Suns: The Epic Story of America's Great Migration* (New York: Random House, 2010), p. 167.

223 **white women may even** Stephanie E. Jones-Rogers, *They Were Her Property* (Yale University Press, 2020).

223 **"'the power behind the wheel'"** Pearl Beasley, "Baby I Need You," letter to family, n.d., on file with author, p. 1.

223 **Her father always sought**   Ibid., p. 3.
224 **"that to get Mr. Terry"**   Ibid.
224 **"twice a month"**   Ibid., pp. 3–4.

CHAPTER 21. NOT RACIST

226 **Granny's great-grandfather John Kinchen**   Court Record, appointment of a tutor (guardian) for John Milton Kinchen, May 12, 1823.

227 **In the said estate**   Court Record, *William Kinchen, Marina Kinchen, John Kinchen, and Mary Kinchen v. William Kinchen and Mary Courtney,* St. Helena Parish Courthouse, Suits in 9th District Court, pp. 64–65, from official transcription photocopied and posted at Ancestry.com.

229 **I soon read in an account**   Henry Parsons, *Parsons Family: Descendants of Cornet Joseph Parsons, Springfield 1636—Northampton, 1655* (New York: Frank Allaben Genealogical Co., 1912), p. 49. See also John Putnam Demos, *Entertaining Satan* (Oxford University Press, 2004), p. 259, Genealogists have speculated about a possible family link between the Pynchons and Parsonses; as Demos puts it, there's "no sure evidence to prove such ties, but they remain a real—and intriguing—possibility." For more on William Pynchon and his later, infamous book, *The Meritorious Price of Our Redemption,* which criticized and was banned by the Puritans, see Daniel Crown, "The Price of Suffering: William Pynchon and the Meritorious Price of Our Redemption," *The Public Domain Review,* Nov. 11, 2015. Crown argues that Pynchon is *"the* forgotten founding father of colonial New England."

230 **"It is probable"**   Henry Martyn Burt, and Albert Ross Parsons, *Cornet Joseph Parsons: One of the Founders of Springfield and Northampton, Massachusetts* (Garden City, N.Y.: Albert Ross Parsons, 1898), p. 45.

230 **"regarded the Pocumtuck"**   Margaret Bruchac, "Revisiting Pocumtuck History in Deerfield: George Sheldon's Vanishing Indian Act," *Historical Journal of Massachusetts,* 39, nos. 1–2, pp. 30–77.

230 **"Wequagon and his wife Awnusk"**   Burt and Parsons, *Cornet Joseph Parsons,* p. 45.

230 **"Indians that were the Inhabitants"**   Ibid., pp. 64–65.

231 **"the last of the Indians"**   Margaret Bruchac, "Sally Maminash: Last of the Indians Here," Historic Northampton website, last accessed May 15, 2021.

232 **I can acknowledge and own this**   For examples of this kind of acknowledgment, see Jill Strauss and Dionne Ford, *Slavery's Descendants: Shared Legacies of Race and Reconciliation* (New Brunswick: Rutgers University Press, 2019). Organizations like Coming to the Table also advocate for acknowledgment as one small tool in, as the website puts it, "working together to create a just and truthful society that acknowledges and seeks to heal from the racial wounds of the past, from slavery and the many forms of racism it spawned." My own efforts to foster what I think of as an "acknowledgment genealogy" movement are also inspired by Native land acknowledgments and Jennifer Mendelsohn's "resistance genealogy" efforts, which tend to focus on the ways right-wing politicans' own family trees fly in the face of their own white supremacist attitudes toward immigration. Acknowledgment genealogy as I envision it invites each of us whose ancestors participated in the harms around this country's origins (or any similar harms) to inform ourselves about that history, be public about it, and commit ourselves to taking up the work that needs to follow.

232 **urges settlers**   "What Else Can I Do?" Manna-hatta Fund website, last accessed May 15, 2021.

CHAPTER 22. DISCONNECTION

233 **"Though I wouldn't know for years"** Sarah Smarsh, *Heartland: A Memoir of Working Hard and Being Broke in the Richest Country on Earth* (New York: Scribner, 2018), p. 33.

234 **"a gene for being left handed"** Emily Raboteau, *Searching for Zion: The Quest for Home in the African Diaspora* (New York: Grove Atlantic, 2013), n.p.

234 **"invulnerable and doomed"** Alexander Chee, "Inheritance," *How to Write an Autobiographical Novel* (New York: W. W. Norton, 2018), p. 178.

234 **"the entire family, the living and"** Ibid., p. 182.

234 **"telling them how angry I was"** Ibid., p. 188.

234 **"could have sent him to jail"** Alexander Chee, "My Family's Shrouded History Is Also a National One for Korea," *The New York Times*, Aug. 27, 2020.

236 **A later resurgence of paganism** The Anglos and the Saxons were two distinct Germanic groups who, along with the Jutes, migrated into England and ultimately coalesced into "a single political realm—the kingdom of England—during the reign of King Æthelstan (924–939)." Julian Harrison, "Who Were the Anglo-Saxons?" British Library website, last accessed May 15, 2021. See also Bede, *Ecclesiastical History of the English Nation* (New York: Fordham University, Internet Medieval Sourcebook, 1996), Book I.

237 **"Cremated remains establish Stonehenge as"** Ben Guarina, "People Buried at Stonehenge 5,000 Years Ago Came from Far Away, Study Finds," *The Washington Post*, Aug. 2, 2018. The massive bluestones at Stonehenge came from somewhere else, possibly a stone circle in Wales. This discovery, in combination with isotopes from cremated remains found at Stonehenge, led the lead researcher to conclude that Stonehenge was constructed to commemorate the ancestors of the original people who lived there. Others scoff at this interpretation of the existing evidence. Alison George, "Stonehenge Was Built with Bits of an Older Welsh Stone Age Monument," *New Scientist*, Feb. 12, 2021. It's hard to imagine what, short of a sign saying, THIS SITE WAS USED FOR ANCESTOR VENERATION, would satisfy skeptics; at the same time, it's true that there is no definitive evidence of the purpose of these particular standing stones in this particular part of the world where these particular remains were carefully moved from elsewhere and buried. For an older foray into the debate, see, for example, M. Parker Pearson and Ramilisonina, "Stonehenge for the Ancestors: The Stones Pass on the Message," *Antiquity*, 72, no. 276 (June 1998) and Pearson and Ramilisonina, "Stonehenge for the Ancestors: Part Two," *Antiquity*, 72, no. 278 (Dec. 1998).

237 **23andMe has amended** Maud Newton, ancestry composition results, 23andMe, Jan. 2021.

238 **By this reasoning, they sanctified** See, for example, Howard Zinn, *A People's History of the United States* (New York: HarperCollins, 1980), n.p. The novelist and expert on Calvinism Marilynne Robinson has a different interpretation of the Puritans' quest. Marilynne Robinson, "Which Way to the City on a Hill?" *The New York Review*, July 18, 2019. See also Paul Corcoran, "John Locke on the Possession of Land: Native Title vs. the 'Principle' of Vacuum Domicilium," *The European Legacy*, 23, no. 3 (Dec. 2017).

238 **"the Indians"** Margaret Bruchac, "Revisiting Pocumtuck History in Deerfield: George Sheldon's Vanishing Indian Act," *Historical Journal of Massachusetts*, 39, nos. 1–2, pp. 58–67.

238 **"the ancestor remained in the midst"** Numa Denis Fustel de Coulanges, *The*

Ancient City: A Study of the Religion, Laws, and Institutions of Greece and Rome, trans. Willard Small (Mineola, N.Y.: Dover, 2006), p. 36.

238 **"I buried you, Proteus"** Euripides, *The Complete Greek Drama,* eds. Whitney J. Oates and Eugene O'Neill, Jr., in Two Volumes, 2, *Helena,* trans. E. P. Coleridge (New York: Random House, 1938), lines 1,165–1,170.

238 **A dialogue attributed to Plato** Plato, *Plato in Twelve volumes,* vol. 9, trans. W.R.M. Lamb (Cambridge, Mass.: Harvard University Press; London: William Heinemann, 1925), line 315(c). But see Deborah Boedeker, "Family Matters: Domestic Religion in Classical Greece," eds. John Bodel and Saul M. Olyan, *Household and Family Religion in Antiquity* (Oxford: John Wiley, 2012), p. 241, arguing that while ancient Greek funerary rites "were conducted by the family and were centered in homes," the "procession, public laments, and burial . . . took place outside it," so Greek practices were "in this respect different from that of some other ancient Mesopotamia . . . [In Greece,] burial places were quite separate from the abodes of the living."

239 **"statistically valid"** Charles W. King, *The Ancient Roman Afterlife* (Austin: University of Texas Press, 2020), p. 129.

239 **In both Greece and Rome** Sarah Iles Johnston, *Restless Dead: Encounters Between the Living and the Dead in Ancient Greece* (Berkeley and Los Angeles: University of California Press, 1999) pp. 39–42; King, *The Ancient Roman Afterlife,* pp. 32–33, 47.

239 **"to benefit the dead"** Johnston, *Restless Dead,* p. 43.

239 **"suffer the consequences of transgressions"** Ibid., p. 54.

239 **"hard to avoid the conclusion"** Ibid., p. 41.

240 **"thrice-fathers"** Ibid., pp. 52–56.

240 **Charles W. King rebuts scholarship** King, *The Ancient Roman Afterlife,* pp. 1–58.

240 **"remove their protection and thus hasten"** Ibid., pp. 8, 44, 46, 93, 124–125.

240 **"was trapped in the vicinity"** Ibid., p. 143.

240 **"presents the heaping of earth"** Ibid., pp. 54–55, 58.

240 **"worship of the new *manes*"** Ibid., pp. 139, 172, 178. Beyond the funeral, the dead were honored at their graves at the festival of Parentalia and at the home shrine during the festival of Lemuria. Home shrines "kept the *manes* perpetually in front of their family's eyes as deities whose powers they could invoke." Ibid.. p. 179.

240 **teraphim, household gods** The Dutch scholar Karel van der Toorn makes a persuasive argument, too intricate and text-based to be discussed in detail here, that biblical teraphim "are more likely to have been ancestor figurines than [non-ancestral] household deities." Karel van der Toorn, "The Nature of the Biblical Teraphim in the Light of the Cuneiform Evidence," *The Catholic Biblical Quarterly,* 52, no. 2 (Apr. 1990), pp. 203–222.

240 **There's substantial evidence** Ibid. See also Diana Edelman, "Hidden Ancestor Polemics in the Book of Genesis?" *Words, Ideas, World: Biblical Essays in Honour of Yairah Amit,* eds. A. Brenner and F. Polak (Sheffield, U.K.: Sheffield Phoenix, 2012), pp. 35–56.

241 **"Return to the land of your"** Genesis 31:3 (RSV).

241 **"longed greatly for"** Genesis 31:30 (RSV).

241 **"the God of your father"** Genesis 31:29 (RSV).

241 **"did you steal my gods"** Genesis 31:30 (RSV).

241 **"Any one with whom you find"** Genesis 31:32 (RSV).

241 **she has her period** Genesis 31:34–35 (RSV).

241 **Susannah Rutherglen makes a strong argument**   Susannah Rutherglen, "Rachel and the Household Gods," Norton Scholar's Prize (W. W. Norton and the Modern Language Association, 2002; originally published on the W. W. Norton website but no longer available there). See also Francesca Stavrakopoulou, *Land of Our Fathers: The Roles of Ancestor Veneration in Biblical Land Claims* (New York: Bloomsbury T&T Clark, 2010), p. 99, discussing the later fate of Laban's/Rachel's teraphim: "As seems likely, these gods are probably best understood as the ancestral figurines . . . belonging to Laban and stolen by Rachel" (Gen., 31:19, 30, 34)," as "deified ancestors whose limited, restricted localization is attested in their ritual abandonment at Shechem, and sharply contrasted with the broader territorial potency of the god of Jacob, who is notably credited with having been with Jacob wherever he has traveled (35:3)." See also Edelman, "Hidden Ancestor Polemics in the Book of Genesis?" p. 33. Another interesting argument is that Rachel took the teraphim to secure her line's position of primacy and that her theft "is part of the original basis for the claim of the house of Joseph to national leadership." Ktziah Spanier, "Rachel's Theft of the Teraphim: Her Struggle for Family Primacy," *Vetus Testamentum*, 42, no. 3 (July 1992), pp. 404–412.

242 **"involves her own blood"**   Rutherglen, "Rachel and the Household Gods," p. 99.

242 **"every man did what was right"**   Judges 17:6 (RSV). The full story, in Judges 17 and 18, is worth considering. In Judges 17, Micah's mother orders a "molten image" that becomes connected with the teraphim in the household shrine. In Judges 18, six hundred men "armed with weapons of war" take the teraphim and the molten image, and various dramatic events (usually construed by evangelical Christians to show that Micah was a "false prophet") ensue, but Micah's mother is not mentioned again. Susan Ackerman sees this erasure as emblematic of the redactors of the Book of Judges and other widespread efforts to obscure the role of women in household and family religion. Not only, she argues, do they "obscure the role that a woman like Micah's mother could play in furnishing her household's shrine, even serving as that shrine's principle patron, they also deny us information regarding women's continuing roles in the life of such a sanctuary." Susan Ackerman, "Household Religion, Family Religion, and Women's Religion in Ancient Israel," eds. Bodel and Olyan, *Household and Family Religion in Antiquity*, p. 141.

242 **In another Old Testament story** I   Samuel 24: 11–17.

242 **Josephus mentioned the custom**   Josephus, *Antiquities of the Jews*, xviii. 9, § 5, quoted in *The Jewish Encyclopedia*, 12 (1906; Wynnewood, Penn: JewishEncyclopedia.com, 2002), pp. 108–109.

242 **may have been a strategy**   Stavrakopoulou, *Land of Our Fathers*, p. 19, arguing that "the powerful role of the dead in the lives of the living likely goes some way towards explaining the biblical condemnation of certain practices associated with the dead." See also Edelman, "Hidden Ancestor Polemics in the Book of Genesis?" p. 49. In summarizing much of the evidence, Edelman argues that Genesis as a whole rests on "hidden polemics" against "divinized ancestors and ancestor worship" as part of an assault on the idea that other deities could coexist with Yahweh.

243 **"many death cultures throughout"**   Stavrakopoulou, *Land of Our Fathers*, p. 15.

243 **"the god of the father"**   Theodore J. Lewis, "Family, Household, and Local Religion at Late Bronze Age Ugarit," eds. Bodel and Olyan, *Household and Family Religion in Antiquity*, p. 61.

243 **"manifest, deify, or merely symbolize"**   Stavrakopoulou, *Land of Our Fathers*, p. 15.

244 **the unacknowledged underpinnings** See generally *Eternal Ancestors: The Art of the Central African Reliquary*, ed. Alisa LaGamma (New York: Metropolitan Museum of Art, 2007).

244 **"'greatest artistic emotions'"** Ibid., p. 7.

244 **"no apparent contradiction to individuals"** "Mitsogo," University of Iowa Stanley Museum of Art website, last accessed May 15, 2021.

245 **"were worthless and were to be"** LaGamma, *Eternal Ancestors*, p. 28. LaGamma also observes that the enthusiasm for these works in the contemporary West "elicits both pride and frustration" in the descendants of the artisans, "given how devoid their own lives are of concrete evidence of their heritage." Ibid., p. 29.

245 **"Fang–Betsi ancestor head"** "Fang–Betsi Ancestor Head Leads $16 Million Clyman Collection of African and Contemporary Art at Sotheby's in New York," *Art Daily*, last accessed May 15, 2021.

245 **"the late-nineteenth-century European colonialists"** Holland Cotter, "Eternal Ancestors: Keeping Watch Over the Dead," *The New York Times*, Oct. 5, 2007.

CHAPTER 23. UNACKNOWLEDGED REMAINS

247 **Some of Max's forebears migrated** Theodore Rudin, Staatsarchive Hamburg (Hamburg Passenger Lists), 1850–1934, Microfilm No. K 1711 (Provo: Ancestry.com, 2008), departure Jan. 6, 1866. For Maria Louise Kestenholz, Theodore Rudin's wife and Max's great-great-grandmother, I haven't been able to locate emigration records, but she was born in Switzerland, married Theodore there, and is listed with him in census documents. See, for example, 1880 U.S. Census, New York (Manhattan), Enumeration Dist. 460, p. 378, image 329. Theodore Rudin, Jr., New York Petition for Naturalization, Common Pleas Court, New York County, arrival date 1871, naturalization date Oct. 21, 1887. I acknowledge that this is Lenape land.

247 **Later, I learned that twenty-five-year leases** Diccon Bewes, "The Secret of Swiss Cemeteries," Diccon Bewes blog, Oct. 31, 2011.

247 **according to the Swiss Center** Beth Zuburchen, President, Swiss Center of North America, email to Maud Newton, on file with author, Feb. 11, 2019.

248 **"the body, as the 'temple'"** Alex Mar, "Rent-a-Grave," *Slate*, Feb. 28, 2011.

248 **"some of the wisest of Native"** Robin Wall Kimmerer, *Braiding Sweetgrass: Indigenous Wisdom, Scientific Knowledge, and the Teachings of Plants* (Minneapolis: Milkweed Editions, 2013), p. 207.

249 **Some of these evangelicals implicitly celebrate** See generally Stephenie Hendricks, *Divine Destruction: Dominion Theology and American Environmental Policy* (New York: Melville House, 2005).

PART SEVEN SPIRITUALITY

CHAPTER 24. THE WITCH

254 **"Historic Parsons House"** "Nathaniel Parsons House," Historic Northampton website, last accessed May 15, 2021.

255 **"not very amiable"** John Homer Bliss, *Genealogy of the Bliss Family in America, from about the Year 1550–1880* (Boston: John Homer Bliss, 1881), p. 37.

255 **"harsh, or openly accusatory"** John Putnam Demos, *Entertaining Satan: Witchcraft and the Culture of Early New England* (Oxford University Press, 2004).

255 **"good-looking woman"** Bliss, *Bliss Family in America*, p. 35.

255 **"relatively meagre"**   Demos, *Entertaining Satan*, p. 262.

255 **trader and businessman, canny and useful**   See Chapter 21.

255 **"was herself deeply affected"**   Demos, *Entertaining Satan*, p. 269.

256 **"frequently and notoriously at odds"**   Ibid., p. 257.

256 **"sought to confine her"**   Ibid., p. 255.

256 **"led by an evil spirit"**   Ibid.

256 **"'would go out in the night'"**   Ibid., p. 257.

256 **"in her fit"**   "The Full Story of the Slander Trial," Historic Northampton website, last accessed May 15, 2021.

257 **"part owner of the first gristmill"**   Demos, *Entertaining Satan*, p. 261.

257 **"occasionally as a defendant"**   Ibid., p. 251.

257 **"admonished"**   Ibid., p. 261.

257 **"the first English child born"**   Madeline Bilis, "Throwback Thursday: When a Northampton Woman Was Saved from the Gallows," *Boston Magazine*, May 12, 2016.

258 **"child of the blind man"**   Demos, *Entertaining Satan*, p. 251.

258 **the "immediate outcome"**   Ibid., p. 249.

258 **"a great blow on the door"**   Testimony of Sarah Bridgman, Northampton's Mary Bliss Parsons Slander and Witch Trial Court Documents, WWLP website, original image reproduced courtesy of East Cambridge Archives via the University of Massachusetts website, Aug. 11, 1656.

258 **"told my girl"**   Ibid. I have translated the language into contemporary English.

258 **"'was in grievous torture'"**   Demos, *Entertaining Satan*, p. 252.

258 **"She said you put them"**   "William Hannum against Mary Parsons," ed. David D. Hall, *Witch Hunting in Seventeenth-Century New England: A Documentary History 1638–1693*, Second Edition (Durham, N.C.: Duke University Press, 2005), p. 102.

258 **"sick as soon as it was born"**   "Ann Bartlett for Mary Parsons," Ibid., p. 104.

259 **"had taken cold"**   Demos, *Entertaining Satan*, p. 254.

259 **"'could not be right'"**   Ibid., p. 255.

259 **"may have tipped the balance"**   Ibid., p. 268.

259 **she "came to her end"**   Ibid., p. 270.

259 **"'she having intimation'"**   Ibid.

260 **"'any marks of witchcraft'"**   Ibid., p. 271.

260 **"Mary Parsons, the wife of"**   Ibid., 272.

260 **"Behold, though human judges"**   Bliss, *Bliss Family in America*, p. 37.

261 **"Betty Negro"**   Demos, *Entertaining Satan*, p. 273.

261 **Nearly a decade later**   "Witchcraft Trial," Historic Northampton website, last accessed May 15, 2021.

CHAPTER 25. GENERATIONAL CURSES

265 **"Faith is the substance of things"**   Hebrews 11:1 (King James Version).

270 **he was a Universalist**   James C. Flanigan, *History of Gwinnett County, Georgia*, Vol. 1 (Hapeville, Ga.: Tyler & Co., 1943), p. 408.

271 **And then it started to rain**   I acknowledge that Granny is buried on Tsalagu-wetiyi (Cherokee)i land.

CHAPTER 26. VENERATION

275 **"Something curious is emerging"** Graham Harvey, "Foreword," *This Ancient Heart: Landscape, Ancestor, Self,* eds. Paul Davies and Caitlin Matthews (Washington, D.C.: Moon Books, 2015), p. 1.

275 **"supposed to have been abandoned"** Ibid., pp. 1–2.

275 **"rejection of the medieval idea"** Ibid., p. 4.

275 **"'lower theologies'"** Erica Hill and Jon B. Hageman, "Leveraging the Dead: The Ethnography of Ancestors," eds. Erica Hill and Jon B. Hageman, *The Archaeology of Ancestors: Death, Memory, and Veneration* (Gainesville, Fla.: University Press of Florida, 2016), p. 9.

276 **"savage"** Edward B. Tylor, "The Philosophy of Religion Among the Lower Races of Mankind," *The Journal of the Ethnological Society of London* (1869–1870), 2, no. 4 (1869–1870), pp. 369–381.

276 **Disagreement soon erupted** Hill and Hageman, *The Archaeology of Ancestors.* pp. 11–12.

276 **"Science, Magic, and Religion"** Courtenay Raia, "History 2D: Science, Magic, and Religion," UCLA, YouTube, 2009.

277 **"worship of the dead and the family"** Claude Lecouteux, *The Return of the Dead: Ghosts, Ancestors, and the Transparent Veil of the Pagan Mind,* trans. John E. Graham (Rochester, Vt.: Inner Traditions, 2009), p. 140.

277 **"the dead back into the family of the living"** Ibid., p. 162.

278 **"bond of faith"** Jill Raitt, "Spiritual Relations, Bodily Realities: Ancestors in the European Catholic Tradition," *Ancestors in Post-Contact Religion: Roots, Ruptures, and Modernity's Memory,* ed. Steven J. Friesen (Cambridge, Mass.: Harvard University Press, 2001), p. 221.

278 **"flesh is literally heir to sin"** Ibid., p. 227. And iterations of Christianity that require believers to renounce kin who stand in the way of their practice essentially demand "renunciation of physical ancestry." Ibid., p. 226.

278 **"the genetic relation of the family"** Ibid., p. 227.

278 **"'born only from above'"** Charles H. Long, "Enlightenment, Ancestors, and Primordiality: A Note on Modernity and Memory," *Ancestors in Post-Contact Religion,* ed. Steven J. Friesen (Cambridge, Mass.: Harvard University Press, 2001), p. 129. And so, Long argues, in our era, the yearning for ancestors bubbles up in twisted form, through "racisms, jingoisms, and nationalisms." Ibid., p. 130. Alexis de Tocqueville, who admired the new democracy in America, wondered about, as Long puts it, "'the long-term viability of a people or a culture that had no ancestors.'" Ibid., p. 128. The danger, de Tocqueville wrote, is that the modern individualism makes "every man forget his ancestors, . . . throws him back forever upon himself alone, and threatens in the end to confine him entirely within the solitude of his own heart." Alexis de Tocqueville, *Democracy in America,* Vol. II, trans. Henry Reeve (New York: D. Appleton, 1904), p. 586.

278 **"there's a veil between"** Jane Brown, email to Maud Newton, Oct. 20, 2020.

278 **"The dead man is just that"** Lecouteux, *The Return of the Dead,* pp. 213–214.

279 **"longest and hardest struggle"** Ronald Hutton, *The Stations of the Sun: A History of the Ritual Year in Britain* (Oxford University Press, 2001), pp. 371–372.

279 **"a prehistoric belief in the danger"** Ibid., p. 366.

279 **"more recent spiritual ancestors"** Ronald Hutton, Afterword, *This Ancient Heart,* p. 184.

279 **"Why should we equate"** Ibid., p. 185.

280 **"'superstitious' contaminations"** Peter Brown, *The Cult of the Saints: Its Rise and Function in Latin Christianity* (University of Chicago Press, 1981), p. 26.

280 **debated "superstition"** Ibid., p. 32.

280 **"most notably the habit of feasting"** Ibid., p. 26.

280 **"an artificial kin group"** Ibid., p. 31.

281 **became law only in 1978** American Indian Religious Freedom Act of 1978, 42 U.S.C. §1996.

281 **one of the most beautiful** Malidoma Patrice Somé, *The Healing Wisdom of Africa: Finding Life Purpose Through Nature, Ritual, and Community* (New York: Tarcher/Putnam, 1999).

281 **"in which I had no say"** Ibid., p. 3.

281 **"the marks of literacy"** Ibid., p. 6.

281 **"a logic that was incompatible"** Ibid., p. 8.

281 **"gradually overshadowed the concepts"** Ibid., p. 7.

281 **"he who makes friends with the stranger"** Ibid., pp. 3, 10.

282 **"'Having been exposed to this,'"** Ibid., p. 12.

282 **"find the deep healing they seek"** Ibid., p. 17.

CHAPTER 27. LINEAGE REPAIR

284 **"I don't identify with"** Honorée Fanonne Jeffers, Twitter direct message, Sept. 28, 2018.

284 **I remember rediscovering an essay** Caitlin Matthews, "Healing the Ancestral Communion: Pilgrimage Beyond Time and Space," *This Ancient Heart: Landscape, Ancestor, Self*, eds. Paul Davies and Caitlin Matthews (Washington, D.C.: Moon Books, 2015).

284 **"continuous sorrow"** Ibid., p. 77.

285 **felt a deep tenderness** Ibid.

285 **"the bright bones of the exposed"** Ibid., pp. 77–78.

285 **"the world's traditional cultures"** Ibid., p. 80.

285 **"ancestral lineage healing intensive"** Ancestral Medicine website, Nov. 16–Nov. 18, 2018. I acknowledge that Black Mountain is on Tsalaguwetiyi (Cherokee), S'atsoyaha (Yuchi), and Catawba land.

286 **ordered *Ancestral Medicine*** Daniel Foor, *Ancestral Medicine: Rituals for Personal and Family Healing* (Rochester, Vt.: Bear & Co., 2017).

286 **"the Earth-honoring ways"** Ibid., pp. 16–17.

286 **"emphasize cross-cultural similarity"** Ibid., p. 18.

287 **a group of students formally training** "Open Letter Regarding Daniel Foor & Ancestral Medicine," Medium, Oct. 19, 2020.

287 **"well" ancestors** Foor, *Ancestral Medicine*, pp. 73–198.

288 **Lindsay Sudeikis** Lindsay Sudeikis, Omnia Sancta website, last accessed May 15, 2021.

290 **Shannon Willis** Shannon Willis, Red Earth Healing website, last accessed May 15, 2021.

291 **"half-breed"** Lyla June Johnston, "The Story of How Humanity Fell in Love with Itself Once Again," Center for Earth Ethics website, Mar. 1, 2018 (originally published on author's Facebook page, Jan. 11, 2016).

291 **Taya Mâ Shere** Taya Mâ Shere, Taya Mâ website, last accessed May 15, 2021.

292 **"prayer for the lineage"** Foor, *Ancestral Medicine*, pp. 113–114.

294 **Langston Kahn** Langston Kahn website, last accessed May 15, 2021. Since then,

Kahn has published his book, *Deep Liberation: Shamanic Tools for Reclaiming Wholeness in a Culture of Trauma* (Berkeley, Calif.: North Atlantic Books, 2021).

295 **"writes his book"** Nick Venegoni, "Emotional Clearing & Spiritual Adulthood with Langston Kahn," the Queer Spirit Podcast, last accessed May 15, 2021.

PART EIGHT CREATIVITY

CHAPTER 28. THE NAMESAKE

299 *The Shadow King* Maaza Mengiste, *The Shadow King* (New York: W. W. Norton, 2019).

299 **"It confirmed what I had always"** Interview with Maaza Mengiste, CBC Radio-Canada, Mar. 20, 2020.

299–300 **"He had the same question mark"** Naomi Alderman, *The Liars' Gospel* (New York: Little, Brown, 2013; Google Books), n.p.

300 **Frank Ching's** *Ancestors* Frank Ching, *Ancestors: 900 Years in the Life of a Chinese Family* (New York: William Morrow, 1988).

300 **"filial sons"** Ibid., pp. 113–114.

300 **"'the root of all virtue'"** Ibid.

301 **"died in disgrace"** Ibid., p. 31.

301 **"the report to the ancestors"** "Keeping up with the Ancestors," *The Guardian*, Jan. 16, 2016.

301 **profile of Maude** James Dickerson, "Car, Driver Are Unique," *Delta Democrat-Times*, May 29, 1977.

302 **"It will be the greatest disappointment"** Albert Bigelow Paine, *A Short Life of Mark Twain* (New York: Harper, 1920), p. 342.

303 **Maude's family was poor** See pp. 39–44 for a discussion of Maude's connection to my Newtons and the family's poverty during her (and my Newton great grand-father's) childhood.

303 **Graduated from Grenada College** Grenada College Annual Register 1919–1920, p. 61.

303 **In the** *Delta Democrat-Times* **profile** Dickerson, *Delta Democrat-Times*, May 29, 1977.

303 **she married Simmons in Elkhart, Indiana** Maude Cor[o]na Newton and Roya[l] Simmons, Marriage Record, Elkhart County (Indiana, Select Marriages 1780–1992, Ancestry.com, Film No. 1845561, p. 331), July 10, 1912.

303 **the architectural firm Simmons & Simmons** Solicitation, *The American Contractor*, Dec. 8, 1915, digitized 2011, p. 74.

304 **his father, John** John Newton, recollections forwarded in email by Mike Newton, on file with author, May 9, 2017.

304 **falsely identifies her as widowed** 1920 U.S. Census, District 0125, Drew, Sunflower County, Mississippi, Roll T625_894, p. 16A.

304 **indicate that she was divorced** 1930 U.S. Census, District 22, Drew, Sunflower County, Mississippi, FHL microfilm 2340901; 1940 U.S. Census, District 67-35, Drew, Sunflower County, Mississippi, Roll M-T06627, p. 8B.

304 **By 1930, her ex-husband, Royal** 1930 U.S. Census, District 15, Elkhart, Elkhart County, Indiana, Roll 584, p. 11A.

305 **"old maids"** John Newton, recollections, May 9, 2017.

305 **"Maude C. (Newton) Simmons collection"** "Simmons (Maude C. Newton) Newspaper Articles [Manuscript]," Manuscript Collections, Mississippi Depart-

ment of Archives and History, Z/2016.000/M/Roll 36602 and Z/2016.000/M/Roll 36602, website collection description last accessed May 15, 2021; Maud Newton, "Great Aunt Maude's . . . Official State Archives," MaudNewton.com, Mar. 1, 2010, quoting the longer description of the archives no longer available on the agency's website and identifying the materials as the "Maude C. (Newton) Simmons collection."

305 **Her "Drew Doings" column**   Ibid. I acknowledge that Drew, Mississippi, is on Chahta Yakni and Ogaxpa Mazho land.

305 **The first article**   Maude Simmons, "Drew," *Enterprise-Tocsin* (Indianola, Miss.), Jan. 4, 1968.

306 **"My walking marathon"**   Ibid., Nov. 14, 1968.

306 **"little Negro boys on the plantation"**   Ibid., Aug. 13, 1970. I acknowledge that the Indianola area, where the Newtons settled in Mississippi, is Chahta Yakni and Ogaxpa Mazho land.

306 **"fuzzy-thinking"**   Maude Simmons, "Dots . . . and Dashes—," No. 126, undated manuscript.

306 **"had the integrity"**   Ibid., No. 127.

306 **"Your little girl will be integrated"**   Ibid., No. 145.

306 **when a Black family**   Constance Curry, "'Silver Rights': One Family's Struggle for Justice in America," *Virginia Quarterly Review*, 68, no. 1 (Winter 1992), digitized Dec. 12, 2003.

306 **"Congress is planning"**   Maude Simmons, "Dots . . . and Dashes—," No. 155, May 20, 1965.

307 **"Many, many years ago"**   Maude Simmons, "Drew," *Enterprise-Tocsin*, Jan. 29, 1970.

307 **a biography I reviewed**   Brad Gooch, *Flannery: A Life of Flannery O'Connor* (New York: Little, Brown, 2009). See also Maud Newton, "Flannery O'Connor's Complex, Flawed Character," NPR, Mar. 31, 2009.

308 **"disingenuous"**   Sadie Stein, "Judging Flannery: Can You Love the Work and Not the Author?" Jezebel, Mar. 31, 2009.

CHAPTER 29. BENEFICIAL AND MALIGNANT CREATIVITY

312 **"I thought he was stupid"**   Sandy Bruce, email to Maud Newton, June 24, 2018.

319 **"Most regrettably we have had"**   Richard Newton, III, letter to Maud Newton and name withheld for privacy, on file with author, Nov. 1, 2004.

319 **"I wanted you to see"**   Richard Newton, III, undated note, on file with author.

320 **"It must be serious"**   Richard Newton, Jr., email to Maud Newton, Aug. 12, 2002.

CHAPTER 30. ROOTS

321 **"February Must Be Met"**   Richard Newton, Jr., "February Must Be Met," undated.

322 **"dire consequences"**   Malidoma Patrice Somé, *The Healing Wisdom of Africa: Finding Life Purpose Through Nature, Ritual, and Community* (New York: Tarcher/Putnam, 1999), p. 107.

INDEX

——

ABOUT THE AUTHOR

MAUD NEWTON is a writer and critic whose work has appeared in *The New York Times Magazine, Harper's, The New York Times Book Review, The Oxford American,* and numerous other publications and anthologies, including *Best American Travel Writing* and the *New York Times* bestseller *What My Mother Gave Me.* Newton was born in Dallas to a Texan mother and Mississippian father. She grew up in Miami and graduated from the University of Florida with degrees in English and law.

maudnewton.com

This book was set in Caslon, a typeface first designed in 1722 by William Caslon (1692–1766). Its widespread use by most English printers in the early eighteenth century soon supplanted the Dutch typefaces that had formerly prevailed. The roman is considered a "workhorse" typeface due to its pleasant, open appearance, while the italic is exceedingly decorative.